Basic Neuroscience

A Structural and Functional Approach

Basic Neuroscience

A Structural and Functional Approach

2nd Edition

Adel K. Afifi, M.D.
Professor of Child Neurology and Anatomy
College of Medicine
The University of Iowa
Iowa City, Iowa

Ronald A. Bergman, Ph.D.
Professor of Anatomy
College of Medicine
The University of Iowa
Iowa City, Iowa

Urban & Schwarzenberg
Baltimore-Munich · 1986

Urban & Schwarzenberg, Inc.
7 E. Redwood Street
Baltimore, Maryland 21202
USA

Urban & Schwarzenberg
Pettenkoferstrasse 18
D-8000 München 2
West Germany

Printed in the United States of America

10   9   8   7   6   5   4   3   2

Library of Congress Cataloging in Publication Data

Afifi, Adel K.
  Basic neuroscience

  Bibliography: p.
  Includes index
  1. Neurology. I. Bergman, Ronald A., 1927–
II. Title. [DNLM: 1. Nervous system. WL'100 A257b]
  QP355.2.A33   1985   612.8   83-26093
  ISBN 0-8067-0102-1   *L9024*

Compositor: EPS Group, Inc.
Printer: John D. Lucas
Copyeditor: Susan Lohmeyer
Indexer: Author
Production and design: Norman Och and Karen Babcock

ISBN 0-8067-0102-1 Baltimore

ISBN 3-541-70102-1 Munich

This work is dedicated to the memory
of
Diana Tamari Sabbagh
and to
Hasib Sabbagh
who continues to encourage the search
for new knowledge

Contents

Preface to the First Edition

Writing an integrated textbook in the field of neuroscience can be likened to walking a tightrope. All of the books in this area can be appreciated for trying to fill one or more needs of the student who is beginning to explore this fascinating and complex subject. The emphasis of a textbook may be toward research and the unknown or toward the clinic where the student will put into practice the facts he has learned. The most difficult problem for textbook authors is to provide a balanced and judicious product that stimulates the student to reach beyond the core text, that uses appropriately the time allotted for the subject, that avoids confusion by stating clearly what is known or thought to be known, and that course-sequences the subject matter without dependence on supporting prerequisites. No book can hope to fulfill all of these goals. We have tried to reach some of these objectives; only through use by students and teachers will we know how many we have achieved.

We believe that a textbook should be complete and balanced, but not exhaustive; it should encourage the search for knowledge beyond its pages; and it should be relevant to the stage of development of the student. The text should be such that it can be assimilated by the student in the time usually allotted for such course work and it should be well illustrated. This is the tightrope we have tried to walk. The contents are forward looking and provide a base on which new and essential information can be added by the student as he continues his studies and develops his expertise and experience in this or in related fields of biomedical science.

We are indebted to many people who allowed us the luxury of time for this effort; most importantly, our families carried much of our personal daily workload with understanding and our colleagues encouraged and supported us.

The illustrations were prepared by Mr. Antranig Chelebian and Mr. Raffi Tokatlian. The slides of the Atlas were prepared by Miss Nadia Bahuth, Miss Artemis Khacherian, and Mrs. Janice Schafer.

The manuscript was typed by Mrs. Fadwa Majdalani-To'mey and Mrs. Shaké Mekhiterian-Tomayan and edited by Mrs. Phyllis Bergman. Their efforts, added to their usual daily burden, cannot be repaid.

We are also indebted to Dr. Raif E. Nassif for taking the photomicrographs of the Atlas; to Dr. Samih Y. Alami for reviewing Chapter 18; to Dr. Suhayl J. Jabbur for helping to shape some of the concepts presented in this book through long years of collaboration in teaching and research; and to Mr. Ara Tekian for his assistance in innumerable tasks.

We are grateful to the editor and staff of Urban & Schwarzenberg, and especially Mr. Braxton Dallam Mitchell, for their interest in this book.

We are solely responsible for errors of fact and expression and we invite suggestions and criticisms by students and teachers to be forwarded to us.

Adel K. Afifi, M.D.
Ronald A. Bergman, Ph.D.
Beirut, 1979

Preface to the Second Edition

This second edition has undergone a number of significant changes which should enhance its usefulness to students of neuroanatomy. The number of illustrations has been increased and the quality of reproduction improved. These new and improved illustrations can be found in the Atlas section, as well as throughout the text. The chapters on higher brain functions and gross topography have been rewritten and expanded. The text has been updated in all chapters to incorporate newer data which have accumulated since the book was originally published. Relevant aspects of applied anatomy and clinical correlation have been included where appropriate. References have been added at the end of each chapter.

We are indebted to numerous colleagues and friends who have helped produce this new edition. Mr. Paul Reimann photographed the brain sections in the Atlas and in the chapter on gross topography. The Armed Forces Institute of Pathology (AFIP) and Dr. Edward R. White, Associate Director of AFIP, gave us permission to photograph human brain sections from the Paul Yakovlev Collection. Mr. Mohamad Haleem, Curator of the Medical Museum of AFIP, assisted in the study and selection of material from the Yakovlev Collection. This Collection is supported by Grant Y01-NS-7-0032-00 from the NINCDS to the AFIP. Dr. Jean Y. Jew contributed significantly to this edition through her constructive criticism and advice on diagrammatic illustrations. These were artistically translated into numerous new figures by Ms. Jennifer Deal. Dr. Kenneth Dolan and Dr. Charles Jacoby, Department of Radiology, The University of Iowa, College of Medicine, and Dr. Jacob Musallam, Department of Radiology, Faculty of Medicine, American University of Beirut, provided the computed axial tomography scans. Dr. Gary Van Hoesen reviewed Chapter 21 and provided the horseradish peroxidase and radioactive amino acid localization illustrations in Chapter 1. Miss Sana Shehadeh produced the photographic prints of the human brain sections. Mrs. Shaké Mekhiterian-Tomayan typed the manuscript, Miss Julliet Vosbigyan provided technical assistance, and Mrs. Phyllis S. Bergman edited the manuscript. The authors are grateful to all those who provided critical and constructive reviews of the first edition; we are especially grateful to our medical students for their input, encouraging comments, and genuine interest.

Adel K. Afifi, M.D.
Ronald A. Bergman, Ph.D.
Iowa City, 1985

Basic Neuroscience

A Structural and Functional Approach

1

Methods in
Neurologic Research

Present knowledge about the structure and function of the nervous system is the result of the ingenious, innovative and painstaking efforts of neuroscientists over the past century to develop more reliable methodologies. The job is far from completed; human curiosity about how the brain works continues to be the impetus for new approaches to understanding the mystery of brain structure and function. The problems encountered in brain research are many and varied in nature. They include the complex interneuronal circuitry within and between brain regions, the variations in cellular and laminar organization of different brain regions, the variations in responses to injury and capacity for repair, peculiarities in staining reactions, species differences and, above all, the difficulty of reaching certain brain regions for study.

The purpose of this chapter is to mention briefly some of the methods used by neuroscientists to elucidate the structure and function of the nervous system.

Neuroanatomic Methods

The following neuroanatomic methods include the older, more classical techniques such as the Weigert and Marchi methods, as well as the more recent techniques used to trace fiber tract pathways in the central nervous system. These are light and electron microscopic techniques. The introduction of new techniques has resulted, in some instances, in a revision of previous concepts about neural connectivity.

Anterograde Degeneration Techniques

Anterograde degeneration techniques delineate the path of degenerated nerve fibers emanating from a region of the nervous system following a lesion placed experimentally or occurring naturally in man in that region.

There are several such techniques. Some of them (Weigert, Marchi) demonstrate the degenerating myelin sheath of nerve fibers; others (Nauta-Gygax, Fink-Heimer) demonstrate the degenerating axons.

Weigert Method   This is a hematoxylin dye method which stains normal myelin sheaths black or dark gray. Any degenerated myelinated tracts in the preparation will remain unstained and can thus be detected (Fig. 1–1).

Luxol Fast Blue Method   This is a simple method for the demonstration of normal myelinated tracts with sulfonated azo dyes. Because of its simplicity, it has largely replaced the earlier methods used for normal myelinated tracts, such as the Weigert method. In addition to its simplicity, the luxol fast blue method can be applied to frozen as well as paraffin sections of material fixed in formaldehyde or almost any other fixative. Furthermore, this method can be combined with counterstains that will demonstrate perikarya and axons. It is thus an ideal method for preparing slides for teaching purposes and for preliminary exploration of the distribution of tracts and nuclear groups.

Marchi Method   This method preferentially demonstrates degenerating myelin with osmium tetroxide. In preparations with degenerating and normal myelinated tracts, only the degenerating tracts will interact with osmium tetroxide and appear black. Normal myelinated tracts remain unstained (Fig. 1–2). A major advantage of the Marchi method, which makes it particularly useful in the study of human postmortem material, is that positive results may be obtained years after degeneration has occurred and in specimens stored in formaldehyde for long periods. A major disadvantage of this method is that it cannot be used to trace nerve fibers to their exact site of termination, since the terminal part of an axon is unmyelinated and cannot be demonstrated by this method.

Nauta-Gygax Method   This silver method preferentially stains degenerating axons (Fig. 1–3). Some normal axons also stain but are easily distinguished from degenerating axons by their appearance. The major advantage of this method over the Weigert and Marchi methods is that it identifies both myelinated and unmyelinated nerve fibers because the axon and not the myelin is stained by this technique. The introduction of this method into brain research in the early fifties resulted in a revision of knowledge about neural connectivity, since previously used methods did not identify thinly myelinated or nonmyelinated fiber tracts. Although the Nauta-Gygax method provides an adequate picture of the connections within a neural system, it gives little if any reliable information about synaptic relationships.

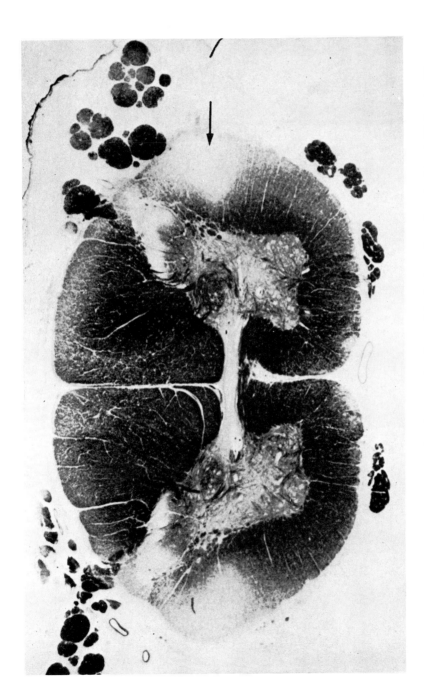

1–1 Photomicrograph of spinal cord showing degeneration (*arrow*) in the lateral corticospinal tract. Weigert × 20.

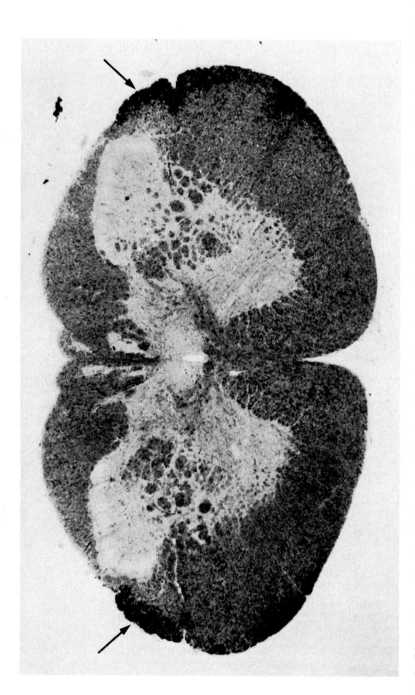

1–2 Photomicrograph of spinal cord-medulla junction showing degeneration (*arrows*) in the spinocerebellar tract. Marchi ×20.

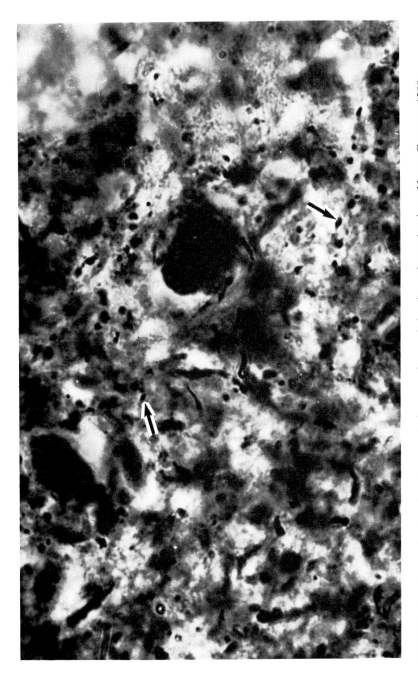

1-3 Photomicrograph showing degenerated axons (*arrows*) in the substantia nigra. Nauta-Gygax ×1200.

Fink-Heimer Method   This is another silver method which delineates not only degenerating axons but also degenerating terminals (Fig. 1–4). Thus, it has an advantage over the Nauta-Gygax method in delineating more precisely the projection pattern of a neural region, including its axonal termination.

Golgi Methods   Since the accidental discovery of the Golgi method in the late 19th century, several modifications of the original technique have been introduced. All these methods impregnate occasional neurons (Fig. 1–5), glia, and blood vessels with a deposit of silver chromate. The methods are particularly suited to young animals, since the presence of myelin interferes with proper impregnation. The unique advantage of the Golgi methods is that they provide a three-dimensional profile of cellular elements and thus are invaluable for both qualitative and quantitative studies of the nervous system. The Golgi methods have been used to estimate the density of postsynaptic dendritic spines and the extent of dendritic fields.

Electron Microscopic Method   This method is of use in identifying degenerating synaptic boutons within a neural system. Following a lesion in a particular brain region, the locus or loci upon which this particular region is believed to project are studied by electron microscopy. The presence of degenerating boutons in these loci will confirm the presence of a synaptic relationship between the two regions. The disadvantages of this method are that it is a highly specialized technique for routine use and it reveals only a minute fraction of the neural system under investigation.

Retrograde Degeneration Technique

The site of neurons giving rise to a neural tract is determined by this method. Such neurons undergo chromatolytic changes in their Nissl substance (Fig. 1–6) or disappear completely if the tract is severed or if the area to which the neurons project is destroyed. Such degenerating neurons are demonstrated by any of the methods that stain ribonucleic acids (Nissl material). The intensity of chromatolysis varies from one site to another within the nervous system, depending upon the type of lesion and the age and species of the animal. Young animals show the most severe chromatolytic changes.

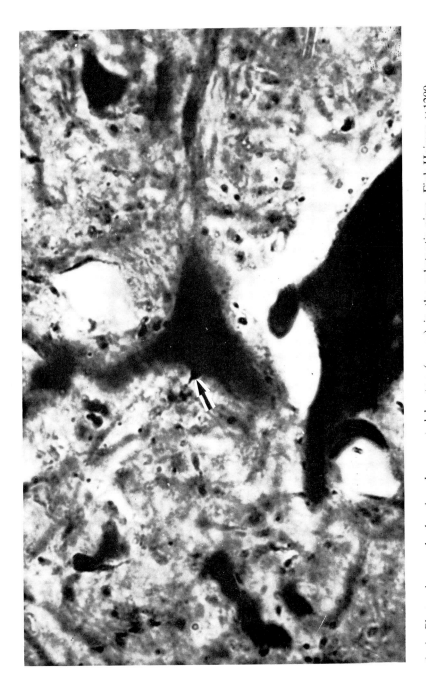

1–4 Photomicrograph showing degenerated bouton (*arrow*) in the substantia nigra. Fink-Heimer ×1200.

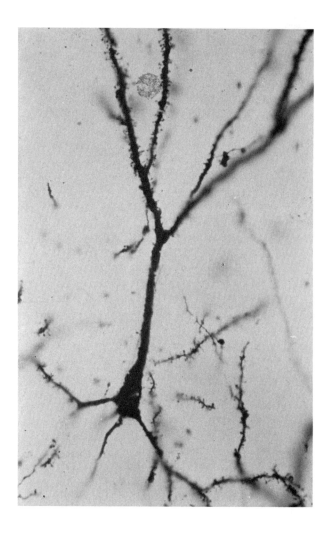

1-5 Photomicrograph showing pyramidal neuron. Golgi ×500.

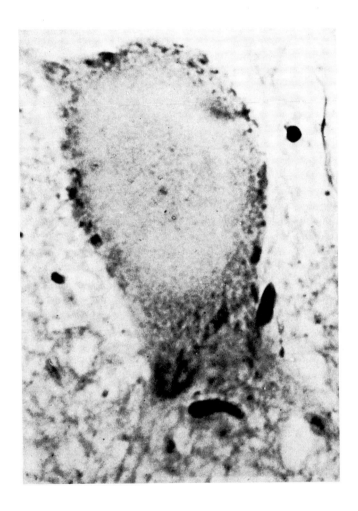

1-6   Photomicrograph of a motor neuron undergoing chromatolysis. Nissl × 1600.

Autoradiography

This is a recent addition to the techniques used in brain research. It relies upon the new and well-documented observation that radioactive amino acids injected in the vicinity of neuronal somata will be taken up by the neuron, incorporated into its macromolecules, and transported down the axon to its terminal. After a certain time following injection, the radioactive amino acids can be demonstrated by autoradiography using light (Fig. 1–7) or electron microscopy. By this method, the path of a neural tract can be identified from its origin to its termination. The most commonly used tritiated amino acids are leucine and proline. In spite of technical difficulties associated with this technique, it nevertheless represents a marked improvement over other anterograde techniques for qualitative and quantitative studies of the nervous system. A major advantage of this method over silver impregnation methods (Nauta-Gygax and Fink-Heimer) is that fibers of passage which do not originate at the site of injection will not take up the tritiated amino acid and thus will not be labeled.

Enzymatic Method

When the enzyme horseradish peroxidase (HRP) is injected at the site of termination of nerve fibers, it is taken up by the terminals and transported retrogradely to the perikaryon, where it is visualized by an enzyme histologic technique as brown granules in the soma and dendrites (Fig. 1–8). The labeling is clearly seen in the light microscope with dark field illumination and in the electron microscope. The major advantages of this method over other retrograde degeneration methods is the relative ease of identification of labeled cells of origin of a neural tract, the absence of a major degree of tissue destruction, and its combined use with such techniques as anterograde tracing (autoradiography), cytochemical staining for acetylcholinesterase, formaldehyde-induced fluorescence, and immunohistochemistry.

Fluorescence Method

This method, originally introduced by Falck and Hillarp in the early sixties, is used to trace the fiber pathways of adrenergic and monaminergic neural systems and relies on the observation that primary amines form fluorescent condensation products when treated with formaldehyde in the presence of protein. These fluorescent condensation products are demonstrated by cells, axons, and terminals by fluorescence microscopy. The application of this method has revealed neural connections which were previously unknown. About 10 groups of noradrenergic neurons have thus been iden-

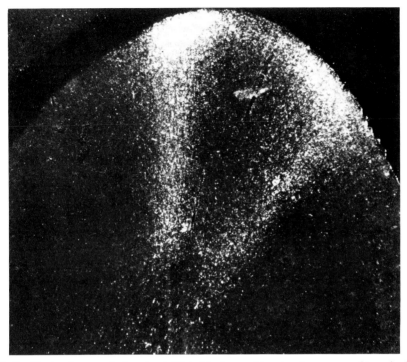

1-7 Photomicrograph showing tritiated lysine and leucine in axons and terminals in the premotor cortex. ×36.

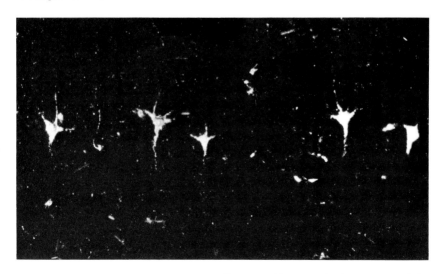

1-8 Photomicrograph showing horseradish peroxidase uptake by neurons of the primary motor cortex. ×250.

tified in the brain stem, the best defined being the nucleus locus ceruleus. Among dopaminergic projections, the one from the substantia nigra to the striatum has been demonstrated unequivocally.

Intracellular Labeling Methods

Intracellular injection of single neurons with fluorescent dyes has been used for a number of years. The method is tedious and the yield of labeled cells is usually low, particularly in mammalian tissues. The most striking success with intracellular labeling has come with a modification of the horseradish peroxidase method. The enzyme has been successfully injected into electrophysiologically identified cells by electrophoresis or air pressure. It has been possible by this method to demonstrate the finest dendritic processes, spines, and axon collaterals of labeled neurons.

Immunohistochemical Methods

The introduction of the histofluorescent technique by Falck and Hillarp for the localization of catecholamines kindled interest in the anatomic localization of other biochemically definable systems. Basically, immunohistochemical methods require that the substance to be localized must be antigenic. Incubation of a tissue section in an antibody-containing solution leads to the development of an immunochemical bond between the specific antibody and the antigen in its original *in vivo* position. The use of a proper marker will aid the visualization of the immunologically bound antigen and antibody. The two markers generally used in neuroanatomic studies are fluorescein isothiocyanate (FITC) and horseradish peroxidase (HRP). The immunohistochemical methods have been successfully used to localize enzymes responsible for the synthesis of neurotransmitters, such as tyrosine hydroxylase, dopamine-B-hydroxylase, phenylethanolamine *N*-methyl transferase, tryptophan hydroxylase, glutamate decarboxylase, and others.

Neurophysiologic Methods

Neurophysiologists rely on stimulation and recording techniques to establish the presence or absence of a structural or functional relationship between two loci in the nervous system. The applied stimulus may be artificial (electric) or natural (receptors of sense organs). The stimulation and recording of the evoked potential may be orthodromic (recording of activity in the terminal projection site of a fiber system) or antidromic (recording of activity in the cells of origin when their axon terminals or axons are stimulated). The latency of the response is used as one criterion to determine the type of relationship between two sites. The determinants of latency include the distance between the points of stimulation and recording, conduction velocity, and the number of intervening synapses. Short latency responses suggest a short pathway, fast-conducting pathway, or oligosynaptic pathway, whereas long latency responses suggest a long pathway, slow-conducting pathway, or multisynaptic pathway. Gross stimulation and recording techniques reflect the relationship between groups of neurons; intracellular recordings reflect the relationship between pairs of neurons. The use of computers and electronic averagers of responses has refined the results obtained by neurophysiologic methods.

Quantitative Methods

These methods are highly specialized and limited in use to special laboratories seeking precise quantitative data. Image analysis by television systems (Quantimat) that scan the microscope field in a linear fashion and record changes in the intensity of transmitted light has been used to count individual grains in autoradiographs and to relate them to underlying structures, *e.g.*, neural laminae. Another device, the computer-assisted pantagraph, permits the morphometric analysis of cross-sectional profiles of cell somata, nuclei, axons, or dendrites in terms of area and diameter. Computer technology has also been used in the analysis of dendritic and axonal length, orientation and branching patterns in an attempt to classify neurons in terms of their three-dimensional organization.

Reference

Heimer, L.; Robards, M.J.: Neuroanatomical Tract-Tracing Methods. Plenum Press, New York, 1981.

2

Neurocytology
and Neurohistology

The cells which comprise the nervous system are vast in number and complexity. As components of peripheral and central nervous systems, they are distributed to reach every part of the body. Their function is to receive stimuli from the external and internal environments and to transmit (by electrochemical processes), modify, coordinate, integrate, and translate these stimuli into meaningful conscious experiences or coordinated motor activity through muscular and glandular tissues.

Cells of the nervous system fall into two general categories; these are nerve cells (neurons) and supporting cells (glia). Nerve cells are intricately linked to each other and to effector organs such as muscle and glands. The different nerve cells influence each other through specialized areas of contact, the synapses. The complexity of the synaptic relationships among the billions of neurons provides the basis for the behavioral complexity of man.

Students of the nervous system have revealed many aspects of the structure and function of cellular components, their organization into functional groups, and the pathways emanating from or projecting upon them. A wide variety of anatomic and physiologic methods have been developed to demonstrate the component parts of the nervous system and their interrelationships in normal and disease states. This chapter is concerned with the structural components of the nervous system.

Cellular Components

Neuron

A neuron or nerve cell consists of a cell body (perikaryon) and all of its processes (axon and dendrites). Neurons vary remarkably in size and shape. The diameter of the cell body may be as small as 4 μm (granule cell of the cerebellum) or as large as 125 μm (motor neuron of the spinal cord). The overall configuration of a cell body may be pyramidal, flask-shaped

15

or stellate, depending upon the number and organization of its processes. The most remarkable feature of the neuron is its processes. In man, the axon may be a meter or more in length, extending from the spinal cord to the fingers or toes or from the cerebral cortex to the distal extent of the spinal cord. The dendrites vary in number and in pattern of branching, which in some instances enormously increases their surface area. Examples of the variation in cell structure are seen in Figures 2–1 and 2–2.

Perikaryon The cell body contains the nucleus and a number of organelles (Fig. 2–3). The nucleus is generally round and usually centrally located. The nucleoplasm is homogeneous and stains poorly with nuclear stains (basic dyes) indicating that the deoxyribonucleic acid (DNA) is in the dispersed or active, euchromatin form. In stark contrast, one deeply stained nucleolus, composed in part of ribonucleic acid (RNA), is normally present within the nucleus. The nuclear contents are enclosed within a distinct nuclear membrane.

The cytoplasm is filled with various organelles and inclusions. Prominent among the organelles is the chromophil substance or Nissl bodies. Nissl bodies are composed of RNA in the form of granules (ribosomes) attached to flattened vesicles. The roles of the nucleus, nucleolus, and cytoplasmic RNA in protein synthesis are well established. The cell body generates the cytoplasmic proteins and other essential constituents which are then distributed throughout the entire neuron. Nissl bodies are found not only in the cell body but also in the dendrites. They are absent from the axon hillock (part of the perikaryon from which the axon arises) and axon. Mitochondria are dispersed throughout the cytoplasm of the nerve cell and play a vital role in the metabolic activity of the neuron. The Golgi apparatus, originally discovered in neurons, is highly developed and is composed of flattened, ovoid, and round agranular vesicles. Small vesicles arising from this organelle may be the source of synaptic vesicles found in axon terminals. Neurofibrils are found in all nerve cells and are continuous throughout all of their processes. They appear to be aggregates of neurofilaments and tubules which are visible only by electron microscopy. Most large nerve cells contain lipochrome pigment granules which appear to accumulate with advancing age of the organism. In addition, certain nerve cells in specific locations in the brain contain melanin granules which are black in color; their function is unknown.

Axon The axon usually arises from the cell body at the axon hillock; it is a slender cylindrical process of variable length. It may be extremely long, as indicated earlier. The axon hillock and axon proper are devoid of Nissl substance; mitochondria, neurofilaments, and tubules are contained within the axoplasm. Axons retain a uniform diameter throughout their

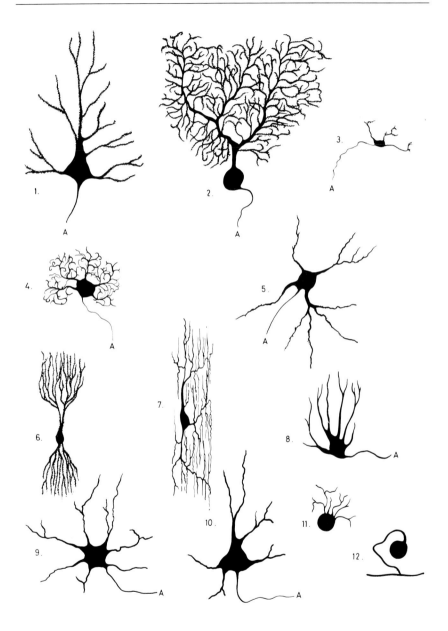

2–1 Schematic diagram illustrating variation in neuronal size, shape, and processes. *1, 4, 5,* and *6* are cortical neurons; *2* and *3* are cerebellar neurons; *7, 9,* and *10* are spinal neurons; *8* is a sympathetic ganglion neuron; *11* is a parasympathetic ganglion neuron; and *12* is a dorsal root ganglion neuron. *A,* axon.

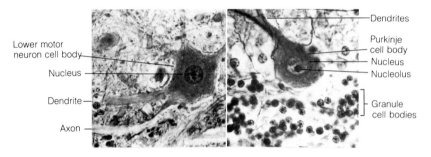

Dendrites

Lower motor neuron cell body

Nucleus

Dendrite

Axon

Purkinje cell body

Nucleus

Nucleolus

Granule cell bodies

2-2 Photomicrographs of neurons of the central nervous system illustrating the extremes in neuronal size. The motor neuron of the spinal cord and the Purkinje cell of the cerebellum are among the largest neurons, whereas the granule cell of the cerebellum is one of the smallest. ×850.

length. They may have collateral branches proximally and usually branch extensively at their distal ends (telodendria) before terminating by synaptic contact with dendrites and cell bodies of other neurons or on effector organs.

Axons may be myelinated or unmyelinated. In either case they are ensheathed by supporting cells; these are Schwann cells in the peripheral nervous system and glia cells in the central nervous system. Myelinated axons are wrapped in multiple layers of the external membrane, or myelin, of these supporting cells. The process of myelin formation will be considered later in this chapter. The sheath is discontinuous at the distal ends of each cell involved in the ensheathing process. This area of discontinuity, termed the node of Ranvier, is believed to be the region in which the axon is in contact with extracellular fluid.

Myelinated axons vary from 1 to 20 μm in diameter, whereas unmyelinated axons are under 2 μm (Fig. 2-4).

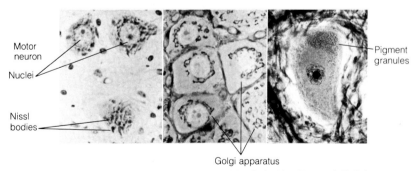

Motor neuron

Nuclei

Nissl bodies

Pigment granules

Golgi apparatus

2-3 Photomicrographs showing cell organelles [Nissl bodies and Golgi apparatus (×200) and pigment granules (×850)].

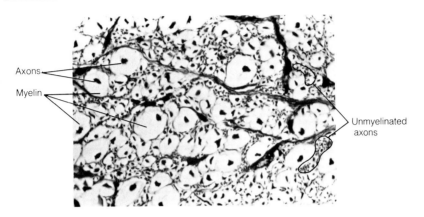

Axons

Myelin

Unmyelinated axons

2-4 Photomicrograph illustrating the wide variety in axon diameter. The space surrounding the large axons represents the myelin sheath extracted during tissue preparation. Note the variation in the size of the axons and sheath. Interspersed among the larger myelinated axons are small clusters of unmyelinated axons. × 680.

Dendrites Although neurons possess only a single axon, they usually have more than one dendrite, which is tapered distally and may be highly branched. The dendrites may increase tremendously the surface area of the cell body from which they arise. They are usually covered by a large number of spines or gemmules, which are small projections representing sites of synaptic contact. They contain all the organelles found within the neuroplasm of the perikaryon except the Golgi apparatus. Neurons which receive axon terminals or synapses from a variety of sources in the nervous system may have an extremely complex dendritic organization, *e.g.*, the Purkinje cell of the cerebellum. Most of the cells of the central nervous system and the autonomic ganglia have dendrites extending from their perikarya. This type of neuron is called multipolar; those which possess only axon-like processes extending from each end of the cell are termed bipolar. Bipolar neurons are found in the retina of the eye and the peripheral ganglia of the vestibulocochlear nerve [cranial nerve (CN) VIII]. Sensory neurons located in the dorsal root of spinal nerves are termed pseudounipolar, because only a single process leaves the cell body before bifurcating to form proximal and distal segments (Fig. 2–5). The processes of bipolar and pseudounipolar neurons are axon-like in structure and have a limited or specific receptive capacity; however, they usually retain the diversified terminal axonal branchings within the central nervous system. Certain cells of the retina, the amacrine cells, are generally regarded as axonless.

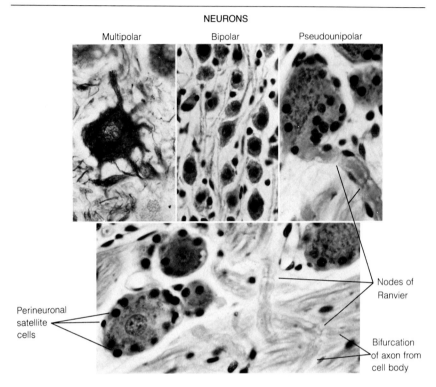

2-5 Photomicrographs showing multipolar (×550), bipolar (×150), and pseudounipolar (×550) neurons. Note the nodes of Ranvier.

Neuroglia

The interstitial supporting cells of the central nervous system are termed neuroglia. They are of several varieties.
1. Astrocytes
    a. Fibrous
    b. Protoplasmic
2. Oligodendroglia
3. Ependymal cells
4. Microglia

Astrocytes The astrocytes, largest of the neuroglia, are branched stellate cells. The nuclei of these cells are ovoid, centrally located and poorly stained, with little heterochromatin and no nucleoli. Their cytoplasm may contain small rounded granules.

Fibrous Astrocytes These cells have thin, spindly processes which radiate from the cell body and terminate with distal expansions or foot plates which are in contact with the walls of blood vessels lying within the central nervous system. The foot processes form a continuous glial sheath, the perivascular limiting membrane, around blood vessels. The cytoplasm of fibrous astrocytes contains filaments which extend throughout the cell, as well as the usual cytoplasmic organelles. Fibrous astrocytes, found primarily within the white matter, are concerned with repair of damaged tissue (scarring).

Protoplasmic Astrocytes These cells have thicker, more numerous branches. They are in close association with neurons and may partially envelop them; thus, they are considered satellite cells. Since they have a close relationship to neurons, they are found primarily in the gray matter of the brain and spinal cord. They may serve as a metabolic intermediary for nerve cells.

Oligodendroglia These small cells have fewer and shorter branches than the astrocytes. The nuclei are round and have condensed, stainable chromatin. The cytoplasm, less extensive than in astrocytes, contains mitochondria, microtubules, and ribosomes, but is devoid of neurofilaments. Oligodendroglia cells are found in both the gray and white matter. They are usally found lying in rows among the axons in the white matter. Electron microscopic studies have implicated the oligodendroglia in central nervous system myelination. Within the gray matter, these cells are closely associated with neurons, as are the protoplasmic astrocytes (perineuronal satellite cells).

Ependymal Cells Ependymal cells line the central canal and the ventricles of the brain. They are cuboidal to columnar in shape, may possess cilia, and line the villi which extend into the ventricles. The cytoplasm contains mitochondria, a Golgi complex, and small granules. These cells are thought to be associated with the formation of cerebrospinal fluid.

Microglia The microglia, unlike other nerve and glial cells, are of mesodermal origin and enter the nervous system early in development. Their cell bodies are small, dense, and elongated. They possess elongated nuclei and have few processes (occasionally two) at either end of the cell. The spindly processes may bear small thorny spines. Under normal conditions the function of the microglia is uncertain. When destructive lesions occur in the nervous system, the cells enlarge and become phagocytic and mobile.

The structure of glial cells as revealed by light microscopy is shown in Figure 2–6.

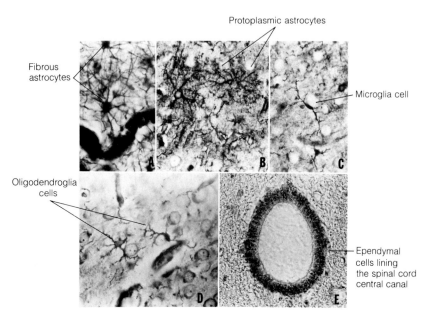

2–6 Photomicrographs showing fibrous astrocytes (*A*), protoplasmic astrocytes (*B*), microglia (*C*), oligodendroglia (*D*), and ependymal cells (*E*). With the exception of the ependymal cells, neuroglia require special stains to reveal their processes. ×680.

Ganglia

Ganglia are collections of nerve cell bodies located outside the central nervous system. There are two types of ganglia, craniospinal ganglia and autonomic ganglia.

Craniospinal Ganglia

The craniospinal ganglia occur in the dorsal roots of the 31 pairs of spinal nerves or in the sensory roots of the trigeminal (CN V), facial (CN VII), vestibulocochlear (CN VIII), glossopharyngeal (CN IX), and vagus (CN X) nerves. The dorsal root ganglia and the cranial nerve ganglia are sensory. They receive stimuli at their distal ends and transmit nerve impulses to the central nervous system. The ganglion cells of the spinal group are pseudounipolar neurons, whereas those of the vestibular and cochlear nerves are bipolar neurons (Fig. 2–5). Dorsal root ganglion cells range in size from 15 to 100 μm in diameter. In general, the cells fall into two size groups. The smaller cells have unmyelinated axons, whereas the larger cells have myelinated axons. Each ganglion cell is surrounded by connective tissue and supporting cells, the perineuronal satellite cells or capsule cells, and from each a single process emerges to bifurcate, forming an inverted T or Y, into proximal and distal axon-like processes. The intracapsular process may be coiled (so-called glomerulus) or relatively straight. The bipolar ganglion cells of the vestibular and cochlear cranial nerves are not encapsulated by satellite cells.

Autonomic Ganglia

Autonomic ganglia are aggregates of neurons extending from the base of the skull to the pelvis, usually in close relationship to and on either side of the vertebral bodies (sympathetic) or as part of the cranial-sacral nerves with ganglia located within the organ innervated (parasympathetic). In contrast to cranial-spinal ganglia, the ganglion cells of the autonomic nervous system are multipolar and receive synaptic input from various levels of the nervous system. Autonomic ganglion cells are surrounded by connective tissue and small perineuronal satellite cells located between the dendrites in close association with the cell body.

Autonomic cells vary in size from 20 to 60 μm in diameter and possess clear spherical or ovoid nuclei; some cells may be binucleated. The cytoplasm contains neurofibrils and small aggregates of RNA, Golgi apparatus, and mitochondria.

The dendritic processes of two or more cells often appear tangled and may form dendritic glomeruli; such cells are enclosed in a single capsule. The terminal arborizations of the ganglionic axons synapse on these dendritic glomeruli as well as on the dendrites of individual ganglion cells. In general, the preganglionic arborization of a single axon brings it into synaptic contact with numerous ganglion cells. The axons of these ganglion cells are of small diameter (0.3 to 1.3 μm).

Autonomic ganglion cells located within the viscera may be few in number and widely distributed. They are not encapsulated, but are contained within connective tissue septa in the organ innervated. The cells of the autonomic ganglia innervate visceral effectors such as smooth muscle, cardiac muscle, and glandular epithelium (Fig. 2–7).

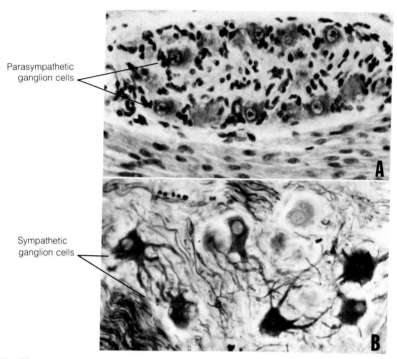

Parasympathetic
ganglion cells

Sympathetic
ganglion cells

2-7 Photomicrographs showing parasympathetic ganglion cells (*A*) and sympathetic ganglion cells (*B*). The stain used in the preparation of *A* does not show cell processes. ×450.

Nerve Fibers

A peripheral nerve is composed of nerve fibers (axons) which vary in size, are myelinated or unmyelinated, and transmit nerve impulses either to or from the central nervous system. A peripheral nerve is often called a mixed nerve because it is composed of both motor and sensory fibers. Nerves containing only sensory fibers are called sensory nerves; those that contain only motor fibers are called motor nerves.

The nerve fibers which constitute a peripheral nerve have been classified according to size and other functional characteristics (Table 2–1). Axons which range in size from 12 to 22 μm are designated as A-alpha, from 5 to 12 μm as A-beta, from 2 to 8 μm as A-gamma and from 1 to 5 μm as A-delta. Preganglionic sympathetic fibers are less than 3 μm in diameter and are designated as B-fibers. All of the above are myelinated nerve

Table 2–1 Some Properties of Mammalian Peripheral Nerve Fibers

Nerve fiber type						
Letter designation	Number designation	Function and/or source	Fiber size (range in μm)	Myelination	Conduction velocity (m/sec)
A-alpha (α)	Ia	Proprioception, stretch (muscle spindle, annulospiral receptor) and motor to skeletal muscle fibers (extrafusal)	12–22	+	70–120
	Ib	Contractile force (Golgi tendon organ)	12–22	+	70–120
A-beta (β)	II	Pressure, stretch (muscle spindle, flower spray receptor), touch and vibratory sense	5–12	+	30–70
A-gamma (γ)	II	Motor to muscle spindle muscle fibers (intrafusal)	2–8	+	15–30
A-delta (δ)	III	Some nerve endings serving pain, temperature and touch	1–5	+	5–30
B		Sympathetic preganglionic axons	<3	+	3–15
C	IV	Other pain, temperature and mechanical receptors; sympathetic, postganglionic axons (motor to smooth muscle and glands)	0.1–1.3	–	0.6–2.0

fibers. The smallest axons (from 0.1 to 3 μm in diameter) are designated as C-fibers and are unmyelinated. Myelinated and unmyelinated nerve fibers are seen in cross-section in Figure 2–4.

A peripheral nerve may contain thousands of axons which are invested in a connective tissue sheath. Three parts are recognized. The outer sheath, the epineurium, is generally thick, is composed of loose connective tissue, and contains blood vessels. It is continuous with the connective tissue of the dura mater. From the epineurium, collagenous septa join with the dense perineurium which separates and encompasses groups of axons in fascicles of differing size. Small blood vessels traverse these septa to reach the nerve fibers. The perineurium is continuous with the pia-arachnoid membrane which extends to the dorsal and ventral roots near the spinal cord. The final subdivision of connective tissue, the endoneurium, invests each individual axon and is continuous with the connective tissue forming

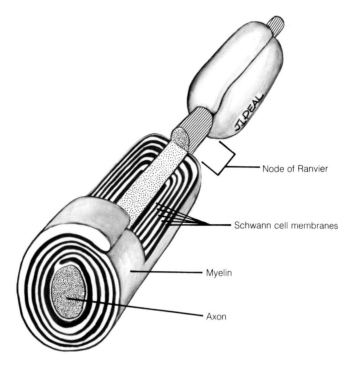

Node of Ranvier

Schwann cell membranes

Myelin

Axon

2-8 Schematic diagram illustrating the wrapping of Schwann cell membranes around the axon to form myelin. Note the node of Ranvier. See also Figure 2-5.

the perineurium and epineurium. This connective tissue provides a tough, protective, tubular sheath for the delicate axons. Within the endoneurium and surrounding each myelinated or unmyelinated axon are the Schwann cells. It is the Schwann cell that produces the myelin sheath (Fig. 2-8). This nucleated sheath of peripheral nerve fibers is also known as the neurolemma or sheath of Schwann.

In general, large axons are myelinated and the smallest axons are unmyelinated. The conduction velocity of axons is directly related to axon diameter and the thickness of the myelin sheath. Conduction is progressively faster in axons with larger diameters and thicker myelin sheaths.

Myelinated Nerve Fibers

Electron microscopic studies have shown that most axons larger than 1 μm are myelinated. The myelin sheath is formed by many concentric double layers of Schwann cell membrane. The cell membrane is tightly wound and the inner or protoplasmic surfaces of the membrane become fused together, forming the dense and thicker lamella of the myelin sheath seen in electron micrographs. The inner, less dense lamella is formed by the outer surfaces of the membrane. The sheath is not continuous but is interrupted at either end of the Schwann cell. A gap always exists between adjacent Schwann cells; this gap is termed the node of Ranvier. The internodal distance varies between 400 and 1500 μm, depending on fiber diameter and species.

Occasionally, areas of incomplete fusion of the Schwann cell membrane occur and small amounts of Schwann cell cytoplasm are trapped between the membranes. These areas of incomplete fusion are called Schmidt-Lanterman clefts. Their significance is not understood; they may be shearing defects in the formation of the myelin or they may represent a kind of distention of the myelin sheath in which Schwann cell cytoplasm is left behind as the cell winds around the axon. Axonal myelin ends near the terminal arborization of the axon.

Myelination within the central nervous system is accomplished by oligodendroglia cells in a manner similar to that of peripheral nerves; however, the internodal distance and gap are smaller.

Unmyelinated Nerve Fibers

Unlike their larger counterparts, several small axons may be contained within the infoldings of a single Schwann cell. The invested axon appears in cross-section to be suspended by a short segment of the invaginated outer membrane which, after encircling it, is folded back and is closely approximated. The similarity in appearance to the intestine within its mesentery has led to the name mesaxon for this membranous arrangement. Within the central nervous system, glia cells serve the same function as Schwann cells by ensheathing the nonmyelinated axons.

Conduction of Nerve Impulses

The cell membrane plays a key role in nerve transmission. In unmyelinated fibers, the impulse is conducted as a spreading wave of change in membrane permeability that moves along the axon and induces the liberation of a transmitter substance at the axon terminal. The change in membrane permeability is associated with an influx of sodium ions and an efflux of potassium ions. In myelinated fibers, permeability changes occur only at the nodes of Ranvier; the insulating effect of myelin along the internodes prevents the propagation of the impulse. The impulse in such nerves jumps from one node to the next. This process is known as saltatory conduction and is faster than the process of continuous conduction of unmyelinated nerves.

Axonal Transport

Proteins synthesized in the perikarya of neurons are transported along the axon to its terminal. There is evidence to suggest that axonal transport flows in two directions: anterograde from the perikarya to the synaptic terminal and retrograde from the terminal to the perikarya. Anterograde transport flows primarily at two rates, a fast rate (100 mm/day) and a slow rate (1 to 3 mm/day).

Synapse

The simplest unit of segmental nerve function requires two neurons; these are a receptor or sensory neuron and a motor or effector neuron, *e.g.*, the patellar tendon reflex or knee jerk. The structural-functional coupling of these two neurons is effected by a synapse. The terminal arborizations of the sensory neuron are dilated into small knobs or boutons which lie on the dendrites, cell body, and axon of the effector neuron (Fig. 2–9). These small bulbs contain synaptic vesicles which vary in size from 300 to 600 Å. The vesicles may appear empty or clear but actually contain acetylcholine. In other kinds of synapses the vesicles may contain a dense particle or core

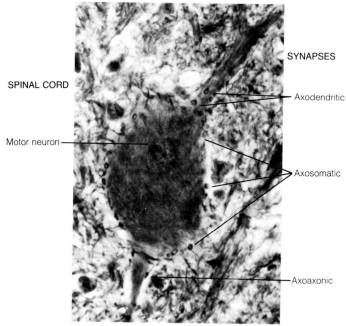

SYNAPSES

SPINAL CORD

Axodendritic

Motor neuron

Axosomatic

Axoaxonic

2–9 Photomicrograph of a lower motor neuron showing synapses on the dendrite, cell body, and proximal portion of the axon (axon hillock). × 800.

which is presumed to be catecholamine. Acetylcholine and catecholamine are among the several chemical transmitter substances which facilitate the transfer of nerve impulses from one neuron to another or to a non-neuronal effector organ. Electron microscopy has revealed a specialized structure for the synapse which consists of thickened presynaptic and postsynaptic membranes separated by a synaptic gap of about 200 A. Besides the synaptic vesicles, the synaptic terminal contains abundant mitochondria and infrequent neurofilaments.

Functionally, synapses may be excitatory or inhibitory; transmission is usually unidirectional and not obligatory, except at the neuromuscular junction. Electron microscopy, however, has shown a wide variety of structural arrangements in synapses, which suggests that in some the transmission may be bidirectional (Fig. 2–10).

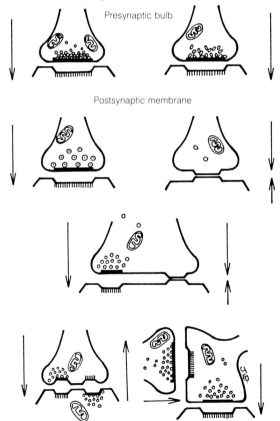

2–10 Schematic diagram illustrating the wide variety of synapses. Note the three types of vesicles (round, flat, and dense core) that characterize chemical synapses. Electrical synapses are devoid of vesicles. *Arrows* indicate the direction of transmission. Redrawn and modified from Bodian, D.: Anat Rec 174 (1972) 73.

Some synapses, termed electrical, have no synaptic vesicles and the adjacent cell membranes are fused. The fused membranes of electrical synapses are called tight junctions or gap junctions. The transmission at these junctions is by electrotonic depolarization; it may be in either direction and is considered obligatory. These are not commonly found in the mammalian nervous system.

Synapses have been classified by their structural association as follows.

1. Axoaxonic, axon to axon
2. Axodendritic, axon to dendrite
3. Axosomatic, axon to cell body
4. Dendrodendritic, dendrite to dendrite
5. Neuromuscular, axon to muscle

In chemical synapses, the following substances have been identified as transmitters.

1. Acetylcholine
2. Monoamines (noradrenaline, dopamine, serotonin)
3. Glycine
4 γ-Aminobutyric acid (GABA)

Neuromuscular Junction

The neuromuscular junction (myoneural junction, motor endplate) is a synapse between a motor nerve terminal and the subjacent part of a muscle fiber. Motor neurons branch extensively near their terminations. One neuron may innervate as few as 10 or as many as 500 or more skeletal muscle fibers. A motor neuron and the muscle fibers innervated by it constitute the motor unit. The motor unit, not the individual muscle fiber, is the basic unit of function. As the nerve fiber approaches the muscle fiber, it loses its myelin sheath and forms a bulbous expansion which occupies a trough on the muscle cell surface (Fig. 2–11). The terminal expansion of the nerve fiber is covered by a cytoplasmic layer of Schwann cells, the neurolemmal sheath, which does not intervene between the nerve ending and the muscle fiber. The endoneurial sheath of connective tissue that surround the nerve fiber outside the neurolemmal sheath is, however, continuous with the connective tissue sheath of the muscle fiber. The endplate is 40 to 60 μm in diameter and is usually located midway along the length of the muscle fiber. The axonal terminal contains synaptic vesicles (filled with acetylcholine) and mitochondria. The synaptic gap (cleft) between the nerve and the muscle is about 500 Å. The postsynaptic membrane of the muscle has numerous infoldings, termed junctional folds (Fig. 2–12). When a motor neuron is fired and the nerve impulse reaches the axon terminals, the contents of the synaptic vesicles (acetylcholine) in the terminal are dis-

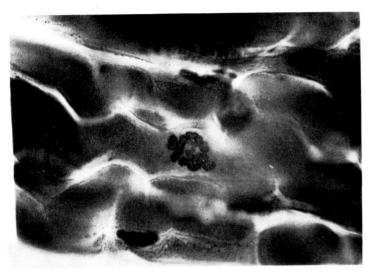

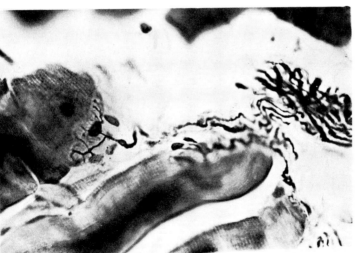

2–11 *Left,* photomicrograph showing terminal arborization of the axon upon a restricted portion of the skeletal muscle (endplate). ×850. *Right,* photomicrograph showing acetylcholinesterase localization in the subneural portion (muscle membrane) of the endplate. ×850.

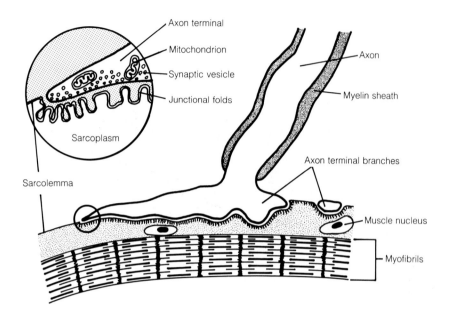

Axon terminal

Mitochondrion

Synaptic vesicle

Junctional folds

Sarcoplasm

Axon

Myelin sheath

Sarcolemma

Axon terminal branches

Muscle nucleus

Myofibrils

2–12 Simplified schematic diagram illustrating the basic components of the obligatory neuromuscular synapse.

charged into the gap between the pre- and postsynaptic membranes. Once acetylcholine is released into the cleft, it diffuses very quickly to combine with acetylcholine receptors in the muscle membrane. This results in the depolarization of the muscle membrane and the appearance of a propagated muscle action potential, leading to muscle contraction. This synaptic activity is always excitatory and is normally obligatory. The subneural sarcolemma or postsynaptic membrane contains the enzyme acetylcholinesterase (Fig. 2–11), which breaks down the depolarizing transmitter, thus allowing the muscle membrane to re-establish resting conditions.

Receptor Organs of Sensory Neurons

The peripheral termination of a sensory neuron is differentiated into specialized dendrites. These dendrites are designed to change or transduce one kind of energy into another, *i.e.*, the electrochemical or nerve impulses. The receptor organs may be classified as free (diffuse) or encapsulated.

Free Nerve Endings

This type of receptor has the widest distribution throughout the body, but is most numerous in the skin. They are also found in mucous membranes, deep fascia, muscles, visceral organs, and elsewhere. The distal arborizations are located in the epithelium between the cells, skin, and mucous membranes lining the digestive and urinary tracts, as well as in all the visceral organs and blood vessels. In addition, they are associated with hair follicles and respond to movement of hair. Certain specialized epithelial cells (neuroepithelium), such as are found in taste buds (Fig. 2–13), olfactory epithelium, and the cochlear and vestibular organs (hair cells), also receive free (receptor) endings. Tendons, joint capsules, periosteum, and deep fascia may also be supplied with this type of ending. These endings probably respond to a wide variety of stimuli, including pain, touch, pressure and tension, and respond indirectly through so-called neuroepithelia to stimuli of sound, smell, taste, and position. The sensory receptor axons may be either myelinated or nonmyelinated.

Encapsulated Endings

Included in this group are the corpuscles of Meissner, Vater-Pacini, Golgi-Mazzoni, and Ruffini; the so-called end bulbs; neuromuscular spindles; and the tendon organ of Golgi.

Meissner's Tactile Corpuscles (Fig. 2–13)   These elongated, rounded bodies are fitted into dermal papillae beneath the epidermis and are about 100 μm in diameter. The corpuscle possesses a connective tissue sheath enclosing stacks of horizontally flattened epithelioid cells. The endoneurium is continuous with the capsule. The myelin sheath terminates and the axon arborizes among the epithelial cells. From one to four myelinated axons, as well as unmyelinated axons, enter the capsule. These receptor organs are widely distributed in the skin, but are found in greatest number in the skin of the fingers, palm of the hand, plantar surface of the foot, and the toes. It is believed that these are touch receptors.

Vater-Pacini Corpuscles (Fig. 2–13)   Pacinian corpuscles are the largest and most widely distributed of the encapsulated receptor organs. They may be as large as 4 mm in length and are the only macroscopic receptor organs of the body. The capsule is elliptical in shape and is composed of concentric lamellae of flattened cells supported by collagenous tissue which invests the unmyelinated distal segment of a large myelinated nerve. The interlamellar spaces are filled with fluid. These corpuscles receive their own blood supply.

Vater-Pacini corpuscles are believed to detect changes that deform the

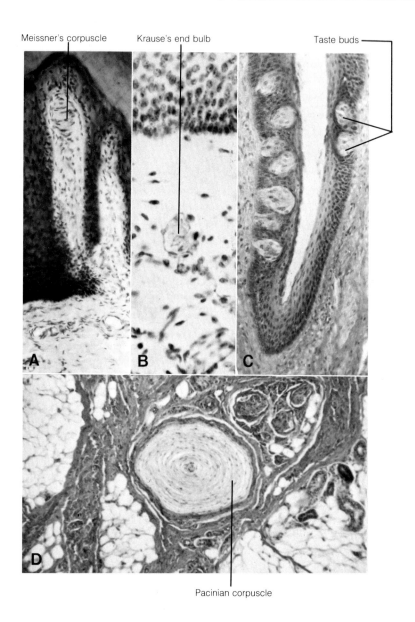

2–13 Photomicrographs showing Meissner's corpuscle (*A*), Krause's end bulb (*B*), taste buds (*C*), and a Pacinian corpuscle (*D*). ×350.

receptor segment of the nerve, such as pressure transients. These ubiquitous receptors are distributed profusely in the subcutaneous connective tissue of the hands and feet. They are also located in the external genitalia, nipples, mammary glands, pancreas and other viscera, mesenteries, linings of the pleural and abdominal cavities, walls of blood vessels, periosteum, ligaments, joint capsules, and muscle.

Golgi-Mazzoni Corpuscles These receptor organs are lamellated (like the Pacinian corpuscle), but instead of a single receptor terminal the unmyelinated receptor is arborized with varicosities and terminal expansions. They are distributed in the subcutaneous tissue of the hands, on the surface of tendons, and elsewhere. Their function is uncertain but is probably related to detection of pressure.

Ruffini Corpuscles These elongated and complex receptors are most readily found in the skin, especially the fingertips, but are widely distributed. The receptor endings within the capsule ramify extensively among the supporting connective tissue bundles. These receptors have been associated with sensations of temperature, particularly heat.

End Bulbs The end bulbs resemble the corpuscles of Golgi-Mazzoni. They have a connective tissue capsule enclosing a gelatinous core in which the terminal, nonmyelinated endings arborize extensively. The end bulbs of Krause (Fig. 2–13) are associated with sensations of temperature (cold) and are strategically located and widely distributed. The structural complexity of these end bulbs varies remarkably, as does their size. It is likely that they serve a wide variety of different functions; their size and distribution, however, preclude easy analysis.

Neuromuscular Spindles These receptors are found in skeletal muscle and are highly organized. They are distributed in both flexor and extensor muscles, but are more abundant in muscles controlling fine movements. Each muscle spindle is less than 1 cm long and contains two to twelve striated fibers (intrafusal fibers) in a connective tissue capsule parallel to the surrounding skeletal muscle fibers (extrafusal fibers).

Histologically, the muscle spindle contains two types of intrafusal muscle fibers (Figs. 2–14 and 2–15). The nuclear chain fiber, smaller in diameter and shorter in length, contains a single row of central nuclei. The nuclear bag fiber, larger and longer, contains a cluster of nuclei in a bag-like dilatation in the central part of the fiber.

Each intrafusal muscle fiber is supplied with both efferent and afferent nerve fibers. The efferent fibers (gamma efferents), which are axons of gamma motor neurons in the anterior horn of the spinal cord, terminate on the polar ends of both the nuclear chain and nuclear bag fibers. The

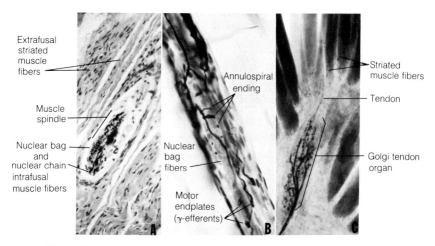

Extrafusal
striated
muscle
fibers

Annulospiral
ending

Striated
muscle fibers

Tendon

Muscle
spindle

Nuclear bag
and
nuclear chain
intrafusal
muscle fibers

Nuclear
bag
fibers

Golgi tendon
organ

Motor
endplates
(γ-efferents)

A   **B**   **C**

2–14   Photomicrographs showing two types of intrafusal muscle fibers within the muscle spindle (*A* and *B*) and a Golgi tendon organ (*C*). *A,* ×200; *B,* ×680; and *C,* ×200.

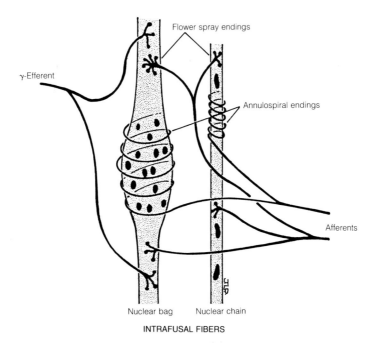

Flower spray endings

γ-Efferent

Annulospiral endings

Afferents

Nuclear bag   Nuclear chain

INTRAFUSAL FIBERS

2–15   The structural organization of the muscle spindle is diagrammed to show the efferent motor innervation of the nuclear bag and nuclear chain fibers. Two sensory (afferent) receptors are shown; these are the annulospiral and flower spray endings.

afferent nerve fibers originate from two types of receptor endings on the intrafusal fibers, the annulospiral (primary) endings and the flower spray (secondary) endings (Fig. 2–15). The annulospiral endings are reticulated branching endings located around the central portion of both the nuclear chain and nuclear bag fibers; they are well developed, however, on the nuclear bag fibers. The flower spray endings are scattered diffusely along the length of the intrafusal fibers, but are found especially on each side of the central portion adjacent to the annulospiral endings. Both nuclear chain fibers and nuclear bag fibers contain this type of ending.

The receptor endings of intrafusal muscle fibers respond to the stretching of extrafusal muscle fibers or their tendons. The activity of the spindle ceases with the relaxation of tension in the spindle when the skeletal muscle contracts. The receptor endings may also be stimulated by the stretching of the intrafusal muscle fibers secondary to gamma motor nerve activity which contracts the polar ends of intrafusal muscle fibers, thus stretching the receptor portions of the fibers.

A static stimulus, such as occurs in sustained muscle stretch, will stimulate both the annulospiral and flower spray endings. On the other hand, only the annulospiral endings respond to a brief stretch of the muscle or vibration.

The afferent nerves emanating from the receptor endings project upon alpha motor neurons in the spinal cord which, in turn, supply the extrafusal muscle fibers. Thus, when a muscle is stretched by tapping its tendon, the stimulated receptor endings initiate an impulse in the afferent nerves which stimulates the alpha motor neurons and results in reflex muscle contraction. As soon as the muscle contracts, the tension in the intrafusal muscle fibers decreases, the receptor response diminishes or ceases, and the muscle relaxes. This is the basis of all monosynaptic stretch reflexes (knee jerk, biceps jerk, etc.). Gamma efferent activity plays a role in sensitizing the receptor endings to a stretch stimulus and helping to maintain muscle tone.

Tendon Organ of Golgi   These receptors are located in tendons close to their junction with skeletal muscles (Fig. 2–14). The organ consists of fascicles of tendon ensheathed by a connective tissue capsule. The capsule encloses the distal end of a large (12 μm) myelinated fiber which divides repeatedly before it splits into unmyelinated (receptor) segments. These branchlets terminate in ovoid expansions that intermingle with and encircle fascicles of collagenous tissue which comprise the tendon. Tendon organs respond to tension in skeletal muscle fibers developed by stretching the muscle or by active contraction of the muscle. The tension thus developed deforms the receptor endings. The function of this receptor is discussed further in the chapter on movement and posture.

Reaction of Neurons to Injury

The reaction of neurons to injury has been studied extensively in experimental animals and confirmed in man; it has actually become one of the methods employed in the study of cell groups and fiber tracts. Responses can be divided into those that occur proximal to the site of injury and those that occur distal to it (Fig. 2–16).

Cell Body and Dendrites

If an axon is severed or crushed, the following reactions can be found in the cell body and dendrites proximal to the site of injury.

1. The entire cell, including the nucleus and nucleolus, swells; the nucleus shifts from its usual central position to the periphery of the cell.
2. The Nissl bodies undergo chromatolysis, *i.e.*, they become diffuse and the normal crisp staining pattern disappears. This process is most marked in the central portion of the cell (perinuclear), but may extend peripherally to involve Nissl bodies located in dendrites.
3. The other organelles, including the Golgi apparatus and mitochondria, proliferate and swell.

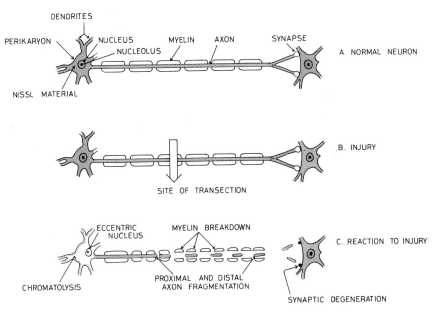

2–16 Schematic diagram of a normal neuron (*A*), site of injury (*B*) and reaction to injury (*C*).

The speed at which these changes occur, as well as their degree, depends on several factors, including the location of the injury, the type of injury, and the type of neuron involved. The closer the injury is to the cell body and the more complete the interruption of the axon, the more severe the reaction and the poorer the chances of full recovery. In general, this reaction is more often seen in motor than in sensory neurons.

The reactions of the cell body and dendrites to axonal injury are termed retrograde cell changes. After about 3 weeks, if the cell survives the injury, the cell body and its processes begin to regenerate. Full recovery takes about 3 to 6 months. The nucleus returns to its central location and is normal in size and configuration. The staining characteristics and structure of the organelles also return to normal. If the regenerative efforts fail, the cell atrophies and is replaced by glia.

Axon

Following injury, the axon undergoes both retrograde (proximal) and anterograde (distal) degeneration. Retrograde degeneration usually involves only a short segment of the axon (a few internodes). Provided the injury to the neuron is reversible, regenerative processes begin with the growth of an axon sprout as soon as new cytoplasm is synthesized and transported from the cell body.

Distal to the site of injury, the severed axon and its myelin sheath undergo what is known as secondary or Wallerian degeneration. The axon, deprived of its continuity with the supporting and nutritive substances from the cell body, begins to degenerate within 12 hours. The axon, which degenerates before its Schwann cell sheath, appears beaded and irregularly swollen within 1 week. The axonal reaction extends distally to involve the synapse. The fragmented portions of the axon are phagocytized by invading macrophages. This process may take considerably longer within the central nervous system.

Along with the degeneration of the axon, the myelin sheath begins to fragment and undergo dissolution within the Schwann cell. Macrophages also play an important role in the removal of myelin breakdown products. The degenerative process occurs within the endoneurium and is soon followed by mitotic activity in the Schwann cells, which form a tube-like sleeve within the endoneurium along the entire length of the degenerated axon.

The growth of axons from the proximal stump begins within 10 hours and may traverse the gap between the proximal and distal ends of the axon and enter the Schwann cell tubes (neurolemma). Although many small axonal sprouts may enter a single tube, only one will develop its normal diameter and appropriate sheath; the others will degenerate. This may occur within 2 or 3 weeks, since regenerative growth normally takes place at a rate of 1.5 to 4 mm/day.

It must be pointed out that chance unfortunately plays an important part in this regenerative activity. If a sensory axon enters a sheath formerly occupied by a motor axon or vice versa, the growing axon will be nonfunctional and the neuron will atrophy. In addition, although the process of degeneration is similar in both the central and peripheral nervous systems, there is a marked difference in the success of the regenerative process in both systems. What has been described above applies to regeneration in the peripheral nervous system.

Neuronal Plasticity

Until a few years ago, it was believed that the mature central nervous system was incapable of recovering its function following injury.

Recent studies have demonstrated that the central nervous system may not be so rigid or static. It has been shown that following lesions the neuronal circuitry may reorganize itself by forming new synapses to compensate for those lost by injury. This property of forming new channels of communication following injury is known as neuronal plasticity.

Neuronal plasticity is most dramatic following partial denervation. In such a situation, the remaining unaffected axons projecting upon the partially denervated region develop axonal sprouts which grow and form new synaptic contacts to replace those that were lost by denervation. The ability of the mature central nervous system to form these sprouts and functional synapses varies from one region to another and from one species to another. The factor or factors that promote sprout formation and synaptogenesis in some, but not all, regions or species are not fully known and are the subject of intensive ongoing research. The identification of factors that promote neuronal plasticity in the injured mature central nervous system may have great impact on the recovery of function in such patients as paraplegics and stroke victims.

The above discussion of plasticity has focused on the regenerative ability of the central nervous system following injury. It should be emphasized, however, that plasticity in its broader sense is an ongoing phenomenon. Although brains are grossly similar anatomically, physiologically, and biochemically, the behavior of humans differs from one individual to another. This difference in behavior reflects the plasticity of the brain in adapting to its environment.

References

Cotman, C.W.: Neuronal Plasticity. Raven Press, New York,1978.

Gershon, M.D.; Schwartz, J.H.; Kandel, E.R.: Morphology of Chemical Synapses and Patterns for Interconnection. In: Principles of Neuroscience, pp. 91–105, Ed. by E.R. Kandel and J.H. Schwartz. Elsevier/North-Holland, New York, 1981.

Gray, E.G.: Synaptic Ultrastructure. In: Neurotransmitter Systems and Their Clinical Disorders, pp.1–16, Ed. by N.J. Legg. Academic Press, London, 1978.

Iversen, L.L.: The Chemistry of the Brain. Sci Am 241, No. 3 (1979) 134–149.

McComas, A.J.: The Neuromuscular Junction. In: Neuromuscular Function and Disorders, pp. 27–34, Ed. by A.J. McComas. Butterworth, London, 1977.

Shepard, G.: The Synaptic Organization of the Brain. An Introduction, pp. 15–34. Oxford University Press, New York, 1974.

Stevens, C.F.: The Neuron. Sci Am 241, No. 3 (1979) 54–65.

Varon, S.S.; Somjen, G.G.: Neuron-Glia Interactions. Neurosci Res Program Bull 17 (1979) 19–41.

Weller, R.O.; Cervõs-Navarro, J.: Pathology of Peripheral Nerves, pp. 30–60. Butterworth, London, 1977.

3

Gross Topography

For didactic purposes, the nervous system is conventionally divided into three major parts. These are the central nervous system, peripheral nervous system, and autonomic nervous system. Although the division simplifies the study of this complex system, the three component parts act in concert in the overall control and integration of the motor, sensory, and behavioral activities of the organism. A great deal of effort has been expended in the elucidation of the structure, connectivity, and function of the nervous system. The methodologic creativity and observational acumen of anatomists, physiologists, psychologists, and physicians have been impressive and rewarding. Their work, however, is far from finished.

The term central nervous system refers to the brain and spinal cord. The term peripheral nervous system refers to cranial nerves, spinal nerves, ganglia associated with cranial and spinal nerves, and peripheral receptor organs. The term autonomic nervous system refers to that part of the nervous system concerned mainly with the regulation of visceral function; its component parts are located partly within the central nervous system and partly within the peripheral nervous system.

This chapter is concerned mainly with the gross features of the central nervous system. Its purposes are to acquaint the student with the terminologic jargon used in the neurologic sciences and to provide orientation to the major components of this system. The autonomic nervous system will be discussed in a separate chapter. The peripheral nervous system is usually covered in standard courses of gross anatomy and microscopic anatomy.

Central Nervous System

The central nervous system is usually considered to have two major divisions, the brain and the spinal cord. The brain is subdivided into the following structures.

1. The two cerebral hemispheres are bilaterally symmetric.

2. The brain stem consists of the diencephalon, mesencephalon (midbrain), pons, and medulla oblongata.
3. The cerebellum.

The cerebral hemispheres and diencephalon are discussed in this chapter. The gross topography of the rest of the brain stem, the cerebellum, and the spinal cord are presented in their respective chapters.

Brain

The brain is semisolid in consistency and conforms to the shape of its container. It weighs approximately 1400 gm in the adult. The male brain is on the average slightly heavier than that of the female, although this has no relationship to intelligence.

The brain is protected from the external environment by three barriers.

1. Skull
2. Meninges
3. Cerebrospinal fluid

The bony skull is the major barrier against physical trauma to the brain.

The meninges are organized into three layers; these are named in order of their proximity to the skull.

1. Dura mater
2. Arachnoid mater
3. Pia mater

The dura mater is a tough, fibrous connective tissue arranged in two layers. An outer parietal layer adheres to the skull and forms its periosteum and an inner meningeal layer is in contact with the arachnoid mater. These two layers of dura are adherent to each other except at sites of formation of dural venous sinuses, such as the superior sagittal and others.

The dura mater has three major reflections which separate components of the brain. The falx cerebri is a vertical reflection between the two cerebral hemispheres. The tentorium cerebelli is a horizontal reflection between the posterior (occipital) parts of the cerebral hemispheres and the cerebellum. The falx cerebelli is a vertical reflection which incompletely separates the two cerebellar hemispheres at the inferior surface.

The arachnoid mater is a nonvascular membrane of an external mesothelium joined with web-like trabeculae to the underlying pia mater.

The pia mater is a thin, translucent membrane intimately adherent to brain substance. Blood vessels of the brain are located on the pia mater. The arachnoid mater and pia mater are collectively referred to as the pia-arachnoid membrane because of their close structural and functional relationships.

The meninges are at times subject to infection. The condition is known as meningitis. This is a serious, life-threatening condition that requires immediate medical treatment. The three layers of meninges are separated from each other and from the bony skull by the following spaces.

1. The epidural space is located between the dura mater and the bony skull. Trauma to the skull with rupture of the middle meningeal artery leads to epidural hemorrhage, which is the accumulation of arterial blood in the epidural space. Because of the pressure produced by such hemorrhage in a closed container such as the skull, epidural hemorrhages are handled as an acute emergency calling for surgical intervention to evacuate the accumulated blood in the epidural space and control the bleeding.

2. The subdural space is located between the dura mater and arachnoid mater. Trauma to the skull may rupture the bridging veins, leading to subdural hemorrhage, the accumulation of blood in the subdural space. This condition also calls for surgical intervention to evacuate the accumulated blood and control the bleeding.

3. The subarachnoid space is located between the arachnoid mater and pia mater. This space contains cerebrospinal fluid and cerebral and spinal blood vessels. Rupture of such vessels leads to subarachnoid hemorrhage, the accumulation of blood in the subarachnoid space. Such a condition may result from trauma to the head, congenital abnormalities in vessel structure or high blood pressure.

The third barrier that protects the brain, the cerebrospinal fluid, is the subject of another chapter in this book.

External Topography of the Brain

For convenience, the topography of the brain will be discussed under three headings: the lateral aspect, the medial aspect, and the ventral aspect.

Lateral Aspect

The lateral aspect of the brain is marked by two principal landmarks that divide the cerebral hemispheres into lobes (Fig. 3–1). The lateral fissure (sylvian fissure) and the central sulcus (rolandic sulcus) divide the cerebral hemisphere into the frontal lobe (dorsal to the lateral fissure and rostral to the central sulcus), temporal lobe (ventral to the lateral fissure), and parietal lobe (dorsal to the lateral fissure and caudal to the central sulcus). If a line were drawn from the parieto-occipital sulcus (best seen on the medial aspect of the hemisphere) onto the lateral aspect of the hemisphere down to the preoccipital notch, it would delineate the boundaries of the parietal lobe rostrally from that of the occipital lobe caudally. Lying deep within the lateral fissure and seen only when the banks of the fissure are separated is the insula or island of Reil (Fig. 3–2). It is concerned primarily with autonomic function.

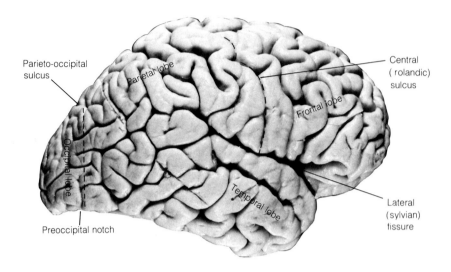

3-1 Photograph of the lateral surface of the brain showing the major fissures and sulci and the four lobes. ×0.9.

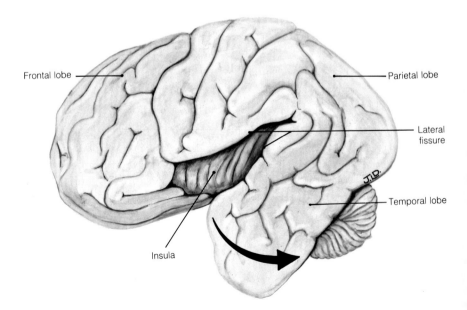

3-2 Schematic diagram showing the insula deep within the lateral fissure.

Frontal Lobe (Fig. 3–3)   Rostral to the central sulcus, between it and the precentral sulcus, is the precentral gyrus (primary motor area), which is one of the most important cortical areas concerned with movement. Although movement can be elicited by stimulation of a number of cortical areas, that developed by stimulation of the precentral gyrus is achieved by a relatively low threshold of stimulation. Body parts are disproportionately and somatotopically represented in the primary motor area. The face representation is lower than the upper extremity representation, followed by the trunk and lower extremity. The leg and foot are represented on the medial surface of the precentral gyrus. In the face area of the precentral gyrus, the lip representation is disproportionately large compared to its actual size in the face. The same applies to the thumb representation in the hand area. This disproportionate representation of body parts in the primary motor cortex is known as motor homunculus.

Stimulation of specific areas of the precentral gyrus results in movement of a single muscle or of a group of muscles in the contralateral part of the body. Lesions of the precentral gyrus result in contralateral paralysis (loss of movement). This is most marked in those muscles used for fine performance, such as buttoning a shirt or writing.

Rostral to the precentral sulcus is the premotor area. This is another important area for movement. Blood flow studies have shown that this

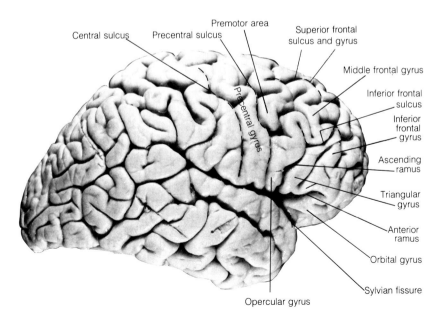

3–3   Photograph of the lateral surface of the brain showing the major gyri and sulci of the frontal lobe. ×0.9.

area plays a role in initiating new programs for movement and in introducing changes in programs in progress.

Rostral to the premotor area, the frontal lobe is divided by two sulci, the superior and inferior frontal sulci, into three gyri. These are the superior, middle, and inferior frontal gyri. The middle frontal gyrus contains an area (area 8 of Brodmann) important for conjugate eye movements. This area is known as the area of frontal eye fields. The inferior frontal gyrus is subdivided by two sulci extending from the lateral (sylvian) fissure, the anterior (horizontal) and ascending rami. Rostral to the anterior ramus is the orbital gyrus; between the two rami is the triangular gyrus and caudal to the ascending ramus is the opercular gyrus. The triangular gyrus and the immediately adjacent part of the opercular gyrus constitute the area of Broca, which, in the dominant (left) hemisphere, represents the motor area for speech. Lesions of this area result in the inability of the individual to express himself in spoken language (aphasia).

Parietal Lobe (Fig. 3–4)   Caudal to the central sulcus, between it and the postcentral sulcus, is the postcentral gyrus, a primary sensory (somesthetic) area which is concerned with general body sensation. Body representation in the primary sensory area is similar to that described for the

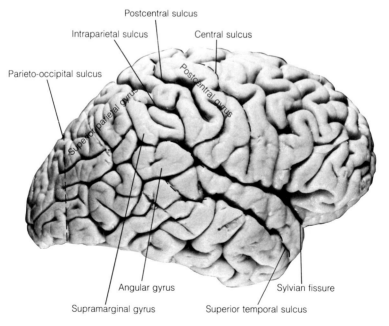

3–4   Photograph of the lateral surface of the brain showing the major gyri and sulci of the parietal lobe. ×0.9.

primary motor area. The disproportionate and somatotopic representation of body parts is known as sensory homunculus. Stimulation of this area in man and other primates elicits sensations of tingling and numbness in the part of the body that corresponds to (and is contralateral to) the area stimulated. Lesions of this area result in loss of sensation contralateral to the site of the brain lesion.

Caudal to the postcentral gyrus, the intraparietal sulcus extends horizontally across the parietal lobe, dividing it into superior and inferior parietal gyri. The inferior parietal gyrus contains two important gyri, the supramarginal and angular gyri. The supramarginal gyrus caps the end of the sylvian fissure, whereas the angular gyrus caps the end of the superior temporal sulcus. Lesions in these two gyri in the dominant hemisphere result in disturbances in language comprehension and object recognition.

Temporal Lobe (Fig. 3–5)   Three gyri comprise the lateral aspect of the temporal lobe. These are the superior, middle, and inferior temporal gyri, separated by the superior and middle sulci. The inferior temporal gyrus extends over the inferior border of the temporal lobe onto the ventral surface of the brain. The superior temporal gyrus contains on its dorsal border (bank of the lateral fissure) the transverse temporal gyri of Heschl (primary auditory area).

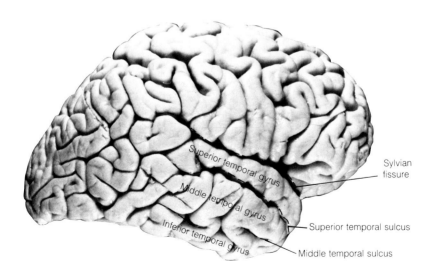

3–5   Photograph of the lateral surface of the brain showing the major gyri and sulci of the temporal lobe. ×0.9.

Occipital Lobe (Fig. 3–1) On the lateral aspect of the brain, the occipital lobe merges with the parietal lobe. The occipital pole contains a
portion of the primary visual area, which is more extensive on the medial
aspect of the occipital lobe.

Medial Aspect (Fig. 3–6)

The corpus callosum, in a midsagittal section of the brain, stands out
prominently as a C-shaped, massive bundle of fibers. The corpus callosum
is generally subdivided into a head (rostrum) at the rostral extremity, a
large body extending across the frontal and parietal lobes, a genu (knee)
connecting the rostrum and body, and a splenium at the caudal extremity.
It consists of fibers that connect the two cerebral hemispheres. Behavioral
studies have shown that the corpus callosum plays an important role in the
transfer of information between the two hemispheres. Lesions in the corpus
callosum disconnecting the right from the left hemisphere result in the
isolation of both hemispheres so that each will have its own learning processes and memories which are inaccessible to the other. The effects of such
isolation are discussed in Chapter 21.

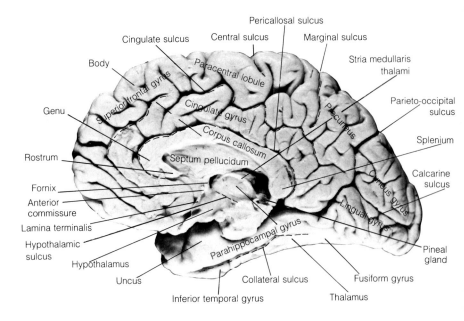

3–6 Photograph of the midsagittal surface of the brain showing major gyri and
sulci. ×0.9.

Dorsal to the corpus callosum, separated from it by the pericallosal sulcus, is the cingulate gyrus, which follows the contours of the corpus callosum and occupies parts of the frontal and parietal lobes. The cingulate gyrus is part of the limbic system, which is concerned with visceral function, emotion, and behavior. The cingulate gyrus is separated from the rest of the frontal and parietal lobes by the cingulate sulcus. Dorsal to the cingulate gyrus, extensions of the pre- and postcentral gyri onto the medial aspect of the brain form the paracentral lobule. The precuneus is the part of the parietal lobe caudal to the paracentral lobule, between the marginal and parieto-occipital sulci. The parieto-occipital sulcus is well delineated on this surface of the brain and defines the boundaries between the parietal and occipital lobes. Extending at approximately right angles from the parieto-occipital sulcus in the occipital lobe is the calcarine sulcus, which divides the occipital lobe into a dorsal cuneus gyrus and a ventral lingual gyrus. The primary visual area is located on each bank of the calcarine sulcus. Lesions of the primary visual area produce loss of vision in the contralateral half of the visual field. This condition is known as hemianopia.

Ventral to the corpus callosum is the septum pellucidum, a thin septum which separates the two lateral ventricles. At the inferior border of the septum pellucidum is another C-shaped fiber bundle, the fornix, which connects the temporal lobe (hippocampal formation) and the diencephalon. In midsagittal sections of the brain, only a small part of the fornix is seen.

Rostral to the anterior extent of the fornix is a small bundle of fibers, the anterior commissure, which connects the two temporal lobes and olfactory or smell structures in both hemispheres. Recent evidence points to a wider distribution of anterior commissure fibers than previously believed. The anterior commissure of man has been shown to be composed of an anterior limb concerned with olfaction and a posterior limb containing neocortical fibers connecting visual and auditory areas in the temporal lobes. There is strong support for the theory that the anterior commissure plays a role in interhemispheric transfer of visual information.

Extending from the ventral border of the anterior commissure to the ventral border of the diencephalon is a thin membrane, the lamina terminalis. This lamina marks the most anterior boundary of the embryologic neural tube.

Behind the rostral extremity of the fornix and extending in an oblique manner caudally is the hypothalamic sulcus. This sulcus divides the diencephalon into a dorsal thalamus and a ventral hypothalamus. The midline area between the two thalami and hypothalami is occupied by the slit-like third ventricle. In some brains, the two thalami are connected across the midline by the interthalamic adhesion (massa intermedia). The thalamus is the gateway to the cerebral cortex. All sensory inputs (except olfaction) pass through the thalamus before they reach the cortex. Similarly, motor inputs to the cerebral cortex pass through the thalamus. The hypothalamus is a major central autonomic and endocrine center. It plays a role in such activities as feeding, drinking, sexual behavior, emotional behavior, and growth.

The dorsal border of the thalamus is the stria medullaris thalami, a thin band which extends caudally to merge with the habenular nuclei. Above the dorsal and caudal part of the diencephalon lies the pineal gland, which is assumed to have an endocrine function. The stria medullaris thalami, habenular nuclei, and pineal gland comprise the epithalamus. The continuation of the cingulate gyrus in the temporal lobe is the parahippocampal gyrus (a component of the limbic lobe). The parahippocampal gyrus is continuous with the uncus (another component of the limbic lobe) in the tip of the temporal lobe. The collateral sulcus separates the parahippocampal gyrus from the inferior temporal gyrus. Along the lateral side of the collateral sulcus is the fusiform (occipitotemporal) gyrus. Extending from the diencephalon caudally are the mesencephalon, pons, and medulla oblongata (Fig. 3–7). The cerebellum occupies a position between the occipital lobe, pons, and medulla oblongata.

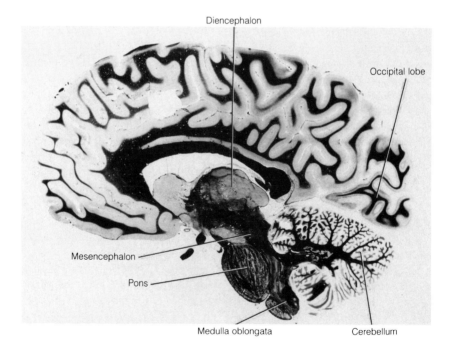

3–7 Photograph of a parasagittal view of the brain showing brain stem components. ×1.1.

The medial aspect of the brain shows to advantage the components of the limbic lobe (Fig. 3–8). These include the subcallosal gyrus, cingulate gyrus, parahippocampal gyrus, and uncus. The limbic lobe forms the core of the limbic system, which is discussed in another chapter.

Parasagittal sections of the brain (Fig. 3–9) show to advantage deeper structures not seen in midsagittal sections, such as the caudate nucleus, putamen, globus pallidus, and internal capsule. Lateral extension of the thalamus is also seen in such sections. The caudate nucleus, putamen, and globus pallidus are known collectively as the corpus striatum. They are basal ganglia of the brain and play a role in regulation of movement. The caudate nucleus and putamen are collectively known as the striatum and are separated by the anterior limb of the internal capsule. The putamen and globus pallidus are collectively known as the lenticular nucleus. Both nuclei are separated from the thalamus by the posterior limb of the internal capsule. The internal capsule carries motor and sensory fibers from the cerebral cortex to lower centers and vice versa. Lesions of the internal capsule result in contralateral motor deficits (paralysis) and sensory deficits.

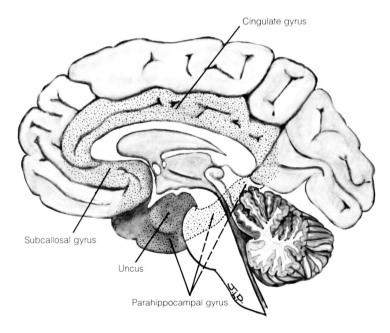

3–8 Schematic diagram of the medial surface of the cerebral hemisphere showing components of the limbic lobe.

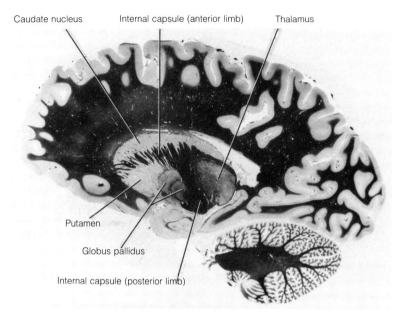

Caudate nucleus Internal capsule (anterior limb) Thalamus

Putamen

Globus pallidus

Internal capsule (posterior limb)

3–9 Parasagittal section of the brain showing the striatum, thalamus and internal capsule and their relationships. × 1.0.

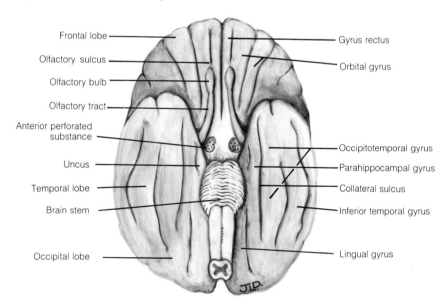

Frontal lobe

Olfactory sulcus

Olfactory bulb

Olfactory tract

Anterior perforated substance

Uncus

Temporal lobe

Brain stem

Occipital lobe

Gyrus rectus

Orbital gyrus

Occipitotemporal gyrus

Parahippocampal gyrus

Collateral sulcus

Inferior temporal gyrus

Lingual gyrus

3–10 Schematic diagram of the ventral surface of the brain showing major gyri and sulci.

Ventral Aspect

Portions of the frontal, temporal, and occipital lobes appear on this aspect of the brain (Fig. 3–10).

Frontal Lobe   The ventral aspect of the frontal lobe shows a longitudinal sulcus, the olfactory sulcus, in which the olfactory tract and bulb are located. Medial to the olfactory sulcus is the gyrus rectus; lateral to the olfactory sulcus is the orbital gyrus. At the caudal extremity of the olfactory tract is the anterior perforated substance, the site of perforating blood vessels passing to deeper regions of the brain.

Temporal Lobe   The ventral aspect of the temporal lobe shows the continuation of the inferior temporal gyrus from the lateral aspect. Medial to the inferior temporal gyrus is the occipitotemporal (fusiform) gyrus. The collateral sulcus separates the latter gyrus from the more medial parahippocampal gyrus and uncus, which constitute parts of the limbic lobe.

Occipital Lobe   The ventral aspect of the occipital lobe shows the continuation of the lingual gyrus from the medial aspect of the brain.

The ventral aspect of the brain shows to advantage the mamillary bodies of the diencephalon, the cranial nerves, and the ventral aspect of the pons, medulla oblongata, and cerebellum (Fig. 3–11). Gross topography of the pons, medulla oblongata, and cerebellum will be discussed in the respective chapters.

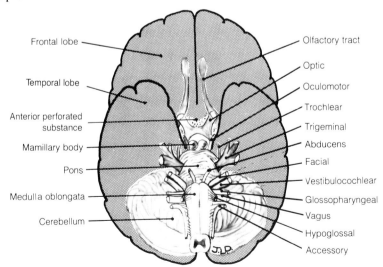

Frontal lobe — Olfactory tract — Optic — Temporal lobe — Oculomotor — Trochlear — Anterior perforated substance — Trigeminal — Mamillary body — Abducens — Facial — Pons — Vestibulocochlear — Medulla oblongata — Glossopharyngeal — Vagus — Cerebellum — Hypoglossal — Accessory

3–11   Schematic diagram of the ventral surface of the brain showing the cranial nerves.

Internal Topography of Brain

Internal brain topography is presented here in a few selective coronal and horizontal sections. A more complete set of sections is shown in the Atlas at the end of this book.

Coronal Sections

Four representative rostrocaudal coronal sections are considered.

Section at Level of Anterior Limb of Internal Capsule   At this level (Fig. 3–12), the anterior limb of the internal capsule separates the caudate nucleus medially from the putamen laterally. The caudate nucleus shows its characteristic bulge into the lateral ventricle. This bulge is lost in degenerative diseases of the caudate nucleus such as Huntington's chorea. The corpus callosum is continuous with the deep white matter of the cerebral hemispheres. The septum pellucidum is ventral to the corpus callosum and forms a partition between the two lateral ventricles.

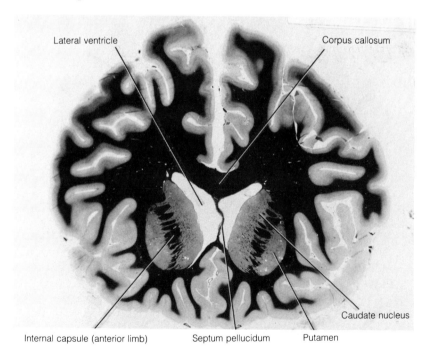

Lateral ventricle   Corpus callosum

Internal capsule (anterior limb)   Septum pellucidum   Putamen

Caudate nucleus

3–12   Photograph of a coronal section of the brain at the level of the anterior limb of the internal capsule. ×0.9.

Section at Level of Anterior Commissure   At this level (Fig. 3–13), the anterior commissure courses ventral to the globus pallidus. Dorsal to the corpus callosum is the cingulate gyrus. The caudate nucleus is smaller and retains its characteristic relationship to the lateral ventricle. The putamen is larger and is lateral to the globus pallidus; the two basal ganglia nuclei are separated from the thalamus by the posterior limb of the internal capsule. The fornix is seen in two sites, ventral to the corpus callosum and ventral to the thalamus.

Section at Level of Optic Tract   At this level (Fig. 3–14), the optic tracts course in the ventral part of the brain on their way to the lateral geniculate nucleus of the thalamus. Each optic tract carries fibers from the ipsilateral and the contralateral retinae. The fornix is located dorsal and medial to the optic tracts, separating the hypothalamus into lateral and medial regions. The anterior commissure is seen beneath the putamen. The thalamus is larger in size and is clearly divided into medial and lateral nuclear groups by the internal medullary lamina. The mamillothalamic tract courses within the thalamus on its way to the anterior nuclear group. The posterior limb of the internal capsule separates the lenticular nucleus (putamen and globus pallidus) from the thalamus. Coursing from the globus pallidus to the thalamus is a bundle of fibers, the ansa lenticularis. Lateral to the putamen

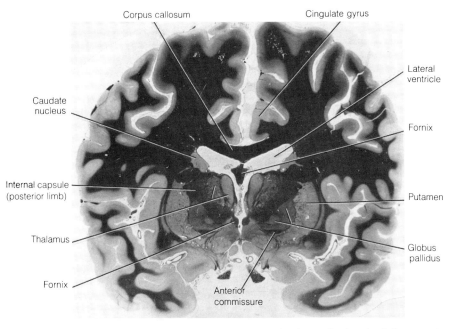

3–13   Photograph of a coronal section of the brain at the level of the anterior commissure. × 1.1.

is the external capsule, one of the efferent cortical bundles. Between the external and extreme capsules lies the claustrum.

Section at Level of Mamillary Bodies   At this caudal diencephalic level (Fig. 3–15), the mamillary bodies occupy the ventral surface of the brain. Emanating from the mamillary bodies are the mamillothalamic tracts on their way to the anterior thalamus. The thalamus at this level is rather large and is separated from the putamen and globus pallidus by the posterior limb of the internal capsule. Medial to the internal capsule and dorsolateral to the mamillary body is the subthalamic nucleus, a component of the diencephalon concerned with movement. Lesions of the subthalamic nucleus give rise to a characteristic involuntary movement disorder contralateral to the lesion known as hemiballismus. The caudate nucleus at this level is small. Between the two diencephalons is the cavity of the third ventricle. The insula (island of Reil) is seen deep within the lateral (sylvian) fissure.

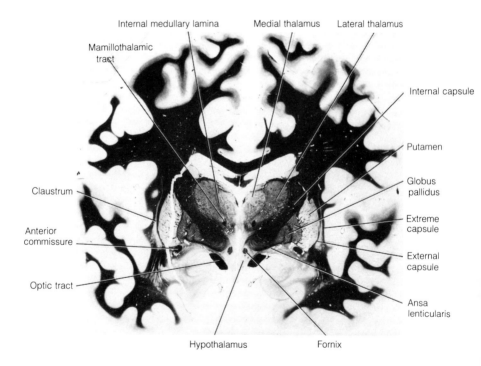

3–14   Photograph of a coronal section of the brain at the level of the optic tracts. × 1.3.

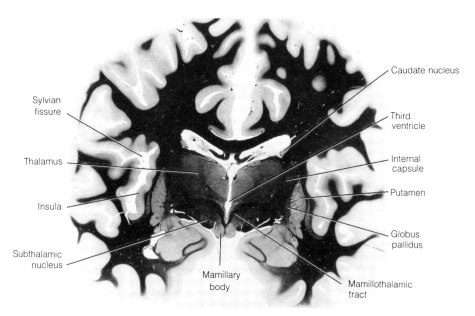

Sylvian fissure

Thalamus

Insula

Subthalamic nucleus

Mamillary body

Caudate nucleus

Third ventricle

Internal capsule

Putamen

Globus pallidus

Mamillothalamic tract

3–15 Photograph of a coronal section of the brain at the level of the mamillary body. ×1.2.

Horizontal Sections

A few representative dorsoventral horizontal sections are presented.

Section at Level of Corpus Callosum At this level (Fig. 3–16), the corpus callosum interconnects the two halves of the brain and is continuous with the white matter core of both hemispheres. The caudate nucleus is shown bulging into the lateral ventricle. The internal capsule is lateral to the caudate and continuous with the white matter core of the hemispheres.

Section at Level of Thalamus and Basal Ganglia At this level (Fig. 3–17), the frontal, temporal, and occipital lobes are seen. The insula (island of Reil) is buried deep within the sylvian fissure. The frontal (anterior) and occipital (posterior) horns of the lateral ventricle are seen in the respective lobes. The septum pellucidum separates the two frontal horns. Ventral to the septum is the fornix. The head of the caudate nucleus is seen bulging into the frontal horn of the lateral ventricle. The tail of the caudate, much smaller than the head, is seen more caudally. Both the anterior and posterior limbs of the internal capsule are seen. The former separates the caudate and putamen nuclei, whereas the latter separates the thalamus and putamen. The rostral part and the caudal part (splenium) of the corpus callosum are also seen.

Lateral
ventricle

Caudate
nucleus

Corpus
callosum

Internal
capsule

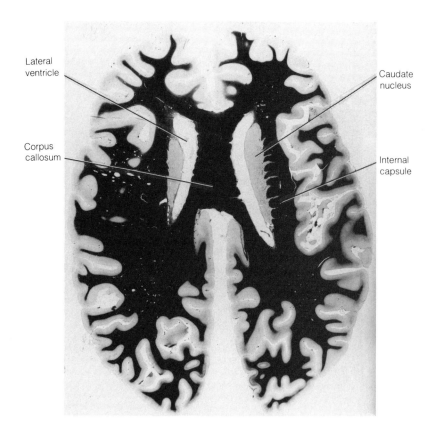

3–16 Photograph of a horizontal section of the brain through the corpus callosum.
× 1.1.

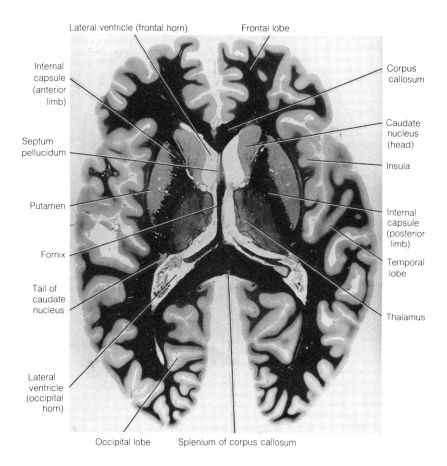

Lateral ventricle (frontal horn) Frontal lobe

Internal capsule (anterior limb)

Corpus callosum

Septum pellucidum

Caudate nucleus (head)

Insula

Putamen

Internal capsule (posterior limb)

Fornix

Temporal lobe

Tail of caudate nucleus

Thalamus

Lateral ventricle (occipital horn)

Occipital lobe Splenium of corpus callosum

3–17 Photograph of a horizontal section of the brain through the thalamus and the basal ganglia. × 1.0.

Section at Level of Anterior Commissure   At this level (Fig. 3–18), the anterior commissure is seen rostral to the putamen, globus pallidus, and the columns of the fornix. The posterior limb of the internal capsule separates the thalamus from the globus pallidus. The hippocampus is seen as an involution into the inferior (temporal) horn of the lateral ventricle. The fimbria of the fornix, containing axons of neurons in the hippocampus, is seen attached to the hippocampus.

Section at Level of Brain Stem   At this level (Fig. 3–19), the cerebellum, mesencephalon, mamillary bodies, and optic chiasma are seen. Rootlets of the oculomotor (CN III) nerve are seen coursing in the mesencephalon. The cerebral peduncles, continuations of the internal capsule, are located in the ventral part of the mesencephalon. Dorsal to the cerebral peduncle is the substantia nigra.

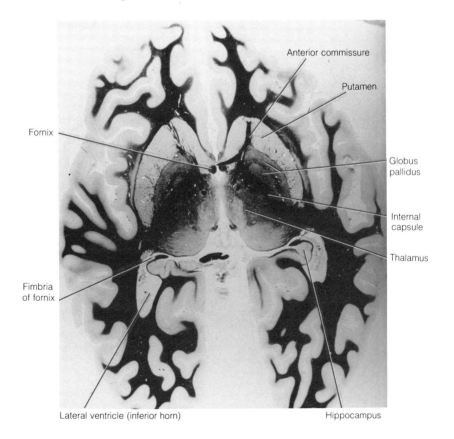

3–18   Photograph of a horizontal section of the brain through the anterior commissure. × 1.4.

The identification of brain structures in horizontal sections has assumed more importance with the introduction of computerized X-ray brain tomography (computerized axial tomography or CAT scans) as a diagnostic tool in neurology. In this procedure, computerized X-ray photographs of horizontal brain sections are taken at a predetermined angle to detect the site and nature of lesions in the brain. This is a highly specialized technique requiring a thorough knowledge of the anatomy of the brain in horizontal sections. For the purpose of this presentation, only four representative CAT scan cuts will be described. The first (Fig. 3–20) is a superficial cut showing the gray and white matter of the hemispheres within the bony skull. The second cut (Fig. 3–21) is through the body and occipital (posterior) horns of the lateral ventricle. The third cut (Fig. 3–22) is through the frontal (anterior) horn of the lateral ventricle and the third ventricle. The caudate nucleus is seen bulging into the anterior horn of the lateral ventricle. The anterior limbs of the internal capsule are seen between the caudate and putamen. The posterior limb of the internal capsule separates the putamen and globus pallidus from the thalamus. Between the two thalami is the third ventricle. The cisterna ambiens is seen caudally. The last and most inferior cut (Fig. 3–23) shows the cerebellum, fourth ventricle, and suprasellar cistern.

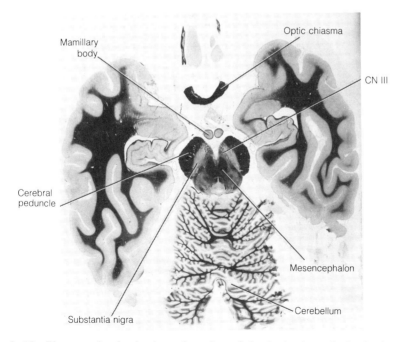

3–19 Photograph of a horizontal section of the brain through the brain stem. × 1.3.

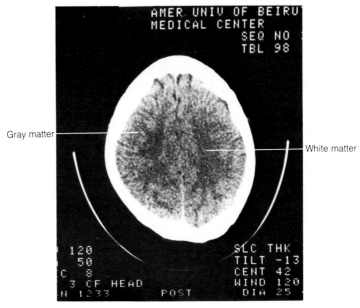

3-20 Photograph of a CAT cut through the upper part of the brain (brain convexity).

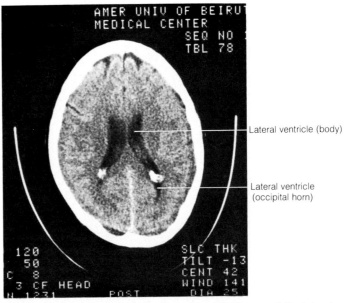

3-21 Photograph of a CAT cut through the body and occipital horns of the lateral ventricle.

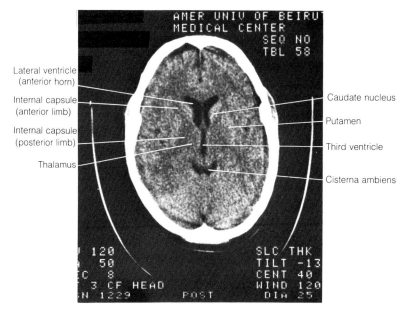

3–22 Photograph of a CAT cut through the frontal horn of the lateral ventricle and the third ventricle.

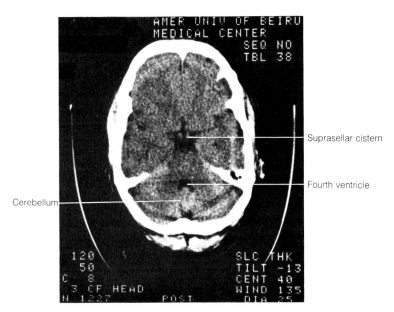

3–23 Photograph of a CAT cut through the fourth ventricle and the cerebellum.

References

Gluhbegovic, N.; Williams, T.H.: The Human Brain. A Photographic Guide. Harper & Row, Hagerstown, 1980.

Haines, D.E.: Neuroanatomy. An Atlas of Structures, Sections, and Systems. Urban & Schwarzenberg, Baltimore, 1983.

Jouandet, M.L.; Gazzaniga, M.S.: Cortical Field of Origin of the Anterior Commissure of the Rhesus Monkey. Exp Neurol 66 (1979) 381–397.

Risse, G.L.; LeDoux, J.; Springer, S.P.; Wilson, D.H.; Gazzaniga, M.S.: The Anterior Commissure in Man: Functional Variation in a Multisensory System. Neuropsychologia 16 (1978) 23–31.

Roberts, M.; Hanaway, J.: Atlas of the Human Brain in Sections. Lea & Febiger, Philadelphia, 1970.

Shipps, F.C.; Jones, J.M.; D'Agostino, A.: Atlas of Brain Anatomy for C.T. Scans, Ed. 2. Charles C Thomas, Springfield, Ill., 1977.

4

Spinal Cord

External Topography

The spinal cord of humans is a cylindrical tube that extends, in the adult, from the foramen magnum to the level of the first or second lumbar vertebra. In embryonic life, the cord occupies the whole length of the vertebral canal; in the newborn, it extends down to the level of the third lumbar vertebra. The variation in the lower level of the cord from fetal life to the adult is explained by the differential growth of the vertebral column and the spinal cord, the former being faster. The spinal cord exhibits two enlargements. These are the cervical and lumbar enlargements, which are sites of neurons that innervate the upper and lower extremities, respectively. The lower end of the cord is tapered to form the conus medullaris from which a pia-glial filament, the filum terminale, extends to the coccyx to anchor the spinal cord. The spinal cord is also anchored to the dura by denticulate ligaments, pial folds stretching from the surface of the cord to the outer dural sheath midway between the dorsal and ventral roots. Denticulate ligaments serve as a useful landmark for the neurosurgeon in identifying the anterolateral segment of the cord when performing operations such as cordotomies for the relief of intractable pain.

The spinal cord of man is considered to have 31 segments, each of which has a pair of dorsal and ventral roots and a pair of spinal nerves. Thus, there are 31 pairs of spinal nerves; they are divided into eight cervical, twelve thoracic (dorsal), five lumbar, five sacral, and one coccygeal. The spinal nerves leave the vertebral canal through the intervertebral foramina. The first cervical nerve emerges above the atlas; the eighth cervical nerve emerges between the seventh cervical (C_7) and the first thoracic (T_1) vertebrae. All other spinal nerves exit beneath the corresponding vertebrae.

Because of the differential rate of growth of the spinal cord and vertebral column, spinal cord segments do not correspond to those of the vertebral column. Thus, in the cervical region, the tip of the vertebral spine corresponds to the level of the succeeding cord segment; that is, the sixth cervical spine corresponds to the seventh spinal cord segment. In the upper thoracic region, the tip of the spine is two segments above the corresponding cord segment; the fourth thoracic spine corresponds to the sixth cord segment. In the lower thoracic and upper lumbar region, the difference between the vertebral and cord level is three segments; the tenth thoracic spine corresponds to the first lumbar cord segment. Because of this, the root filaments of spinal cord segments have to travel progressively longer distances from cervical to sacral segments to reach the corresponding intervertebral foramina from which the spinal nerves emerge. The crowding of lumbosacral roots around the filum terminale is known as the cauda equina.

The spinal cord is covered by three meningeal coats; these are the pia, arachnoid, and dura mater. The spinal cord terminates at the level of L_1-L_2 vertebrae, whereas the dura mater extends down to the level of S_1-S_2 vertebrae. A sac filled with cerebrospinal fluid and devoid of spinal cord is formed in the subarachnoid space. This sac is a favorable site for clinicians to introduce a special spinal needle to obtain cerebrospinal fluid for examination or to inject drugs or dyes into the subarachnoid space for purposes of treatment or diagnosis. This procedure is called a lumbar puncture or spinal tap.

Cross-Section Topography

In cross-section, the spinal cord is composed of a centrally placed, butterfly- or H-shaped area of gray matter surrounded by white matter. The two wings of the butterfly are connected across the midline by the dorsal and ventral gray commissures above and below the central canal, respectively (Fig. 4–1). The gray part of the cord contains primarily the cell bodies of neurons and glia. The white part of the cord contains primarily fiber tracts.

The two halves of the spinal cord are separated by the dorsal (posterior) median septum and the ventral (anterior) median fissure (Fig. 4–2). The site of entrance of dorsal root fibers is marked by the dorsolateral (posterolateral) sulcus; similarly, the site of exit of ventral roots is marked by the ventrolateral (anterolateral) sulcus (Fig. 4–2). These landmarks divide the white matter of each half of the cord into a dorsal (posterior) funiculus, a lateral funiculus, and a ventral (anterior) funiculus (Fig. 4–2). Furthermore, the dorsal (posterior) funiculus is partially divided into two unequal parts by the dorsal (posterior) intermediate septum (Fig. 4–2).

The H-shaped gray matter is also divided into a smaller dorsal (posterior) horn or column and a larger ventral (anterior) horn or column. The thoracic and upper lumbar cord segments, in addition, exhibit a wedge-shaped intermediolateral horn or column (Fig. 4–3).

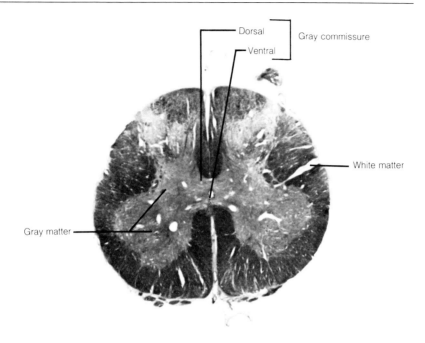

4–1 Photomicrograph of the spinal cord showing the central butterfly-shaped gray matter and the surrounding white matter.

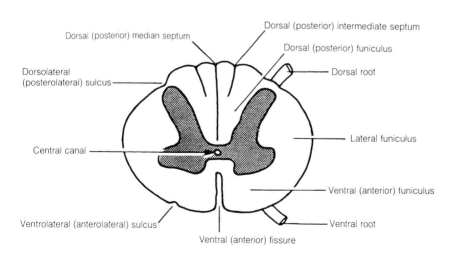

4–2 Cross-sectional diagram of the spinal cord showing the sulci and fissure that delineate the funiculi.

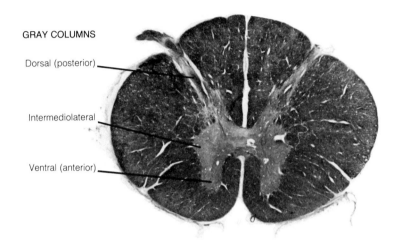

GRAY COLUMNS

Dorsal (posterior)

Intermediolateral

Ventral (anterior)

4–3 Photomicrograph of the spinal cord showing the division of gray matter into columns.

Microscopic Anatomy

Gray Matter

Older Terminology Prior to 1952, the organization of the gray matter of the spinal cord was viewed in the following way.

Dorsal Horn The dorsal (posterior) horn or column contains the following cell clusters, all of which are concerned with sensory function and receive axons of the dorsal root ganglia via the dorsal root. These cell clusters are the posteromarginal nucleus, the substantia gelatinosa, and the nucleus proprius.

Intermediolateral Horn The intermediolateral horn or column, which is limited to the thoracic and upper lumbar segments of the cord, contains cell bodies of the sympathetic nervous system, the axons of which leave the spinal cord via the ventral root.

Ventral Horn The ventral horn or column contains multipolar motor neurons, the axons of which comprise the major component of the ventral root.

Intermediate Zone This zone contains the nucleus dorsalis of Clarke and a large number of interneurons.

The above organizational pattern is illustrated diagrammatically in Figure 4–4.

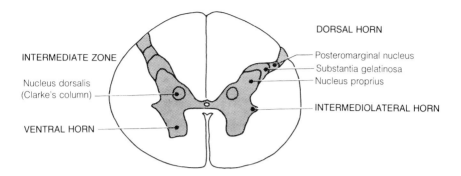

4-4   Cross-sectional diagram of the spinal cord showing the major nuclear groups within the gray columns.

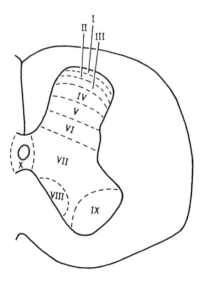

4-5   Schematic diagram of half of the spinal cord showing the location of Rexed laminae.

Rexed Terminology   In 1952, Rexed investigated the cytoarchitectonics, or cellular organization, of the spinal cord in the cat and found that cell clusters in the cord are arranged with extraordinary regularity into 10 zones. His observations have subsequently been confirmed in other species, including the monkey. Figure 4-5 is a diagrammatic representation of the location of the 10 laminae of Rexed. Table 4-1 compares the older terminology with the more recent Rexed terminology.

Table 4–1 Cellular Organization of Spinal Cord

Rexed terminology	Older terminology
Lamina I	Posteromarginal nucleus
II	Substantia gelatinosa
III, IV	Nucleus proprius
V	Neck of posterior horn
VI	Base of posterior horn
VII	Intermediate zone, intermediolateral horn
VIII	Commissural nucleus
IX	Ventral horn
X	Grisea centralis

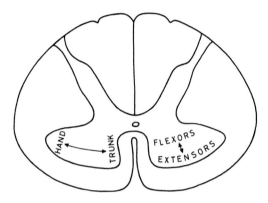

4–6 Schematic diagram of the spinal cord showing somatotopic organization of ventral horn neurons.

Laminae I to IV are concerned with exteroceptive sensations, whereas laminae V and VI are concerned primarily with proprioceptive sensations, although they respond to cutaneous stimuli. Lamina VII acts as a relay between midbrain and cerebellum. Lamina VIII modulates motor activity, most probably via the gamma neuron. Lamina IX is the main motor area of the spinal cord. It contains large alpha and smaller gamma motor neurons. The axons of these neurons supply the extrafusal and intrafusal muscle fibers, respectively. Alpha motor neurons in this lamina are somatotopically organized in such a way that neurons supplying flexor musculature are dorsally placed, whereas neurons supplying extensor muscle groups are ventrally placed. In addition, neurons supplying trunk musculature are medially placed, whereas neurons supplying extremity musculature are laterally placed (Fig. 4–6).

Physiologic studies have demonstrated two types of alpha motor neurons, the tonic and the phasic. The tonic variety are characterized by a lower rate of impulse firing and slower axonal conduction. No anatomic criteria are available to distinguish tonic from phasic alpha motor neurons.

Physiologic studies have also demonstrated two types of gamma motor neurons, the static and the dynamic.

The static variety is related to the nuclear chain type of intrafusal muscle fiber concerned with the static response of the muscle spindle, whereas the dynamic variety is related to the nuclear bag type of intrafusal muscle fiber concerned with the dynamic response of the spindle. As is the case with alpha motor neurons, no anatomic criteria are available to differentiate static from dynamic gamma motor neurons.

In addition to alpha and gamma motor neurons, lamina IX contains interneurons. One of these interneurons, the Renshaw cell, has received much attention from neuroscientists. The Renshaw cell is interposed between the recurrent axon collateral of an alpha motor neuron and the dendrite or cell body of the same alpha motor neuron. The axon collateral of the alpha motor neuron excites the Renshaw cell and in turn the axon of the Renshaw cell inhibits the parent alpha motor neuron. Through this feedback loop, a parent alpha motor neuron may influence its own activity. Recent studies have shown that Renshaw cell axons project to near as well as distant sites, including laminae IX, VIII and VII.

Quantitative studies of the dendritic organization of spinal motor neurons have shown that approximately 80% of the receptive area of a neuron is formed of dendrites; although dendrites extend up to 1000 μm from the cell body, the proximal third contains most of the synapses and is most effective in reception of incoming stimuli. Lamina X surrounds the central canal and contains neuroglia.

Neurons in the gray matter of the spinal cord have been classified into two general categories on the basis of their axonal course. Tract neurons have axons which contribute to the formation of a tract. Examples of such neurons include the dorsal column of Clarke, which gives rise to the dorsal spinocerebellar tract, and neurons in the dorsal horn that give rise to the spinothalamic tract. In contrast, root neurons have axons which contribute to the formation of the ventral root. Examples of such neurons include alpha and gamma motor neurons in the anterior horn and the autonomic neurons in the intermediolateral horn.

White Matter

The white matter of the spinal cord is organized into three funiculi (Fig. 4–7).

1. Posterior funiculus
2. Lateral funiculus
3. Anterior funiculus

Each of these funiculi contains one or more tracts or fasciculi. A tract

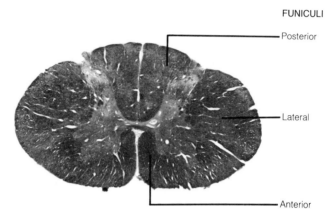

4-7 Photomicrograph of the spinal cord showing the division of white matter into three funiculi.

is composed of nerve fibers sharing a common origin, destination, and function. In general, the name of a tract denotes its origin and destination; the spinocerebellar tract connects the spinal cord and cerebellum, the corticospinal tract connects the cortex and spinal cord, etc.

Posterior Funiculus Nerve fibers in this funiculus are concerned with two general modalities. These are kinesthesia (sense of position and movement) and discriminative touch (precise localization of touch, including two-point discrimination).

Lesions of this funiculus will therefore be manifested clinically by loss or diminution of the following sensations.

1. Vibration sense
2. Position sense
3. Two-point discrimination
4. Touch
5. Weight perception

The presence or absence of these different sensations is tested by the neurologist as follows.

1. Vibration is tested by placing a vibrating tuning fork over a bony prominence.
2. Position sense is tested by moving the tip of the patient's finger or toe dorsally and ventrally and asking the patient (whose eyes are closed) to identify the position of the part moved.
3. Two-point discrimination is tested by simultaneously pricking the patient in two adjacent areas of skin. Under normal conditions, a person is able to recognize these two simultaneous stimuli as separate stimuli if the distance between them is not less than 5 mm on the fingertips using pins and not less than 10 cm on the shin using fingertips.

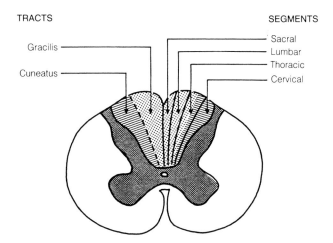

TRACTS   SEGMENTS

Sacral
Gracilis   Lumbar
                                          Thoracic
Cuneatus   Cervical

4-8 Schematic diagram of the spinal cord showing spatial arrangement of fibers in the posterior white funiculus.

4. Touch is tested by placing a cotton ball gently over the skin.
5. Weight perception is tested by asking the patient (whose eyes are closed) to estimate roughly a weight placed in his hand.

The nerve fibers that contribute to the posterior funiculus have their cell bodies in the dorsal root ganglia. The peripheral receptors contributing to this system are those located in joint surfaces or joint capsules, which convey information about position of body parts, and Pacinian corpuscles, which are concerned with vibration.

Nerve fibers of the posterior funiculus are thickly myelinated and occupy the medial part of the dorsal root. Those that enter the spinal cord below the sixth thoracic segment are located medially in the posterior funiculus and form the gracile tract. Fibers that enter the spinal cord above the sixth thoracic segment are located more laterally and form the cuneate tract. Thus, the nerve fibers in the posterior funiculus are laminated or layered in such a way that those arising from the sacral region are most medial, whereas those from the cervical region are most lateral (Fig. 4–8). It should be pointed out that the lamination in the posterior funiculus is both segmental (sacral, lumbar, etc.) and modality-oriented. Physiologic studies have shown that fibers conducting impulses from hair receptors are superficial and are followed by fibers mediating tactile and vibratory sensations in successively deeper layers.

The fibers forming the posterior funiculus ascend throughout the spinal cord and synapse on the posterior column nuclei in the medulla oblongata. Axons of these nuclei then cross in the midline and ascend to the thalamus and from there to the sensory cortex.

Recent studies suggest that only 25% of the fibers entering the posterior funiculus reach the posterior column nuclei. There is also evidence to suggest the presence, in the posterior funiculus, of postsynaptic fibers arising from laminae V and VI of Rexed; these fibers constitute 9% of the posterior funiculus and are located in the gracile tract. Physiologic studies suggest that these postsynaptic fibers are polymodal since they respond both to nociceptive and non-nociceptive stimuli.

Some of the fibers in the posterior funiculus send collateral branches that terminate upon neurons in the posterior horn of gray matter. Thus, these collaterals give the posterior funiculus a role in modifying sensory activity in the posterior horn. As is discussed later, this role is inhibitory to pain impulses.

Stimulation of the posterior funiculus has been used in the treatment of chronic pain. In one large study, 47% of treated patients responded initially to this stimulation, but the percentage dropped to 8% after 3 years. None of the patients studied had complete relief from pain.

There are reports in the literature of lesions in the posterior funiculus in man and animals without concomitant deficit in the modalities presumably carried by this system. This is explained by the presence of another system, the spinocervical thalamic, located in the lateral funiculus, which may compensate for posterior funiculus deficits.

Lateral and Anterior Funiculi   The posterior funiculus contains only one ascending fiber system, whereas the lateral and anterior funiculi contain several ascending and descending tracts. Only those tracts with established functional or clinical relevance will be discussed.

Ascending Tracts   All of the following tracts have their cells of origin in dorsal root ganglia.

Dorsal spinocerebellar tract   This ascending fiber system conveys to the cerebellum proprioceptive impulses from receptors located in muscles, tendons, and joints. The impulses arising in muscle spindles travel via Ia and II nerve fibers, whereas those arising in Golgi tendon organs travel via Ib nerve fibers. Central processes of neurons in dorsal root ganglia (DRG) enter the spinal cord via the dorsal root and either ascend or descend in the posterior funiculus for a few segments before reaching the spinal nucleus or they may reach the nucleus directly. Nerve cells, the axons of which form this tract, are located in the nucleus dorsalis of Clarke (also known as Clarke's column) within lamina VII of Rexed (Fig. 4–9). This nucleus is not found throughout the extent of the spinal cord, but is limited to the spinal cord segments between the eighth cervical and second lumbar. Because of this, the dorsal spinocerebellar tract is not seen below the second lumbar segment. Nerve fibers belonging to this system and entering below L_2 ascend to the L_2 level, where they synapse with cells located in the

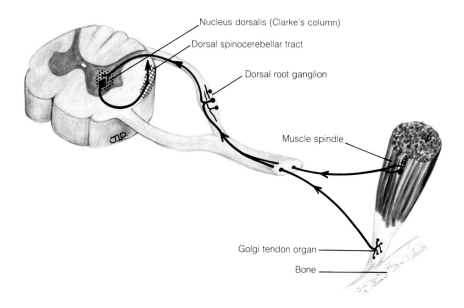

Nucleus dorsalis (Clarke's column)

Dorsal spinocerebellar tract

Dorsal root ganglion

Muscle spindle

Golgi tendon organ

Bone

4-9 Schematic diagram of the spinal cord showing the formation of the dorsal spinocerebellar tract.

nucleus. Similarly, nerve fibers entering above the upper limit of the nucleus ascend in the cuneate tract to reach the accessory cuneate nucleus in the medulla oblongata, which is homologous to the nucleus dorsalis (Fig. 4-10). Fibers in this tract are segmentally laminated in such a way that fibers from lower limbs are superficially placed. The fibers in this tract reach the cerebellum via the inferior cerebellar peduncle (restiform body) and terminate upon the rostral and caudal portions of the vermis. The dorsal spinocerebellar tract conveys to the cerebellum information pertaining to muscle contraction, including phase, rate, and strength of contraction.

There is evidence to suggest that some of the fibers forming this tract arise from neurons in laminae V and VI of Rexed, as well as from the nucleus dorsalis of Clarke.

Ventral spinocerebellar tract This fiber system conveys impulses almost exclusively from Golgi tendon organs via Ib afferents. Dorsal root fibers destined for this tract synapse with neurons in laminae V to VII of Rexed. Axons arising from these neurons then cross to form the ventral spinocerebellar tract, which ascends throughout the spinal cord, medulla oblongata and pons before entering the contralateral cerebellum via the superior cerebellar peduncle (brachium conjunctivum). Thus, the fibers of

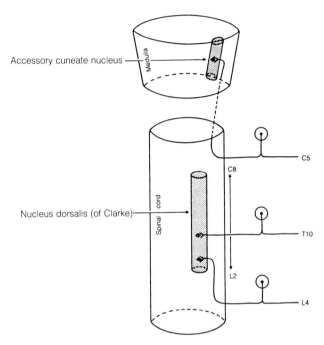

4-10 Schematic diagram of the spinal cord showing the homology of the accessory cuneate nucleus and the nucleus dorsalis of Clarke.

this tract undergo double crossing, one in the spinal cord and another in the cerebellum. The majority of fibers in this tract terminate in the vermis and intermediate lobe, mostly homolateral to the limb of origin, but also contralateral. The ventral spinocerebellar tract transmits to the cerebellum information related to interneuronal activity and the effectiveness of the descending pathways.

In addition to the above classic spinocerebellar pathways, there are at least two other indirect pathways from the spinal cord to the cerebellum.

1. Spino-olivocerebellar, with an intermediate station at the inferior olive in the medulla oblongata
2. Spinoreticulocerebellar, with an intermediate synapse in the lateral reticular nucleus of the medulla.

The impulses traveling via the indirect spinocerebellar pathways reach the cerebellum after a longer latency than that observed with the more direct spinocerebellar pathways. It is thus postulated that impulses traveling via the classic direct pathway reach the cerebellum sooner and will condition it for the reception of impulses arriving later via the indirect pathways.

Spinocervical thalamic tract Nerve fibers destined to form the spinocervical tract are central processes of DRG. They enter the spinal cord

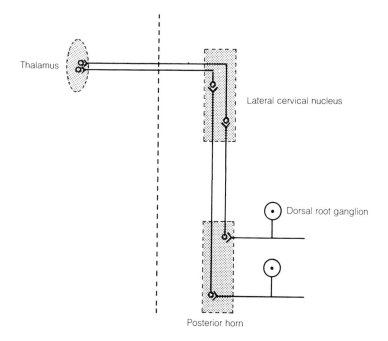

Thalamus

Lateral cervical nucleus

Dorsal root ganglion

Posterior horn

4–11   Schematic diagram showing the formation of the spinocervical thalamic tract.

with the thickly myelinated fibers of the medial division of the dorsal root. They travel within the posterior funiculus for several segments before entering the posterior horn gray matter to synapse on neurons there. Axons of neurons in the posterior horn ascend in the lateral funiculus to the upper two cervical segments, where they synapse on neurons of the lateral cervical nucleus. Axons of this nucleus cross to the opposite lateral funiculus and ascend to the thalamus (Fig. 4–11).

The spinocervical thalamic tract accounts for the presence of kinesthesia and discriminative touch after total interruption of the posterior funiculus. Although this tract has not been demonstrated in man, its presence has been assumed because of the persistence of posterior funiculus sensations after total posterior funiculus lesions. Thus, the older concept of the necessity of the posterior funiculus for discriminatory sensation is being challenged. Instead, a newer concept is evolving which attributes to the posterior funiculus a role in the discrimination of those sensations that must be actively explored by the animal and to the spinocervical thalamic system a role in the discrimination of sensations that are passively impressed on the animal.

Lateral spinothalamic tract   This ascending fiber tract is located medial to the dorsal and ventral spinocerebellar tracts (Fig 4–12) and is concerned

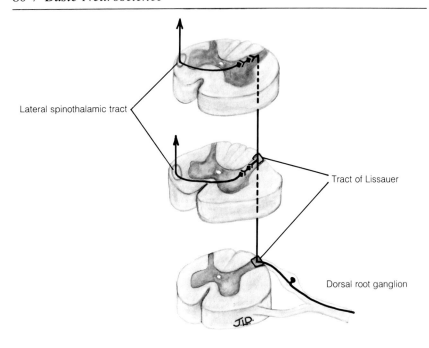

Lateral spinothalamic tract

Tract of Lissauer

Dorsal root ganglion

4–12 Schematic diagram showing the formation of the lateral spinothalamic tract.

with transmission of pain and temperature sensations. Root fibers contributing to this tract (C-fibers and A-delta fibers) have their neurons of origin in the dorsal root ganglion. They are unmyelinated and thinly myelinated fibers that generally occupy the ventrolateral region of the dorsal root as it enters the spinal cord. Incoming root fibers establish synapses in laminae I to VI of Rexed. Axons of neurons in these laminae in turn establish synapses with neurons in laminae V to VIII. Axons of tract neurons in laminae V to VIII, as well as some axons arising from neurons in lamina II, cross to the opposite lateral funiculus in the anterior white commissure within one to two segments above their entry level to form the lateral spinothalamic tract. Fibers of sacral origin are located most laterally and those of cervical origin more medially in the tract. This segmental lamination is useful clinically in differentiating lesions within the spinal cord from those compressing the spinal cord from outside. In the former, the cervical fibers are affected early, whereas the sacral fibers are affected either late or not at all. This condition, known clinically as sacral sparing, is characterized by preservation of pain and temperature sensations in the sacral dermatomes and their loss or diminution in other dermatomes. In addition to this segmental lamination, the lateral spinothalamic tract exhibits modality lamination, in which fibers conveying pain sensations are anteriorly located and those conveying thermal sense are most posteriorly located. This segregation of fibers in a modality pattern, however, is incomplete. Once formed, this tract ascends throughout the length of the spinal cord and brain stem to reach the thalamus, where it synapses upon neurons in the posteroventral lateral nucleus.

Lesions of this tract result in loss of pain and thermal sense in the contralateral half of the body beginning one or two segments below the level of the lesion. In contrast to this pattern of pain and thermal loss, lesions of the dorsal root result in segmental loss of pain and temperature ipsilateral to the lesion, whereas lesions of the crossing fibers in the anterior white commissure result in bilateral segmental loss of pain and temperature in dermatomes corresponding to the affected spinal segments. This last pattern is often noted in syringomyelia, a disease in which the central canal of the spinal cord encroaches upon, among other sites, the anterior white commissure.

The lateral spinothalamic tract may be sectioned surgically for the relief of intractable pain. In this procedure, known as cordotomy, the surgeon uses the ligamentum denticulatum of the spinal meninges as a landmark and orients his knife anterior to the ligament to reach the tract.

There has been increased interest in pain pathways and pain mechanisms in recent years. These extensive studies have shown that the lateral spinothalamic tract is only one of several pathways carrying pain impulses. Other pathways conveying this modality include a multisynaptic pathway associated with the reticular system and a spinotectal pathway. These studies have also developed the concept of an inhibitory input into the posterior horn from the thickly myelinated fibers of the dorsal root and posterior column. This has led clinicians to stimulate these inhibitory fibers traveling in the posterior column in an attempt to relieve intractable pain.

Out of these recent studies on pain mechanisms has evolved the gate control theory of pain proposed by Melzack and Wall (Fig. 4–13). According to this theory, two afferent inputs related to pain enter the spinal cord. One input is via small fibers which are tonic and adapt slowly with a continuous flow of activity, thus keeping the gate open. Impulses along these fibers will activate an excitatory mechanism which increases the effect of arriving impulses. The second input is via large, thickly myelinated fibers which are phasic, adapt rapidly, and fire in response to a stimulus. Both types of fibers project into lamina III of Rexed, which suggests that this lamina is the modular center for pain. The thin fibers inhibit, whereas the thick fibers facilitate, neurons in this lamina. Both types of fibers also project into laminae V to VIII of Rexed where the tract cells are located. Both thin and thick fibers are facilitatory to neurons in these laminae. Furthermore, axons of neurons in lamina III have a presynaptic inhibitory effect on both small and large axons projecting on laminae V to VIII. These different relationships (Fig. 4–13) can be summarized as follows:

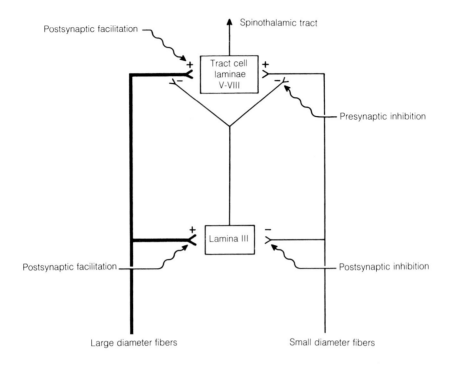

4–13 Schematic diagram of the gate control theory of pain.

1. Ongoing activity which precedes a stimulus is carried by the tonic, slowly adapting fibers that tend to keep the gate open.
2. A peripheral stimulus will activate both small and large fibers. The discharge of the latter will initially fire the tract cells (T-cells) through the direct route, then partially close the gate through their action via lamina III (facilitation of presynaptic inhibition).
3. The balance between large and small fiber activation will determine the state of the gate. If the stimulus is prolonged, large fibers will adapt, resulting in a relative increase in small fiber activity which will open the gate further and increase T-cell activity. If large fiber activity is increased, however, by a proper stimulus (vibration), the gate will tend to close and T-cell activity will diminish.

Since its publication, the gate control theory has been modified and further clarified. It is now recognized that inhibition occurs by both presynaptic and postsynaptic inputs from the periphery, as well as by descending cortical influences. While it is generally agreed that a gate control for pain exists, its functional role and detailed mechanism need further exploration.

Ongoing research in pain mechanisms has given rise in recent years to much interesting data, some of which are summarized below.

1. Two types of pain receptors have been identified: unimodal nociceptors responding to nociceptive stimuli and polymodal nociceptors responding to nociceptive, chemical, and mechanical stimuli.
2. Three types of spinothalamic neurons have been identified in the dorsal horn: low threshold mechanoreceptors in laminae VI to VII, high threshold nociceptors in lamina I, and wide dynamic range neurons in lamina V responding to both mechanoreceptor and nociceptor stimulation. The wide dynamic range neurons receive inputs from both low threshold mechanoreceptors and high threshold nociceptors and are probably concerned with visceral and referred pain.
3. Only the nociceptor neurons are inhibited by serotonergic fibers from the nucleus raphe magnus.
4. Several neurotransmitter substances have been identified in the dorsal horn: noradrenalin and serotonin in the substantia gelatinosa, and substance P, somatostatin, and enkephalins in laminae I to III. Substance P has been found to be excitatory, whereas enkephalins are inhibitory.
5. C-fibers entering via the dorsal root terminate on marginal zone (lamina I) and substantia gelatinosa (lamina II) neurons. They excite neurons in all these laminae via axodendritic synapses. Axons of substantia gelatinosa neurons in turn inhibit marginal zone neurons via axosomatic synapses.
6. A-delta fibers establish excitatory synapses on substantia gelatinosa and nucleus proprius (laminae III and IV) neurons. Since substantia gelatinosa neurons inhibit marginal zone neurons, repetitive stimulation of the A-delta fibers can significantly inhibit marginal zone neurons. In common practice, this is probably what happens when pain from a cut on the finger is reduced by local pressure (stimulation of A-delta fibers).
7. About 24% of sacral and 5% of lumbar originating fibers in the lateral spinothalamic tract project to the ipsilateral thalamus.

Anterior spinothalamic tract   This is a tract concerned with light touch. Fibers contributing to this tract in the dorsal root establish synapses in laminae VI to VIII. Axons of neurons in these laminae cross to the opposite side of the anterior white commissure for several segments and gather in the lateral and anterior funiculi to form the tract. Somatotopic organization in this tract is similar to that in the lateral spinothalamic tract. The course of this tract in the spinal cord and brain stem is similar to that of the lateral spinothalamic. Unilateral lesions of this tract are not detectable clinically because light touch is also carried by other ascending systems, such as the posterior column. Bilateral lesions, however, result in disturbances in itching and tickling responses and libidinal sensations.

Recent evidence suggests the following. This tract conveys pain impulses in addition to touch; some of its fibers ascend ipsilaterally all the way to the midbrain where they cross in the posterior commissure and project primarily upon intralaminar neurons in the thalamus, with some fibers reaching the periaqueductal gray matter in the midbrain. It is believed to convey the aversive and motivational, nondiscriminative pain sensations, in contrast to the lateral spinothalamic tract, which is believed to convey the well-localized discriminative pain sensations.

Other ascending tracts Other ascending tracts of less clinical significance include the spino-olivary, spinotectal and spinocortical. The functional significance of these multisynaptic pathways is not very well delineated; they may play a role in feedback control mechanisms.

Descending Tracts The ascending tracts originate in dorsal root ganglia neurons; the descending tracts, in contradistinction, originate from several sites. As with the ascending tracts, only the descending tracts of clinical or functional significance will be discussed.

Corticospinal tract The cells of origin of this tract are located in the cerebral cortex. From their site of origin, axons of the corticospinal tract descend throughout the whole length of the neuraxis (brain stem and spinal cord). At the caudal end of the medulla oblongata, the majority of corticospinal fibers cross (pyramidal decussation) to form the lateral corticospinal tract, located in the lateral funiculus of the spinal cord. The uncrossed fibers remain in the anterior funiculus as the anterior corticospinal tract (Fig. 4–14). The majority of fibers in the corticospinal tract are small in caliber, ranging in diameter from 1 to 4 μm. Only about 3% of the fiber population are large caliber fibers (>10 μm in diameter). The large caliber fibers arise from the giant cells of Betz in the motor cortex. In the spinal cord, corticospinal fibers project upon interneurons in laminae IV to VII of Rexed. There is evidence also for a direct projection of a small number of fibers upon motor neurons in lamina IX in the monkey and possibly man. The impulses conveyed via this system are facilitatory to flexor moto neurons. The termination of the corticospinal tract in laminae IV to VI (which also receive sensory impulses from the periphery) suggests that thi tract plays a role in modulation of sensory input to the spinal cord.

Lesions of the corticospinal tract result in paralysis. If the lesion occurs above the level of decussation, paralysis is contralateral to the side of the lesion. If the corticospinal lesion is below the decussation (*i.e.*, in the spinal cord), the paralysis is homolateral to the side of the lesion. In addition to paralysis, lesions in the corticospinal tract result in a conglomerate of neurologic signs which include spasticity (resistance to the initial phase of passive movement of a limb or muscle group), hyperactive myotatic reflexes (exaggerated response of knee jerk and other deep tendon reflexes), Babinski sign (abnormal flexor reflex in which stroking the lateral aspect of

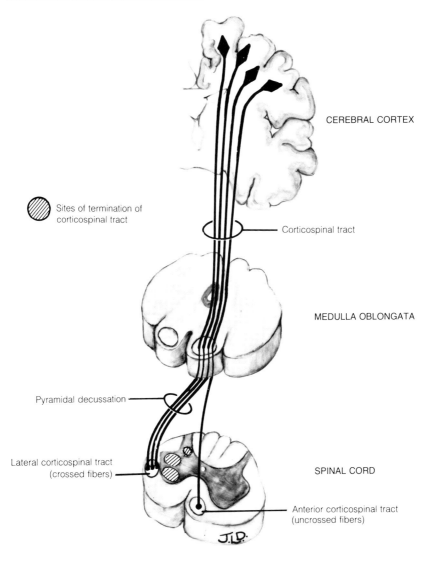

CEREBRAL CORTEX

Sites of termination of
corticospinal tract

Corticospinal tract

MEDULLA OBLONGATA

Pyramidal decussation

Lateral corticospinal tract
(crossed fibers)

SPINAL CORD

Anterior corticospinal tract
(uncrossed fibers)

J.L.D.

4–14 Composite diagram of the origin, course, and termination of the lateral and anterior corticospinal tracts.

the sole of the foot results in dorsiflexion of the big toe and fanning out of the other toes), and clonus (an alternating contraction of antagonistic muscles resulting in a series of extension and flexion movements). Collectively, this conglomerate of signs is referred to by clinicians as "upper motor neuron signs."

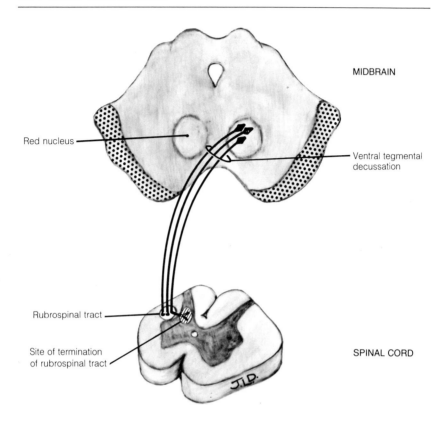

MIDBRAIN

Red nucleus

Ventral tegmental decussation

Rubrospinal tract

Site of termination of rubrospinal tract

SPINAL CORD

4–15 Composite schematic diagram of the origin, course, and termination of the rubrospinal tract.

Rubrospinal tract Neurons of origin of this tract are located in the posterior two-thirds of the red nucleus in the midbrain. Fibers forming this tract cross in the ventral tegmental decussation of the midbrain and descend throughout the whole length of the neuraxis to reach the lateral funiculus of the spinal cord, in close proximity to the corticospinal tract (Fig. 4–15). They terminate in the same laminae in the base of the dorsal horn as the corticospinal tract fibers and similarly facilitate flexor motor neurons. Because of the similarity in the site of termination of both tracts and because the red nucleus receives an input from the cortex, the rubrospinal tract has been considered by some as an indirect corticospinal tract (Fig. 4–16). The two tracts constitute the dorsolateral pathway for movement, in which the corticospinal tract initiates movement and the rubrospinal corrects the errors in movement.

Lateral vestibulospinal tract The neurons of origin of this tract lie in the lateral vestibular nucleus located in the pons. From their site of origin,

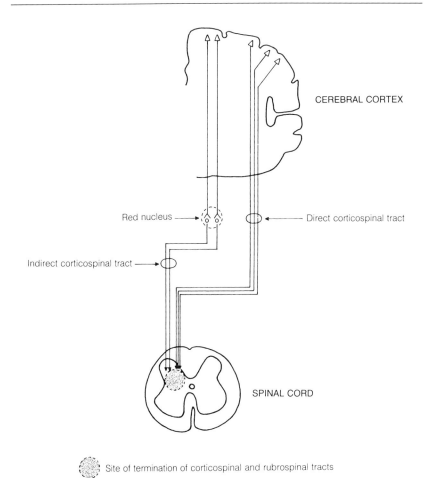

CEREBRAL CORTEX

Red nucleus

Direct corticospinal tract

Indirect corticospinal tract

SPINAL CORD

Site of termination of corticospinal and rubrospinal tracts

4–16 Composite schematic diagram comparing the origin, course, and termination of the corticospinal and rubrospinal tracts.

fibers descend uncrossed and occupy a position in the lateral funiculus of the spinal cord (Fig. 4–17). The fibers in this tract terminate on interneurons in laminae VII and VIII, with some direct terminations on alpha motor neuron dendrites in the same laminae. The impulses conducted in this system facilitate extensor motor neurons.

Medial vestibulospinal tract The neurons of origin of the medial vestibulospinal tract are located in the medial vestibular nucleus. From their neurons of origin, fibers join the medial longitudinal fasciculus and terminate on neurons in laminae VII and VIII. They have a facilitatory effect on flexor motor neurons.

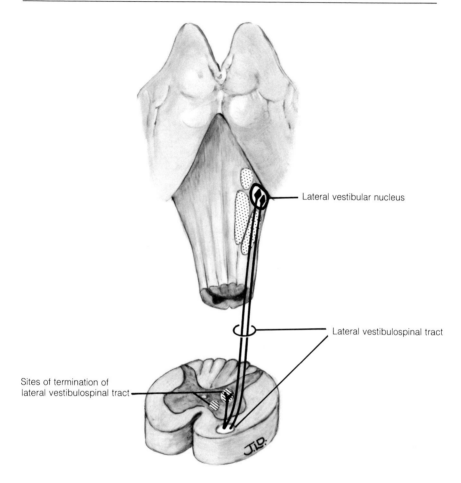

Lateral vestibular nucleus

Lateral vestibulospinal tract

Sites of termination of
lateral vestibulospinal tract

4–17 Composite schematic diagram of the origin, course, and termination of the lateral vestibulospinal tract.

Reticulospinal tracts The neurons of origin of these tracts are located in the reticular formation of the pons and medulla oblongata. The pontine reticulospinal tract is located in the anterior funiculus of the spinal cord, whereas the medullary reticulospinal tract is located in the lateral funiculus. Both tracts descend predominantly ipsilaterally, but both have, in addition, some crossed components. The pontine reticulospinal tract is facilitatory to extensor motor neurons, whereas the medullary reticulospinal tract facilitates flexor motor neurons.

Earlier studies suggested that reticulospinal fibers arise from large reticular neurons in the medial two-thirds of the medulla and pons. Recent studies show that these fibers originate from many smaller cells. Physiologic

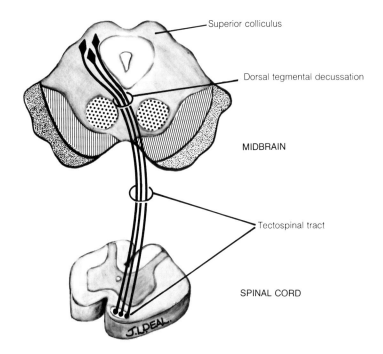

Superior colliculus

Dorsal tegmental decussation

MIDBRAIN

Tectospinal tract

SPINAL CORD

J.L.DEAL

4–18   Composite schematic diagram of the origin and course of the tectospinal tract.

studies suggest that the rostrally originating (pons and rostral medulla) fibers are fast conducting and elicit monosynaptically postsynaptic potentials in spinal motoneurons, whereas the caudally originating fibers (caudal medulla) elicit longer latency postsynaptic potentials in spinal motoneurons. The pontine fibers terminate in laminae VII and VIII of Rexed, whereas the medullary fibers terminate primarily in lamina VII, with some reaching lamina IX through their interaction with motoneuron dendrites in laminae VII and VIII. Besides influencing motor neurons, descending reticular fibers modify sensory activity at spinal cord levels through interaction with spinothalamic tract neurons in the dorsal horn.

Tectospinal tract   From their neurons of origin in the superior colliculus of the midbrain, fibers of this tract cross in the dorsal tegmental decussation in the midbrain and descend throughout the neuraxis to occupy a position in the anterior funiculus of the cervical spinal cord (Fig. 4–18). Fibers of this tract terminate on neurons in laminae VI, VII, and VIII. The function of this tract is not well understood; it is believed to play a role in the turning of the head in response to light stimulation.

Descending autonomic pathway   Fibers belonging to this descending system originate predominantly from the hypothalamus. They are small caliber fibers that follow a polysynaptic route and are diffusely scattered in the anterolateral funiculus of the spinal cord. They project on the intermedio-lateral cell column. Lesions of this system result in autonomic disturbances. If the lesion involves the sympathetic component of this system at or above T_1 level, a characteristic syndrome known as Horner's syndrome will result. This syndrome is manifested by 1) miosis (small pupil), 2) pseudoptosis (minimal drooping of the eyelid), 3) anhidrosis (absence of sweating) of the face, and 4) enophthalmos (slight retraction of the eyeball). All of these signs occur on the same side as the lesion and are due to interruption of sympathetic innervation to the dilator pupillae, tarsal plate, sweat glands of the face, and retro-orbital fat, respectively.

Functional Overview of Spinal Cord

From the above it is evident that the spinal cord is organized into three major functional zones: the dorsal horn, the intermediate zone, and the ventral horn.

1. The dorsal horn receives several varieties of sensory information from receptors in the skin surface (exteroceptive), as well as from deeper lying receptors in joints, tendons, and muscles (interoceptive). Cell characteristics in the dorsal horn vary greatly with respect to extent of receptive fields and the degree of specificity of the modality received. Information received from the periphery is not merely relayed in this zone, but is modified by virtue of the various peripheral inputs received, as well as by descending influences from the cerebral cortex and sub-cortical areas. The sum total of this interaction in the dorsal horn is then mediated to the motor neurons in lamina IX, to interneurons, or to ascending tracts (Fig. 4–19).

2. The intermediate zone receives a variety of inputs from the dorsal root and dorsal horn, as well as from cortical and subcortical areas. The information received here is integrated and modified before being pro-jected to other zones.

3. The ventral horn receives an input from the dorsal root (monosynaptic reflex connections) or from the dorsal horn, the intermediate zone, or the descending tracts. The descending tracts influence motor neurons either directly or indirectly through interneurons in the intermediate zone. They selectively facilitate flexor motor neurons (corticospinal, rubrospinal and medullary reticulospinal tracts) or extensor motor neu-rons (vestibulospinal and pontine reticulospinal tracts). The output (Fig. 4–20) from the ventral horn is via either the alpha motor neurons to influence striated musculature or the gamma motor neurons to influence intrafusal muscle fibers.

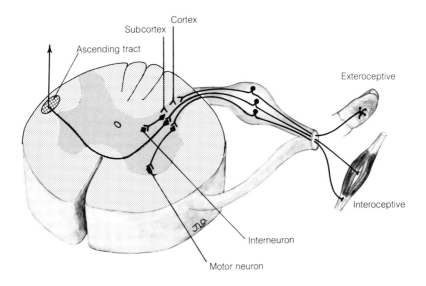

4–19 Composite schematic diagram of the spinal cord showing the input and output of the dorsal horn.

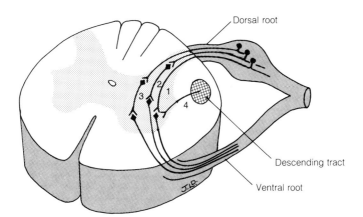

1 = Direct dorsal root fiber establishing monosynaptic reflexes
2 = Axon of neuron in dorsal horn
3 = Axon of neuron in intermediate zone
4 = Axon from descending tract

4–20 Composite schematic diagram of the spinal cord showing the input and output of the ventral horn.

Blood Supply

The spinal cord receives its blood supply from the following arteries.

1. Subclavian artery via the following branches: vertebral artery, ascending cervical artery, inferior thyroid artery, deep cervical artery, and superior intercostal artery.
2. Aorta via the following branches: intercostal arteries and lumbar arteries.
3. Internal iliac artery via the following branches: iliolumbar artery and lateral sacral artery.

Branches of the subclavian artery supply the cervical spinal cord and the upper two thoracic segments; the rest of the thoracic spinal cord is supplied by the intercostal arteries. The lumbosacral cord is supplied by the lumbar, iliolumbar, and lateral sacral arteries.

The vertebral arteries give rise to anterior and posterior spinal arteries in the cranial cavity. The two anterior spinal arteries unite to form a single anterior spinal artery which descends in the anterior median fissure of the spinal cord. The posterior spinal arteries, smaller than the anterior, remain paired and descend in the posterolateral sulci of the spinal cord. All other arteries send branches which enter the intervertebral foramina, penetrate the dural sheath, and divide into anterior and posterior branches (radicular arteries) that accompany the anterior and posterior nerve roots. These radicular arteries contribute to the three major spinal cord arteries: the anterior spinal and the paired posterior spinal arteries. Since most of the radicular arteries contributing to the anterior spinal artery are small, blood supply is mainly dependent on the four to ten of these which are large. In contrast, the posterior spinal arteries receive from 30 to 40 well-developed radicular arteries. Anastomoses between the anterior and posterior spinal arteries occur caudally around the cauda equina. There is very little anastomosis at each segmental level.

The anterior spinal artery gives off a sulcal branch in the anterior median fissure. This branch turns either right or left to enter the spinal cord; only in the lumbar and sacral cords are there both right and left branches. The sulcal arteries are most numerous in the lumbar region and fewest in the thoracic region. Sulcal arteries supply the anterior and intermediolateral gray horns, the central gray matter and Clarke's column, *i.e.*, all the gray matter except the dorsal horn. They also supply the bulk of the white matter of the anterior and lateral funiculi. Thus the anterior two-thirds of the spinal cord is fed from the anterior spinal artery; the remaining third, including the posterior funiculus and posterior horn, is supplied by the two posterior spinal arteries. The outer rim of the spinal cord is supplied by coronal branches which arise from the anterior spinal artery, pass laterally around the cord, and form imperfect anastomoses with the posterior spinal artery branches.

Certain segments of the spinal cord are more vulnerable than others to a compromise in blood flow. The segments that are particularly vulnerable are T_1 to T_4 and L_1. These are regions of the spinal cord which derive their blood supply from two different sources. At the level of T_1 to T_4, for example, the anterior spinal artery becomes small and its sulcal branches are not adequate to provide the necessary blood supply. These segments are dependent for their blood supply on the radicular branches of the intercostal arteries. If one or more of the intercostal vessels are compromised, the T_1 to T_4 spinal segments could not be adequately supplied by the small sulcal branches of the anterior spinal artery. As a result, the segment or segments affected would be damaged.

Venous drainage of the spinal cord corresponds to the arterial supply with the following differences.

1. There is only one posterior spinal vein.
2. Anastomoses between the anterior and posterior spinal veins are more frequent than between the arteries.
3. The territorial drainage from the anterior two-thirds of the spinal cord by the anterior spinal vein and from the posterior one-third by the posterior spinal vein is generally maintained but not immutable.
4. Venous tributaries within and around the spinal cord are much more numerous than arterial tributaries, so that venous obstruction rarely damages the spinal cord.

Applied Anatomy

Sensory Disturbances

Lesions of the spinal cord that involve the posterior or lateral funiculus will result in sensory signs and symptoms. Posterior funiculus lesions will be manifested by diminution or loss of vibration sense, position sense, two-point discrimination, and deep touch. Light touch will not be affected because it is also carried by the anterior spinothalamic tract. These sensory deficits will appear on the same side as the spinal cord lesion in dermatomes at and below the level of the spinal cord lesion (Fig 4–21).

Lesions of the lateral funiculus will result in disturbances in pain and temperature sensations because of involvement of the lateral spinothalamic tract. The disturbances in pain and temperature will occur contralateral to the side of the spinal cord lesion in dermatomes beginning one or two levels below the lesion. If the spinal cord lesion is at T_8 on the right side, the diminution or loss of pain and temperature will be found on the left side in dermatomes supplied by T_{10} or T_{11} and below (Fig. 4–22).

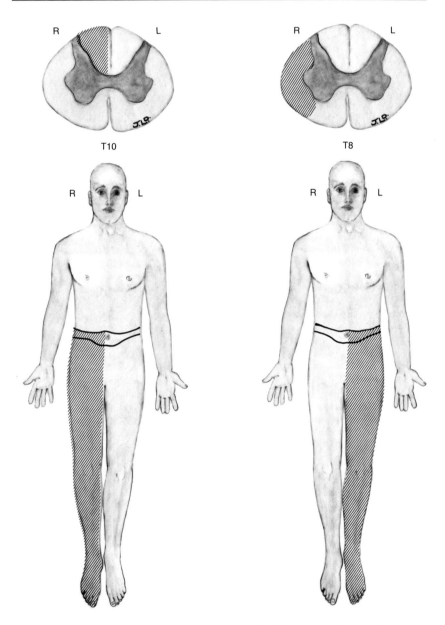

4-21 Schematic diagram showing the distribution of sensory deficit resulting from lesions in the posterior funiculus.

4-22 Schematic diagram showing the distribution of sensory deficit resulting from lesions in the lateral funiculus.

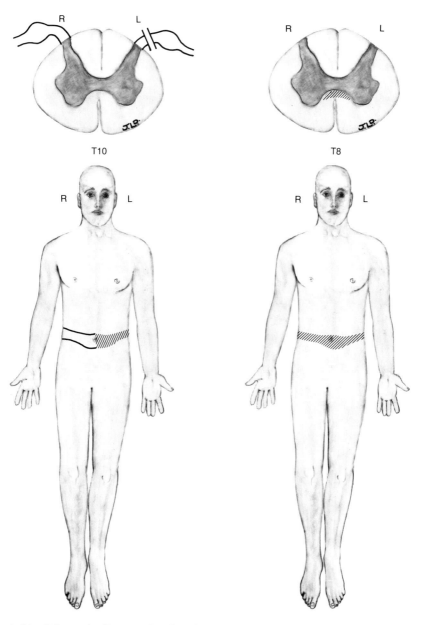

4–23 Schematic diagram showing the distribution of sensory deficit resulting from lesions of the dorsal root.

4–24 Schematic diagram showing the distribution of sensory deficit resulting from lesions of the anterior white commissure.

Tract, Dorsal Root, and Anterior White Commissure

Lesions involving an ascending tract, the dorsal root or the anterior white commissure will be manifested by different sensory deficits. If the lateral spinothalamic tract on the right side is affected, the sensory deficit will involve the left half of the body supplied by fibers one or two segments below the level of the spinal cord lesion (Fig. 4–22). Lesions of the dorsal root, however, will be manifested by loss of sensations in only the dermatome or dermatomes supplied by the affected dorsal roots. Thus, if a lesion involves dorsal root T_{10}, then the sensory deficit will be limited to the corresponding dermatome on the same side as the dorsal root affected (Fig. 4–23).

On the other hand, lesions affecting the anterior white commissure will be manifested by bilateral dermatomal loss of pain and temperature one or two segments below the level of the spinal cord lesion (Fig. 4–24). In this situation, only pain and temperature sensations will be affected, since they are the only modalities that cross in the anterior white commissure and are not represented by other tracts. Light touch fibers which also cross in this commissure will be affected; however, since light touch is also represented in the posterior column, no deficit in light touch will occur.

Motor Disturbances

Deficits in motor function are usually associated with spinal cord lesions resulting from involvement of motor neurons in the anterior horn or of the descending corticospinal tract. The deficits resulting from each are distinct and are clinically known as lower motor neuron and upper motor neuron paralysis, respectively.

Lower motor neuron paralysis is characterized by 1) paresis (weakness) or paralysis (loss of movement), 2) decreased muscle tone (flaccidity), 3) decreased or absent deep tendon (myotatic) reflexes, 4) fibrillations and/ or fasciculations (spontaneous activity of muscle fibers at rest), and 5) muscle atrophy. All of these signs occur ipsilateral to the spinal cord lesion in the part of the body supplied by the spinal cord segments involved. The paralysis that occurs with poliomyelitis is an example of such a lesion. Similar signs will result from lesions of the ventral root.

Upper motor neuron paralysis is characterized by 1) weakness or loss of movement, 2) exaggerated deep tendon reflexes, 3) clonus, 4) abnormal superficial reflexes such as Babinski reflex, and 5) spasticity. Although upper motor neuron paralysis is associated clinically with lesions of the corticospinal tract, recent anatomic and physiologic studies have pointed out the possibly important role of other descending fiber systems in this type of paralysis. The paralysis that occurs in strokes is an example of such a lesion.

Spinal Cord Syndromes

Hemisection

The following signs will be detected in hemisection of the spinal cord. The nuclear group or tract giving rise to these signs is indicated.

Ipsilateral Signs   Signs ipsilateral to the spinal cord lesion are as follows.

Corticospinal Tract Signs   The following upper motor neuron signs occur below the level of the hemisection.

1. Muscle paralysis
2. Spasticity
3. Hyperactive myotatic reflexes
4. Babinski sign
5. Clonus

Posterior Column Signs   These include loss of the following sensations below the level of the hemisection.

1. Vibration
2. Position
3. Two-point discrimination
4. Deep touch

Ventral Horn Signs   The following lower motor neuron signs are found in muscles supplied by the affected cord segment.

1. Muscle paralysis
2. Muscle atrophy
3. Loss of myotatic reflexes
4. Fibrillations and fasciculations

Contralateral Signs   Signs contralateral to the spinal cord lesion are as follows.

Lateral Spinothalamic Tract Signs   Loss of pain and thermal sense in the contralateral half of the body beginning one or two segments below the level of hemisection.

Anterior Spinothalamic Tract Signs   Diminution of light touch in the contralateral half of the body beginning several segments below the lesion.

Bilateral Signs   Segmental loss of pain and thermal sense occurs one or two segments below the level of the hemisection due to interruption of spinothalamic fibers crossing in the anterior white commissure.

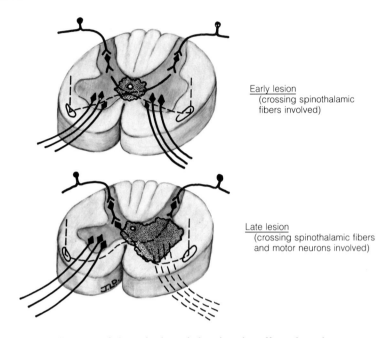

Early lesion
(crossing spinothalamic
fibers involved)

Late lesion
(crossing spinothalamic fibers
and motor neurons involved)

4-25   Schematic diagram of the spinal cord showing the affected cord structures in syringomyelia.

Lesions around Central Canal (Syringomyelia)

Lesions in or around the central canal (Fig. 4–25) will encroach first on the fibers conveying pain and temperature in the anterior white commissure. The effect will be segmental and bilateral loss of temperature and pain sensations in the dermatomes involved. Such a lesion is characteristic of the clinical condition known as syringomyelia. This type of lesion usually affects the cervical spinal segments but may affect other segments of the spinal cord as well. In some patients, the lesion (syrinx) may involve the brain stem (syringobulbia). In most instances, the original lesion may progress to involve, in addition to the anterior white commissure, the anterior, lateral, and/or posterior columns of the spinal cord, with symptoms and signs corresponding to the affected column as detailed above.

Anterior Horn and Lateral Corticospinal Tract Syndrome

This syndrome is known clinically as motor neuron disease or amyotrophic lateral sclerosis. It is a degenerative disease affecting the anterior horn and the lateral corticospinal tract bilaterally. It is thus manifested by a combination of lower and upper motor neuron signs, including paralysis, muscular atrophy, fasciculation and fibrillation, exaggerated myotatic reflexes, and a Babinski sign. This is a progressive condition which involves the spinal cord as well as motor nuclei of cranial nerves in the brain stem.

Combined System Degeneration Syndrome

In this syndrome, there is bilateral degeneration of the posterior and lateral column tracts with loss of kinesthesia and discriminative touch, as well as upper motor neuron signs. It is seen in patients with pernicious anemia. A hereditary form of this syndrome is known as Friedreich's ataxia, in which the dorsal spinocerebellar tract is also bilaterally involved in the degenerative process.

Spinal Shock

Complete transection of the spinal cord results in disturbances of motor, sensory, and autonomic functions. The manifestations of such a lesion in the immediate and early stages (2 to 3 weeks) differ from those in later stages.

Motor Manifestations   In the immediate and early stages following transection, there is flaccid paralysis of all muscles innervated by the spinal cord segments affected by the lesion, as well as those below the level of the lesion bilaterally. The paralysis of muscles below the level of the lesion will change into the spastic variety in later stages. Flaccid paralysis of muscles innervated by the affected spinal cord segments is attributed to the injury of motor neurons in the anterior horn or their ventral roots. The early flaccid paralysis below the level of the lesion is attributed to the sudden withdrawal of a predominantly facilitating or excitatory influence from supraspinal centers. The spastic type paralysis that follows is attributed to release of segmental reflexes below the level of the lesion from supraspinal inhibitory influences. This spastic paralysis results in the development of flexor spasms which eventually change into extensor spasms. During the stage of flexor spasm, the patient's paralyzed limbs are kept in almost permanent hip and knee flexion (paraplegia-in-flexion). In the extension spasm stage, the limbs are kept extended at the knee and ankle (paraplegia-in-extension). Experience with war victims has shown that paraplegia-in-flexion occurs in complete cord transection, whereas paraplegia-in-extension occurs in incomplete cord lesion.

Sensory Manifestations   All sensations are lost at and below the level of the lesion bilaterally. In addition, there is a hyperpathic zone at the border of the lesion and for one or two dermatomes above it. In this hyperpathic zone, the patient complains of pain of burning character.

Bladder Function   In the immediate and early stages following transection, all volitional or reflex functions of the urinary bladder are lost, resulting in urinary retention. This may last from 8 days to 8 weeks. Subsequently, a state of automatic bladder emptying develops. Once a sufficient degree of bladder distention occurs, sensory receptors in the bladder wall evoke reflex contraction of the detrusor muscle, thus emptying the bladder.

Bowel Function   Similar to bladder function, the immediate and early effect of cord transection is paralysis of bowel function and fecal retention. This is changed in later stages to intermittent automatic reflex defecation.

Sexual Function   Erection and ejaculatory functions are lost in males in the immediate and early stages. Later on, reflex erection and ejaculation appear as a component of the automatic activity of the isolated cord and are evoked by extrinsic and intrinsic stimuli. In the female, there may be temporary cessation of menstruation and irregularities in the menstrual cycle.

References

Angaut-Petit, D.: The Dorsal Column System. I. Existence of Long Ascending Post-Synaptic Fibers in the Cat's Fasciculus Gracilis. Exp Brain Res 22 (1975) 457–470.

Applebaum, A.E.; Leonard, R.B.; Kenshalo, D.R.; Martin, R.F.: Nuclei in Which Functionally Identified Spinothalamic Tract Neurons Terminate. J Comp Neurol 188 (1979) 575–586.

Bishop, B.: Pain: Its Physiology and Rationale for Management. Part I. Neuroanatomical Substrate of Pain. Phys Ther 60 (1980) 13–20.

Boivie, J.: An Anatomical Reinvestigation of the Termination of the Spinothalamic Tract in the Monkey. J Comp Neurol 186 (1979) 343–370.

Craig, A.D.; Burton, H.: The Lateral Cervical Nucleus in the Cat: Anatomic Organization of Cervicothalamic Neurons. J Comp Neurol 185 (1979) 329–346.

Guttmann, L.: Clinical Symptomatology of Spinal Cord Lesions. In: Handbook of Clinical Neurology, Vol. 2, pp. 178–216, Ed. by P.J. Vinken and G.W. Bruyn. North-Holland Publishing Co., Amsterdam, 1978.

Hall, J.G.: Supraspinal Inhibition of Spinal Neurons Responding to Nociceptive Stimulation. Neurosci Lett 14 (1979) 165–169.

Hughes, J.T.: Vascular Disorders. In: Pathology of the Spinal Cord, Vol. VI, Major Problems in Pathology, pp. 61–90. W.B. Saunders Co., Philadelphia, 1978.

Jankowski, E.; Lindström, S.: Morphological Identification of Renshaw Cells. Acta Physiol Scand 81 (1971) 428–430.

Kerr, F.W.L.; Fukushima, T.: New Observations on the Nociceptive Pathways in the Central Nervous System. In: Pain: Research Publication: Association for Research in Nervous and Mental Diseases, Vol. 58, pp. 47–61, Ed. by J.J. Bonica. Raven Press, New York, 1980.

Matsushita, M.; Hosoya, Y.; Ikeda, M.: Anatomical Organization of the Spinocerebellar System in the Cat as Studied by Retrograde Transport of Horseradish Peroxidase. J Comp Neurol 184 (1979) 81–106.

Rustioni, A.; Hayes, N.L.; O'Neill, S.: Dorsal Column Nuclei and Ascending Spinal Afferents in Macaque. Brain 102 (1979) 95–125.

Scheibel, M.E.; Scheibel, A.B.: Inhibition and the Renshaw Cell: A Structural Critique. Brain Behav Evol 4 (1971) 53–93.

Van Keulen, L.C.M.: Axon Trajectories of Renshaw Cells in the Lumbar Spinal Cord of the Cat as Reconstructed after Intracellular Staining with Horseradish Peroxidase. Brain Res 167 (1979) 157–162.

Wall, P.D.: The Role of Substantia Gelatinosa as a Gate Control. In: Pain: Research Publication: Association for Research in Nervous and Mental Diseases, Vol. 58, pp. 205–231, Ed. by J.J. Bonica. Raven Press, New York, 1980.

Willis, D.: The Case for the Renshaw Cell. Brain Behav Evol 4 (1971) 5–52.

Willis, W.D.; Leonard, R.B.; Kenshalo, D.R.: Spinothalamic Tract Neurons in the Substantia Gelatinosa. Science 202 (1978) 986–988.

Willis, W.D.: Studies of the Spinothalamic Tract. Tex Rep Bio Med 38 (1979) 1–45.

Willis, W.D.; Kenshalo, D.R.; Leonard, R.B.: The Cells of Origin of the Primate Spinothalamic Tract. J Comp Neurol 188 (1979) 543–574.

Young, R.F.: Evaluation of Dorsal Column Stimulation in the Treatment of Chronic Pain. Neurosurgery 3 (1978) 373–379.

5

Medulla Oblongata

Gross Topography

Ventral (Anterior) Surface (Fig. 5–1)

The anterior median fissure of the spinal cord continues on the ventral (anterior) surface of the medulla. On each side of this fissure are the medullary pyramids. The medullary pyramids carry descending cortico-spinal and corticobulbar fibers from the cerebral cortex to the lateral and anterior corticospinal tracts in the spinal cord and cranial nerve nuclei. In the lower part of the medulla, the corticospinal fibers in the pyramid partly cross to the opposite side to form the lateral corticospinal tract. This decussation or crossing forms the basis for the motor control of one cerebral hemisphere over the contralateral half of the body and is known as the motor or pyramidal decussation. The pyramids are bounded laterally by the anterolateral (ventrolateral) sulcus, a continuation of the same structure in the spinal cord. Lateral to this sulcus, in about the middle of the medulla, are the inferior olives. Lateral to each olive is the posterolateral (dorso-lateral) sulcus. Rootlets of the hypoglossal (CN XII) nerve exit between the pyramids and olives in the anterolateral sulcus. Rootlets of the accessory (CN XI), vagus (CN X), and glossopharyngeal (CN IX) cranial nerves exit lateral to the olives.

Dorsal (Posterior) Surface (Fig. 5–2)

The posterior (dorsal) median sulcus and posterolateral (dorsolateral) sulcus of the spinal cord continue on the dorsal surface of the medulla. Between these two surface landmarks are the rostral prolongations of the gracile and cuneate tracts and their nuclei. On the dorsal surface of the medulla, the gracile and cuneate nuclei form protuberances known, re-

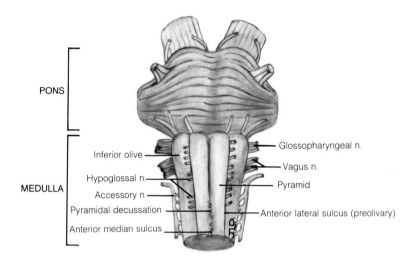

5-1 Schematic diagram showing the major structures seen on the ventral surface of the medulla oblongata.

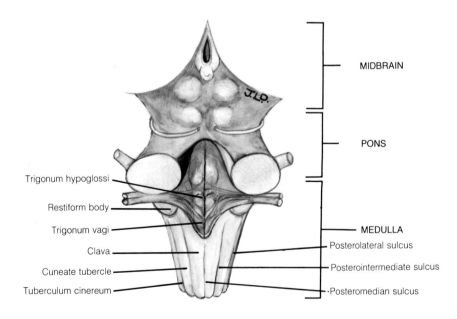

5-2 Schematic diagram showing the major structures seen on the dorsal surface of the medulla oblongata.

spectively, as clava and cuneate tubercles. Lateral to the cuneate tubercle, between it and the posterolateral sulcus, is the tuberculum cinereum, which represents the surface marking of the spinal nucleus of the trigeminal (CN V) cranial nerve.

Fourth Ventricle

Floor (Fig. 5–3)   The rostral part of the dorsal surface of the medulla oblongata forms the caudal part of the floor of the fourth ventricle; the rostral part of the floor is formed by the pons. The medullary and pontine parts of the floor comprise a diamond-shaped structure.

The medullary part of the floor has the following surface landmarks.

Posterior Median Fissure   This is a continuation of the posterior median sulcus of the spinal cord.

Hypoglossal Trigone   This is a protuberance of the hypoglossal (CN XII) cranial nerve nucleus into the floor of the fourth ventricle.

Vagal Trigone   This is a protuberance of the dorsal motor nucleus of the vagus (CN X) cranial nerve into the floor of the fourth ventricle.

The pontine part of the floor contains the facial colliculus, which represents the surface markings of the subependymal bundle of the facial (CN VII) cranial nerve making a loop around the nucleus of the abducens (CN VI) nerve.

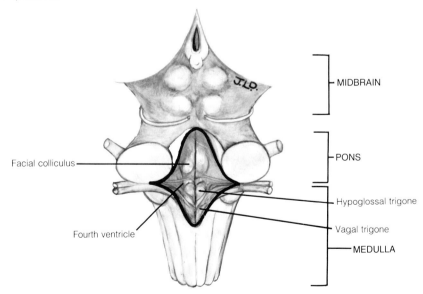

5–3   Schematic diagram showing the major structures seen in the floor of the fourth ventricle.

Between the rostral (pontine) and caudal (medullary) parts of the floor of the fourth ventricle is an intermediate zone containing the stria medullaris, a fiber bundle which courses laterally. This is the surface landmark of fibers from the arcuate nucleus of the medulla oblongata on their way to the cerebellum.

Roof (Fig. 5–4)   Three structures form the roof of the fourth ventricle. These are the anterior medullary velum, cerebellum, and tela chorioidea, which is formed by the neural ependyma [the original posterior (inferior) medullary velum] covered by a mesodermal pia mater.

From the tela chorioidea in the posterior part of the roof of the fourth ventricle, the choroid plexus projects as two vertical and two lateral ridges forming a T-shaped structure with a double vertical stem.

Lateral Boundaries   The lateral boundaries of the fourth ventricle (Fig. 5–5) are formed from rostral to caudal by the following structures.

Brachium Conjunctivum   This structure connects the cerebellum and midbrain.

Restiform Body   This structure connects the medulla oblongata and cerebellum.

Clava and Cuneate Tubercles   These are the surface markings of the gracile and cuneate nuclei, respectively.

The lateral angles of the fourth ventricle are the lateral recesses.

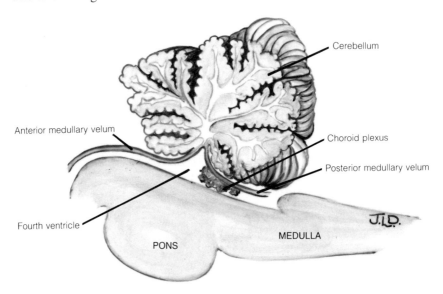

5–4   Schematic diagram showing structures that form the roof and floor of the fourth ventricle.

Characteristic Levels

The internal structure of the medulla is best understood when examined at three caudorostral representative levels: the level of motor (pyramidal) decussation, the level of sensory (lemniscal) decussation, and the level of inferior olive.

Level of Motor (Pyramidal) Decussation

The two main distinguishing features of this level (Fig. 5–6) are pyramidal decussation and dorsal column nuclei.

Pyramidal Decussation Although the concept of control of one side of the body by the contralateral hemisphere (law of cruciate conduction) has been known since the time of Hippocrates, the actual crossing of the pyramids was not observed until 1709; it was described the following year. This description was ignored, however, until Gall and Spurzheim called attention to it in 1810. Many anatomists denied the existence of the pyramidal decussation until 1935, when Cruveilhier traced the pyramidal bundles to the opposite side.

The pyramids contain two types of descending cortical fibers, the corticobulbar and the corticospinal. As they descend in the medulla oblongata,

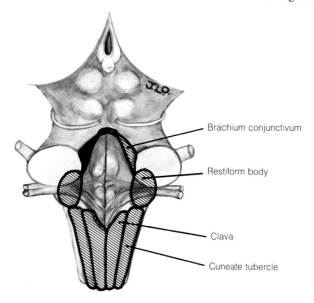

5–5 Schematic diagram showing structures that comprise the lateral wall of the fourth ventricle.

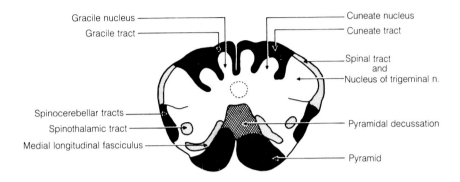

5–6 Schematic diagram showing the major structures seen in the medulla oblongata at the level of the pyramidal decussation.

the corticobulbar fibers leave the pyramid to project on nuclei of cranial nerves. Near the caudal border of the medulla, roughly 75 to 90% of the corticospinal fibers in the pyramid decussate to the opposite side to form the lateral corticospinal tract. The rest of the corticospinal fibers descend homolaterally to form the anterior corticospinal tract. It has been observed that the left pyramid decussates first in 73% of humans; this, however, bears no relationship to handedness of the individual. The corticospinal fibers conveying impulses to the neck and upper extremity musculature cross first. These fibers are separate from, and rostral to, those conveying impulses to the lower extremities; they are also more superficially located and are identified in the lower medulla in close proximity to the odontoid process of the second cervical vertebra. Because of this anatomic location, fractures of the odontoid process or mass lesions in that location will result in paralysis of muscles of the upper extremities but may spare muscles of the lower extremities. On the other hand, paralysis of an ipsilateral arm and a contralateral leg (hemiplegia cruciata) can occur as the result of a lesion in the lower medulla that injures the crossed fibers to the arm as well as the uncrossed fibers to the leg.

The pyramidal decussation constitutes the anatomic basis for the voluntary motor control of one half of the body by the opposite cerebral hemisphere. As the pyramidal fibers decussate, the fibers of the medial longitudinal fasciculus are displaced laterally.

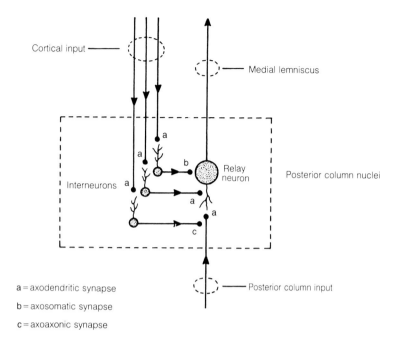

Cortical input

Medial lemniscus

a

a

b

Relay
neuron

Posterior column nuclei

Interneurons a

a

a

c

a = axodendritic synapse

b = axosomatic synapse

c = axoaxonic synapse

Posterior column input

5–7 Schematic diagram depicting the major input and output of the posterior column nuclei, as well as their internal neural circuitry.

Dorsal Column Nuclei In the dorsal (posterior) column, two nuclei appear. These are the nucleus gracilis in the tractus gracilis and the nucleus cuneatus in the tractus cuneatus. The gracile nucleus appears and disappears caudal to the cuneate nucleus. Caudally, both the nuclei and the tracts capping them are seen; rostrally, only the nuclei are seen. The surface projections of these two nuclei into the dorsal (posterior) surface of the medulla form the clava and cuneate tubercles.

The dorsal column nuclei contain clusters of round sensory relay neurons separated by interneurons. The dorsal column nuclei receive two inputs. One input is from the gracile and cuneate tracts, which project on the gracile and cuneate nuclei, respectively, and form axodendritic synapses upon the dendrites of the round sensory relay neurons (Fig. 5–7). The other input is from the cerebral cortex, which reaches the dorsal column nuclei via the pyramid and projects upon interneurons. Axons of interneurons, in turn, establish axodendritic and axosomatic synapses with the round sensory relay neurons, as well as axoaxonic synapses with axons of the gracile and cuneate tracts (Fig. 5–7). The latter type of synapse forms the anatomic basis for the presynaptic inhibition known to occur in the dorsal column nuclei.

The dorsal column nuclei are organized both for spatial origin and stimulus specificity of afferent fibers. Afferent fibers from C_1-T_7 project to the nucleus cuneatus, whereas fibers below T_7 project to the nucleus gracilis. It has been shown in animal experimentation that overlapping terminations are more extensive and irregular in the gracile nucleus than in the cuneate nucleus, with less autonomous terminal representation of individual dorsal roots. Cortical afferents to the dorsal column nuclei originate from the primary sensory and motor cortices and are somatotopically organized. Forelimb cortical areas project upon the cuneate nucleus and hindlimb cortical areas project upon the gracile nucleus. In addition to this somatotopic organization, the dorsal column nuclei exhibit modal specificity. A neuron in the dorsal column nuclei may respond to hair movement alone or to vibration alone. The peripheral receptive fields of the dorsal column nuclei are generally small and have an excitatory center with an inhibitory surround.

The main efferent projection of the dorsal column nuclei is the medial lemniscus, which terminates in the thalamus. Other projections, confirmed recently, include those to the inferior olive and the cerebellum. The cerebellar fibers originate mainly from the cuneate nucleus with minor contributions from the gracile nucleus.

Another feature seen at the level of the motor decussation is the spinal nucleus of the trigeminal nerve. This nuclear mass occupies a dorsolateral position in the medulla and is capped by the descending (spinal) tract of the trigeminal nerve. The spinal trigeminal nucleus extends throughout the medulla oblongata and descends caudally to the level of C_3 of the cervical spinal cord. It is continuous caudally with the substantia gelatinosa of the spinal cord and rostrally with the main sensory nucleus of the trigeminal nerve in the pons. The spinal tract and nucleus of the trigeminal nerve are concerned with exteroceptive sensations (pain, temperature, and light touch) from the ipsilateral face. The spinal nucleus is divided into three parts along its rostrocaudal extent. The caudal part is the caudalis nucleus, which extends from the obex of the medulla oblongata rostrally to the substantia gelatinosa of the spinal cord, with which it is continuous caudally. It mediates pain and temperature sensations from the ipsilateral side of the face. Rostral to the obex is the nucleus interpolaris, which is distinct cytologically from the nucleus caudalis. It mediates dental pain. Rostral to the interpolar nucleus and just caudal to the main sensory nucleus of the trigeminal is the nucleus oralis, which mediates tactile sensations from the oral mucosa.

Fibers of the spinal tract originating from the mandibular region of the face project down to the third and fourth cervical segments. Those from the perioral region project to lower medullary levels. Those originating

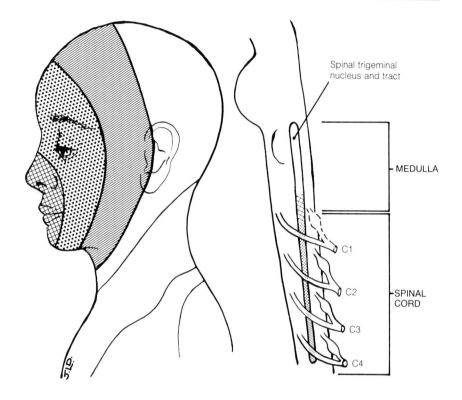

Spinal trigeminal
nucleus and tract

MEDULLA

C1

C2   SPINAL
CORD

C3

C4

5-8 Schematic diagram illustrating the spatial organization in the medulla and spinal cord of afferent exteroceptive fibers from the face.

between the mandible and the perioral region terminate in the upper cervical region (Fig. 5–8). Evidence in support of the above distribution pattern is found in patients in whom the spinal tract of the trigeminal is cut (tractotomies) for relief of pain. Thus, tractotomies that spare the lower medulla will spare pain and temperature sensations around the mouth. In contrast to the above onion skin pattern of distribution of exteroceptive sensations on the face, described by Dejerine in 1914, some recent observations suggest that all fibers carrying pain impulses from the face, and not only those from the mandible, reach lower cervical levels. Pain neurons in the spinal trigeminal nucleus, like their counterparts in the spinal cord, have been classified physiologically into high threshold (HT), low threshold (LT), and wide dynamic range (WDR) neurons. Specific thermoreceptive neurons have been localized on the outer rim of the nucleus. In addition to the major input from exteroceptors in the face, the spinal trigeminal nucleus has been shown to receive an input from the nucleus locus ceruleus in the pons and to send fibers back to the locus ceruleus. The locus ceruleus input is inhibitory. It should be pointed out that the spinal tract of the trigeminal conveys, in addition to exteroceptive sensations from the face, general somatic fibers belonging to facial (CN VII), glossopharyngeal (CN IX), and vagus (CN X) cranial nerves.

The following ascending tracts are also seen at the level of the motor decussation. The spinothalamic tracts traverse the medulla in close proximity to the spinal nucleus and tract of the trigeminal (Fig. 5–6). Lesions of the medulla in this location will therefore produce sensory loss of pain and temperature on the face ipsilateral to the medullary lesion (spinal tract and nucleus of trigeminal), as well as loss of the same sensations on the body contralateral to the medullary lesion (spinothalamic tract). Although the lateral and anterior spinothalamic tracts retain their spinal cord positions in the caudal medulla, the position of the anterior spinothalamic tract in the rostral medulla has not been definitely delineated in man and its fibers probably run along with the lateral spinothalamic tract.

The spinal cord positions of the dorsal and ventral spinocerebellar tracts remain unchanged in the medulla (Fig. 5–6).

Other ascending and descending tracts encountered in the spinal cord traverse the medulla on their way to higher or lower levels.

Level of Sensory (Lemniscal) Decussation

The distinguishing feature of this level (Fig. 5–9) is the crossing of second order neurons of the dorsal column system. Axons of relay neurons in the dorsal column nuclei course ventromedially (internal arcuate fibers) and cross to the opposite side (sensory decussation) above the pyramids to form the medial lemniscus. In the decussation, fibers derived from the gracile nucleus come to lie ventral to those derived from the cuneate nucleus. The medial lemniscus thus carries the same modalities of sensation carried by the dorsal column. Lesions of the medial lemniscus will result in loss of kinesthesia and discriminative touch contralateral to the side of the lesion in the medulla. The sensory decussation provides part of the anatomic basis for sensory representation of one-half of the body in the contralateral hemisphere. The other part is provided by the crossing of the spinothalamic system in the spinal cord.

Medial Longitudinal Fasciculus   The medial longitudinal fasciculus (MLF), which is displaced dorsolaterally by the pyramidal decussation, is pushed further upward by the sensory decussation so that it comes to lie dorsal to the medial lemniscus (Fig. 5–9). It retains this position throughout the extent of the medulla oblongata.

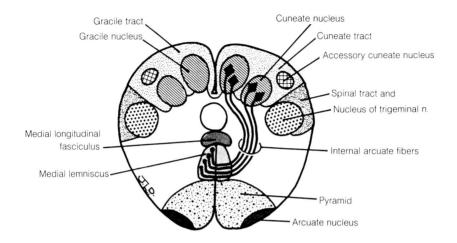

Gracile tract
Gracile nucleus
Cuneate nucleus
Cuneate tract
Accessory cuneate nucleus
Spinal tract and Nucleus of trigeminal n.
Medial longitudinal fasciculus
Internal arcuate fibers
Medial lemniscus
Pyramid
Arcuate nucleus

5–9   Schematic diagram showing the major structures encountered in the medulla oblongata at the level of the sensory decussation.

Accessory Cuneate Nucleus   A group of large neurons located dorsolateral to the cuneate nucleus is known as the accessory (lateral or external) cuneate nucleus. Although this nucleus shares its name with the cuneate nucleus, it does not belong functionally to the dorsal column system. Instead, it is part of the spinocerebellar system. Fibers of the spinocerebellar system entering the spinal cord above the level of C_8 (upper extent of the dorsal nucleus of Clarke) ascend with the posterior column fibers and terminate upon neurons of the accessory cuneate nucleus. Second order neurons course dorsolaterally as dorsal external arcuate fibers and reach the cerebellum (cuneocerebellar fibers) via the restiform body. Like the spinocerebellar system, the cuneocerebellar tract is concerned with unconscious proprioception. Recently, neurons in the accessory cuneate nucleus have been shown to receive fibers from the glossopharyngeal (CN IX) and vagus (CN X) nerves, as well as from the vasopressor and cardioacceleratory areas of the posterior hypothalamus. Stimulation of the accessory cuneate nucleus has been shown to produce bradycardia and hypotension. This response has been shown to be due to vagal stimulation. It is suggested that hypertension triggers the accessory cuneate nucleus, via cardiovascular reflexes, to produce bradycardia and hypotension.

Arcuate Nuclei   A group of neurons located on the anterior (ventral) aspect of the pyramid is known as the arcuate nucleus. The arcuate nuclei increase in size significantly in rostral levels of the medulla and become

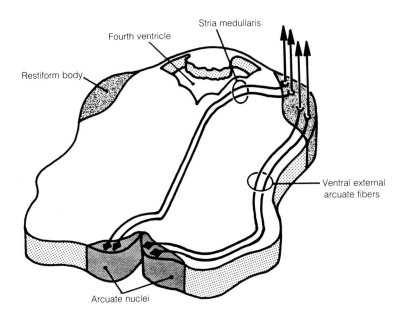

5–10 Schematic diagram illustrating the course (on one side only) of arcuato-cerebellar fibers within the medulla oblongata.

continuous with the pontine nuclei in the pons. The afferent and efferent connections of the arcuate nuclei are identical with those of pontine nuclei. Their major input is from the contralateral cerebral cortex. Their major output is to the homolateral and contralateral cerebellum via the restiform body. The arcuatocerebellar fibers reach the restiform body via two routes (Fig. 5–10). One route courses along the outer surface of the medulla (ventral external arcuate fibers). The other route courses along the midline of the medulla and turns laterally in the floor of the fourth ventricle, forming the stria medullaris of the floor of the fourth ventricle.

Level of Inferior Olive

The distinguishing feature of this level (Fig. 5–11) of the medulla is the appearance of the inferior olivary nuclei, which are convoluted laminae of gray matter dorsal to the pyramids. They project from the ventrolateral surface of the medulla as olive-shaped structures (Fig. 5–1). The inferior olivary nuclear complex consists of three nuclear groups.

1. Principal olive (the largest of the complex)
2. Dorsal accessory olive
3. Medial accessory olive

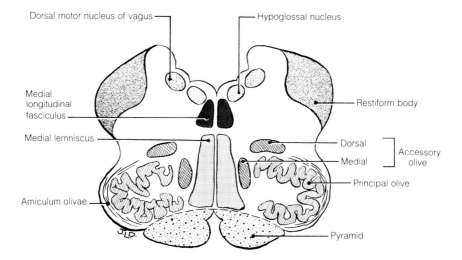

5-11 Schematic diagram showing the major structures encountered in the medulla oblongata at the level of the inferior olive.

The olivary complex in man is estimated to contain 0.5 million neurons. The complex is surrounded by a mass of fibers known as the amiculum olivae.

The inferior olives receive fibers from the following sources (Fig. 5-12).

1. Cerebral cortex via the corticospinal tract to both principal olives
2. Basal ganglia to both principal olives via the central tegmental tract
3. Periaqueductal gray matter of the midbrain to the homolateral principal olive via the central tegmental tract
4. Red nucleus to the homolateral principal olive via the central tegmental tract
5. The two principal olives across the midline
6. Spinal cord to the accessory olives of both sides via the spino-olivary tract

The following additional inputs have been described recently.

7. Dorsal column nuclei to contralateral accessory olives
8. Deep cerebellar nuclei, via the superior cerebellar peduncle, to the principal and accessory olives
9. Vestibular nuclei to both inferior olives

The major output of the inferior olivary complex is to the cerebellum (olivocerebellar tract). Olivocerebellar fibers arise from both olivary complexes, but are primarily from the contralateral complex. They pass through the hilum of the olive, traverse the medial lemniscus, and course through

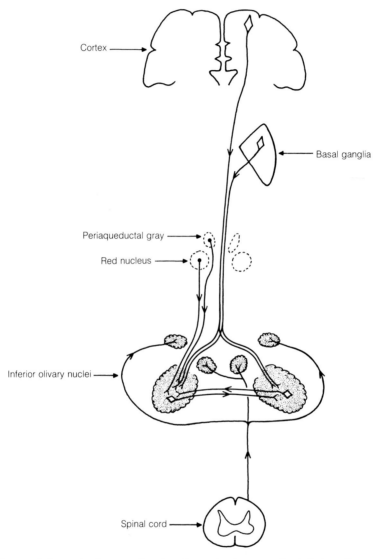

5–12 Schematic diagram showing the major input to the inferior olivary nuclei.

the opposite olive to enter the restiform body on their way to the cerebellum. Olivocerebellar fibers constitute the major component of the restiform body and are localized in the ventromedial part. Olivocerebellar
fibers originating from the accessory olives and the medial parts of the
principal olives project onto the vermis of the cerebellum, whereas fibers
originating from the rest of the principal olive project to the cerebellar

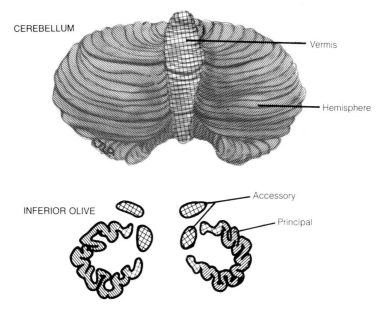

5–13   Schematic diagram illustrating the spatial relationships between the inferior olivary nuclei and the cerebellum.

hemispheres (Fig. 5–13). The deep cerebellar nuclei also receive fibers from the olivocerebellar tract.

Thus, the inferior olivary complex is a relay station between the cortex, subcortical structures, spinal cord, and cerebellum.

The ascending and descending fiber tracts, as well as the nuclear complexes encountered in more caudal levels of the medulla, are present at this level. Cranial nerve nuclei of the medulla will be discussed later.

Medullary Reticular Formation

The medullary reticular formation is characterized by a wealth of neurons of various sizes and shapes intermingled with a complex network of fibers. It spans the area between the pyramids (ventrally) and the floor of the fourth ventricle (dorsally). It is phylogenetically old and in lower forms constitutes the major part of the central nervous system. Caudally, the reticular formation appears about the level of the pyramidal decussation. Rostrally, it is continuous with the reticular formation of the pons. Physiologically, the reticular formation is a polysynaptic system, rich in collateral fibers for dispersion of impulses.

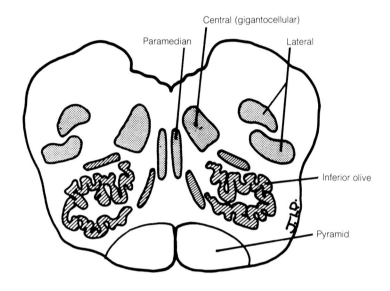

5-14 Schematic diagram showing the major subdivisions of the reticular nuclear complex in the medulla oblongata.

Although the reticular formation was previously considered an unorganized network of neurons and fibers, more recent studies suggest that it is organized into well-defined subdivisions with known afferent and efferent connections. In general, the medullary reticular formation is organized into three subgroups (Fig. 5–14).

1. Paramedian (raphe) nuclear group (caudal nucleus of the raphe)
2. Central group (gigantocellular and ventral reticular nuclei)
3. Lateral group (lateral reticular nucleus and parvicellular nucleus)

The caudal nucleus of the raphe is a small-celled, slender structure, continuous from the medulla to the lower pons. It produces the neurotransmitter serotonin and has connections to the spinal cord which inhibit dorsal horn neurons that give rise to the spinothalamic tract.

The gigantocellular nucleus lies in the rostral medulla and is characterized by large neurons. The ventral reticular nucleus contains small neurons and is located caudal to the gigantocellular nucleus.

The lateral reticular nucleus is located dorsal to the inferior olive. The parvicellular nucleus contains both large and small neurons and is located lateral to the gigantocellular nucleus.

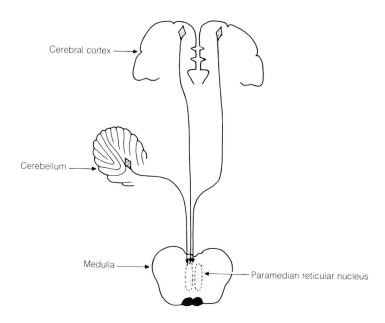

5-15 Schematic diagram illustrating the major inputs to the paramedian group of reticular nuclei.

Afferent Connections

The paramedian nuclear group (Fig. 5-15) receives fibers from the following.

1. Cerebral cortex (homolateral and contralateral)
2. Homolateral cerebellum

The central nuclear group (gigantocellular nucleus) (Fig. 5-16) receives fibers from the following.

1. Homolateral and contralateral cerebral cortex
2. Lateral nuclear group (parvicellular nucleus)
3. Spinal cord (spinoreticular tract)

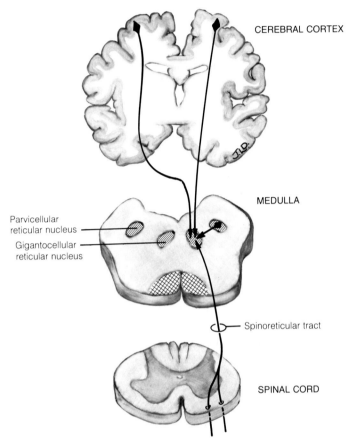

CEREBRAL CORTEX

MEDULLA

Parvicellular
reticular nucleus

Gigantocellular
reticular nucleus

Spinoreticular tract

SPINAL CORD

5–16 Schematic diagram illustrating the major inputs to the gigantocellular (magnocellular) group of reticular nuclei.

The lateral nuclear group (Fig. 5–17) receives fibers from the following.

1. Contralateral red nucleus (lateral reticular nucleus)
2. Spinothalamic tract (lateral reticular nucleus)
3. Spinoreticular tract (lateral reticular nucleus)
4. Second order neurons of some sensory systems (trigeminal, auditory and vestibular) (parvicellular nucleus)

As a rule, the medullary reticular formation receives no fibers from the medial lemniscus.

Figure 5–18 is a composite diagram of the afferent connections of the medullary reticular formation. In summary, the afferent connections of the medullary reticular formation come from the following.

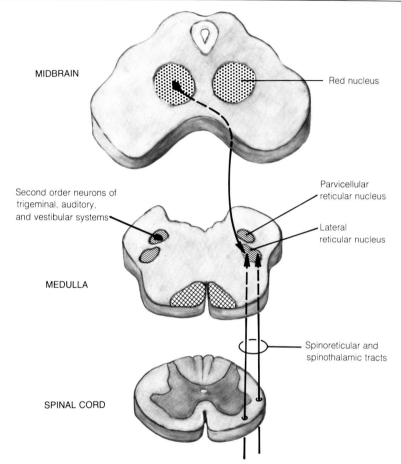

MIDBRAIN

Red nucleus

Second order neurons of
trigeminal, auditory,
and vestibular systems

Parvicellular
reticular nucleus

Lateral
reticular nucleus

MEDULLA

Spinoreticular and
spinothalamic tracts

SPINAL CORD

5–17 Schematic diagram illustrating the major inputs to the lateral group of reticular nuclei.

1. Cerebral cortex
2. Red nucleus
3. Cerebellum
4. Spinal cord
5. Second order neurons of some sensory systems

Efferent Connections

The major efferent flow from the paramedian nuclear group is to the cerebellum (vermis) via the restiform body. The cerebellum receives fibers from the homo- and contralateral paramedian groups. The caudal nucleus of the raphe (raphe magnus) has been shown to project to the dorsal horn

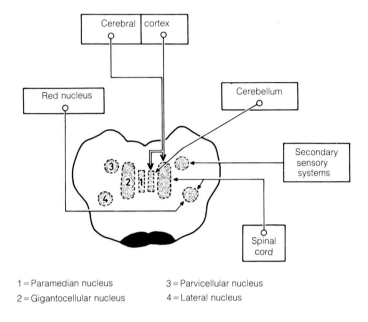

1 = Paramedian nucleus   3 = Parvicellular nucleus
2 = Gigantocellular nucleus   4 = Lateral nucleus

5–18 Composite schematic diagram of the afferent connections of the medullary reticular formation.

of the spinal cord. The transmitter in this projection is serotonin, which inhibits spinothalamic tract neurons.

The central nuclear group has two major outputs. These are mostly to the homolateral thalamus (intralaminar nuclei and reticular nucleus) via the central tegmental tract, but also to the spinal cord (the medullary reticulospinal tract). The medullary reticulospinal tract recently has been shown to originate from both the ventral reticular and gigantocellular nuclei and to be topographically organized. Fibers originating from the dorsal parts of the above nuclei project to the cervical spinal cord and supply upper extremity neurons; fibers originating from the ventral parts of the nuclei project to the lower thoracic and lumbar spinal cord and supply lower extremity neurons.

The lateral nuclear group projects to both cerebellar hemispheres, but mostly to the homolateral one (lateral reticular nucleus), as well as to the central nuclear group (parvicellular nucleus).

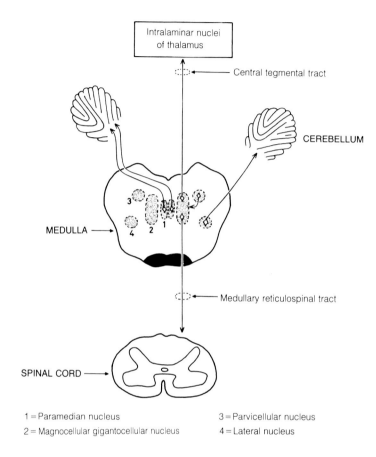

1 = Paramedian nucleus   3 = Parvicellular nucleus
2 = Magnocellular gigantocellular nucleus   4 = Lateral nucleus

5–19 Composite schematic diagram of the efferent connections of the medullary reticular formation.

Figure 5–19 is a composite diagram of the efferent connections of the medullary reticular formation. In summary, the efferent connections of the medullary reticular formation are to the following.

1. Thalamus (part of the reticular activating system which is important in the arousal response)
2. Spinal cord
3. Cerebellum

Various studies suggest that the reticular formation is concerned with 1) somatic motor functions, 2) visceral motor functions, and 3) consciousness, sleep, and attention. Stimulation of the medullary reticular formation facilitates flexor motor neurons and inhibits extensor motor neurons. It also results in visceral changes, such as an increase in blood pressure and an increase or decrease in heart rate (depending on the area stimulated). The connection between the central group of reticular neurons and the thalamus belongs to the reticular activating system concerned with sleep, wakefulness, and attention.

Inferior Cerebellar Peduncle (Restiform Body)

The brain stem and cerebellum are connected by three peduncles.

1. The inferior cerebellar peduncle (Fig. 5–20), between the medulla and cerebellum
2. The middle cerebellar peduncle (brachium pontis), between the pons and cerebellum
3. The superior cerebellar peduncle (brachium conjunctivum), between the cerebellum and midbrain

The inferior cerebellar peduncle (restiform body) contains a group of fiber tracts and is located on the dorsolateral border of the medulla oblongata. It appears rostral to the clava and cuneate tubercles and forms a distinct bundle at about the midolivary level. The fiber tracts contained within the inferior cerebellar peduncle include the following afferent and efferent tracts.

1. Olivocerebellar tract (the largest component of this peduncle)
2. Dorsal spinocerebellar tract
3. Reticulocerebellar and cerebelloreticular tracts
4. Cuneocerebellar tract
5. Arcuatocerebellar tract
6. Cerebello-olivary tract

A small inner part of the restiform body is known as the juxtarestiform body. It contains the following fiber tracts.

1. Cerebelloreticular tract
2. Cerebellovestibular tract (from nucleus fastigi of cerebellum to vestibular nuclei)
3. Direct vestibular nerve fibers to the cerebellum
4. Cerebellospinal tract (from nucleus fastigi of cerebellum to motor neurons of cervical spinal cord)
5. Secondary vestibular fibers from vestibular nuclei to the cerebellum

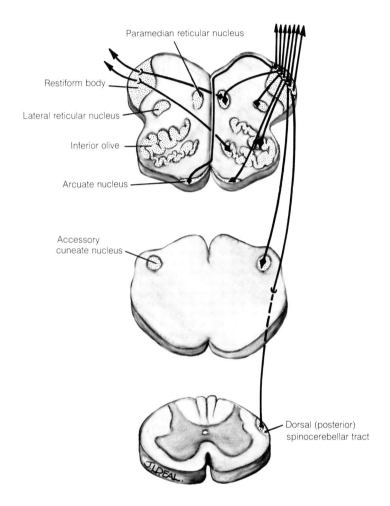

5–20 Composite schematic diagram of the components of the inferior cerebellar peduncle.

Lesions of the inferior cerebellar peduncle result in the following symptoms and signs.

1. Ataxia (lack of coordination of movement), with tendency to fall toward the side of the lesion
2. Nystagmus (involuntary rapid eye movement)
3. Some muscular hypotonia

Cranial Nerve Nuclei of Medulla

The following cranial nerves have their nuclei located in the medulla oblongata: 1) hypoglossal (CN XII) nerve, 2) accessory (CN XI) nerve, 3) vagus (CN X) nerve, 4) glossopharyngeal (CN IX) nerve, and 5) vestibulocochlear (CN VIII) nerve.

Hypoglossal (CN XII) Nerve

The hypoglossal nerve contains primarily somatic motor nerve fibers that innervate the intrinsic and extrinsic muscles of the tongue. It also contains afferent proprioceptive fibers from the muscle spindles of tongue muscles.

The nucleus of the hypoglossal nerve extends throughout the medulla oblongata, except for its most rostral and caudal levels. It is divided into cell groups corresponding to the tongue muscles they supply. The surface markings of the nucleus in the floor of the fourth ventricle are known as trigonum hypoglossi. The nucleus receives both crossed and uncrossed corticoreticulobulbar fibers. The root fibers of the nerve course in the medulla oblongata lateral to the medial lemniscus and emerge on the ventral surface of the medulla between the pyramid and the inferior olive (Fig. 5–21).

A number of nuclear masses in close proximity to the hypoglossal (CN XII) nucleus are believed to be reticular neurons which project to the cerebellum and thalamus and do not contribute fibers to the hypoglossal nerve. They are known as its satellite nuclei (nucleus intercalatus, nucleus prepositus, and nucleus of Roller).

Lesions of the hypoglossal nerve will result in lower motor neuron paralysis of the tongue musculature homolateral to the lesion (Fig. 5–22, A).

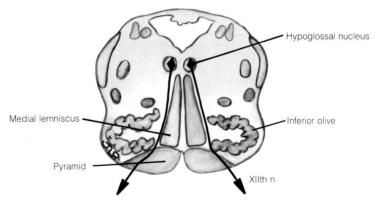

5–21 Schematic diagram of the origin and intramedullary course of filaments of the hypoglossal nerve.

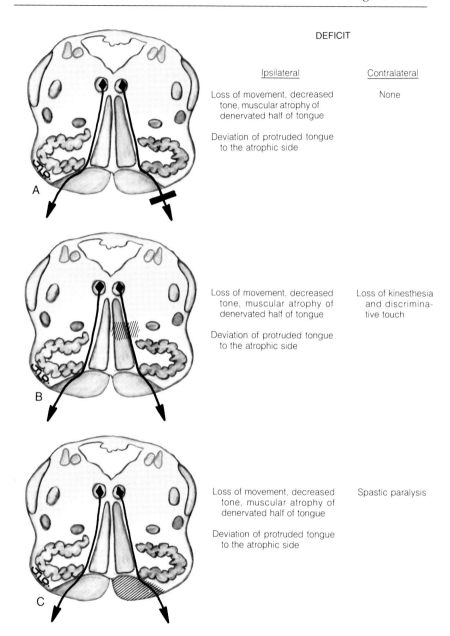

DEFICIT

	Ipsilateral	Contralateral
A	Loss of movement, decreased tone, muscular atrophy of denervated half of tongue Deviation of protruded tongue to the atrophic side	None
B	Loss of movement, decreased tone, muscular atrophy of denervated half of tongue Deviation of protruded tongue to the atrophic side	Loss of kinesthesia and discriminative touch
C	Loss of movement, decreased tone, muscular atrophy of denervated half of tongue Deviation of protruded tongue to the atrophic side	Spastic paralysis

5–22 Schematic diagram illustrating lesions of the hypoglossal nerve in its extra- and intramedullary course and the resulting clinical deficits of each.

This is manifested by the following.

1. Loss of movement
2. Loss of tone
3. Muscular atrophy
4. Deviation of the protruding tongue to the atrophic side (by action of the normal genioglossus muscle)

Lesions involving the rootlets of the hypoglossal nerve and the adjacent medial lemniscus within the medulla will result in signs and symptoms of hypoglossal nerve lesion and contralateral loss of kinesthesia and discriminative touch (Fig. 5–22, B).

Lesions involving the rootlets of the hypoglossal nerve and the adjacent pyramid within the medulla will be manifested by signs and symptoms of hypoglossal nerve lesion and contralateral paralysis (Fig. 5–22, C).

Accessory (CN XI) Nerve

The accessory nerve (Fig. 5–23) has two roots, the spinal and the cranial.

The spinal root arises from the accessory nucleus, which is a collection of motor neurons in the anterior horn of the upper five or six cervical spinal segments and the caudal part of the medulla. From their cells of origin, the rootlets course dorsolaterally and exit from the lateral part of the spinal cord between the dorsal and ventral roots. The spinal root of the accessory nerve enters the cranial cavity through the foramen magnum and leaves it through the jugular foramen. The spinal root contains somatic motor fibers that supply the sternocleidomastoid and the upper part of the trapezius muscles.

The cranial root arises from the caudal pole of the nucleus ambiguus in the medulla oblongata. The cranial root emerges from the lateral surface of the medulla, joins rootlets of the vagus nerve (forming its recurrent laryngeal branch), and supplies the intrinsic muscles of the larynx. Thus, the cranial root of the accessory nerve is in essence a part of the vagus nerve.

The following are manifestations of unilateral lesions of the accessory nerve.

1. Downward and outward rotation of the scapula on the same side
2. Moderate sagging of the shoulder on the same side
3. Weakness on turning the head to the side opposite the lesion
4. No observable abnormality of head position in repose

Vagus (CN X) Nerve

The vagus nerve (Fig. 5–24), a mixed nerve containing both afferent and efferent fibers, is associated with four nuclei in the medulla oblongata.

The efferent components of the nerve are related to two medullary nuclei.

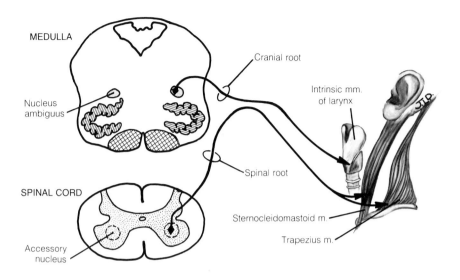

5–23 Schematic diagram illustrating the neurons of origin of the accessory nerve and muscles supplied by the nerve.

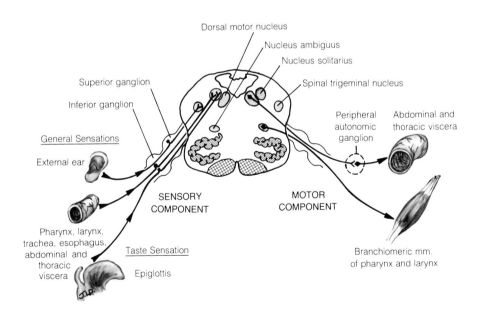

5–24 Schematic diagram of the components of the vagus nerve and the areas they supply.

Dorsal Motor Nucleus of the Vagus   This is a column of cells located dorsolateral or lateral to the hypoglossal nucleus that extends, both rostrally and caudally, a little beyond the hypoglossal nucleus. Axons of neurons in this column course ventrolaterally in the medulla and emerge from the lateral surface of the medulla between the inferior olive and the inferior cerebellar peduncle. Axons arising from this nucleus are preganglionic parasympathetic fibers that convey general visceral efferent impulses to the viscera in the thorax and abdomen. Postganglionic fibers arise from terminal ganglia located in the thorax and abdomen within or upon the innervated viscera. The dorsal motor nucleus of the vagus receives fibers from the vestibular nuclei; thus, excessive vestibular stimulation (*e.g.,* motion sickness) results in nausea, vomiting, and a change in heart rate.

Nucleus Ambiguus   This is also known as the ventral motor nucleus of the vagus. It is a column of cells located about half-way between the inferior olive and the nucleus of the spinal tract of the trigeminal nerve. Axons of neurons in this nucleus course dorsomedially and then turn ventrolaterally to emerge from the lateral surface of the medulla between the inferior olive and the inferior cerebellar peduncle. These axons convey special visceral efferent impulses to the branchiomeric muscles of the pharynx and larynx (pharyngeal constrictors, cricothyroid, intrinsic muscles of the larynx, levator veli palatini, palatoglossus, palatopharyngeus, and uvula).

The afferent components of the vagus nerve are related to two medullary nuclei.

Nucleus of the Spinal Tract of the Trigeminal   This nucleus receives general somatic afferent fibers from the external ear. Neurons of origin of these fibers are in the superior ganglion of the vagus nerve. The general somatic afferent component of the vagus nerve is small and its ganglion contains relatively few neurons.

Nucleus Solitarius   This nucleus receives two types of visceral afferent fibers.

General Visceral Afferent Fibers   These fibers convey general visceral sensations from the pharynx, larynx, trachea, and esophagus, as well as the thoracic and abdominal viscera.

Special Visceral Afferent Fibers   These fibers convey taste sensations from the region of the epiglottis.

The neurons of origin of both types of afferent fibers reside in the inferior ganglion of the vagus. Central processes of neurons in this ganglion enter the lateral surface of the medulla oblongata, course dorsomedially and form the tractus solitarius, which projects on cells of the nucleus solitarius. Neurons in the latter nucleus are organized in such a way that those receiving general visceral afferent fibers are located in the caudal and medial part of the nucleus, whereas those receiving special visceral afferent fibers (taste) are located in the rostral and lateral part.

Bilateral lesions of the vagus nerve are fatal, due to complete laryngeal paralysis and asphyxia.

Unilateral vagal lesions result in ipsilateral paralysis of the soft palate, pharynx, and larynx, manifested by hoarseness of voice, dysphagia (difficulty in swallowing), and dyspnea (difficulty in breathing).

Glossopharyngeal (CN IX) Nerve

The glossopharyngeal nerve (Fig. 5–25), also a mixed nerve (containing both afferent and efferent components), is associated with four nuclei in the medulla.

The efferent components of the glossopharyngeal nerve are related to two nuclei.

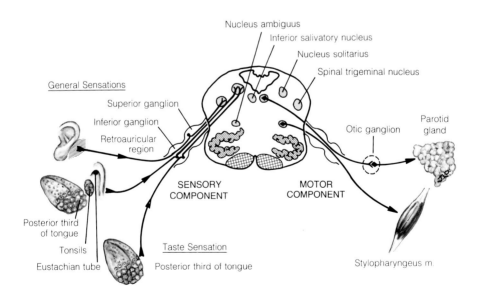

5–25 Schematic diagram of the components of the glossopharyngeal nerve and the structures they supply.

Nucleus Ambiguus Axons of neurons that travel with the glossopharyngeal nerve arise from the rostral part of this nucleus and supply special visceral efferent fibers to the stylopharyngeus muscle. This efferent component of the glossopharyngeal nerve is small.

Inferior Salivatory Nucleus This is a group of neurons that are difficult to distinguish from reticular neurons in the dorsal aspect of the medulla. Axons of neurons in this nucleus leave the medulla from its lateral surface. They are preganglionic general visceral efferent fibers conveying secretomotor impulses to the parotid gland. They travel via the lesser petrosal nerve to the otic ganglion from which postganglionic fibers supply the parotid gland.

The afferent components of the glossopharyngeal nerve are related to the same two nuclei associated with the vagus nerve.

Nucleus of the Spinal Tract of the Trigeminal This nucleus receives general somatic afferent fibers from the retroauricular region. Neurons of origin of these fibers are located in the superior ganglion within the jugular foramen.

Nucleus Solitarius This nucleus receives two types of visceral afferent fibers.

General Visceral Afferent Fibers These fibers convey tactile, pain, and thermal sensations from the mucous membranes of the posterior third of the tongue, the tonsils, and the eustachian tube.

Special Visceral Afferent Fibers These fibers convey taste sensations from the posterior third of the tongue.

Neurons of origin of the visceral afferent fibers are located in the inferior ganglion. Within the medulla, they form the tractus solitarius and project upon the nucleus solitarius in a manner similar to that described for the vagus nerve.

The glossopharyngeal nerve also contains a special afferent branch, the carotid sinus nerve. This branch innervates the carotid sinus, which is a baroreceptor center. Elevation of carotid arterial pressure will stimulate the carotid sinus nerve, which, upon reaching the medulla, sends collaterals to the dorsal motor nucleus of the vagus. General visceral efferent components of the vagus nerve then reach ganglion cells in the wall of the heart to slow down the heart rate and reduce blood pressure. This glossopharyngeal-vagal reflex is especially sensitive in elderly people. Extreme care should be taken when manipulating the carotid sinus region in such people.

Unilateral lesions of the glossopharyngeal nerve are manifested by the following signs.

1. Loss of pharyngeal (gag) reflex
2. Loss of carotid sinus reflex
3. Loss of taste in posterior third of tongue
4. Deviation of uvula to the unaffected side

Vestibulocochlear (CN VIII) Nerve

The vestibular component of the vestibulocochlear nerve will also be discussed in the chapter on the pons. The two vestibular nuclei that appear at rostral levels of the medulla are the inferior vestibular nucleus and the medial vestibular nucleus.

The inferior vestibular nucleus is located medial to the restiform body and is characterized in histologic preparations by the presence of dark-staining bundles of fibers coursing through it.

The medial vestibular nucleus, located medial to the inferior nucleus, is poorly stained in myelin preparations.

Blood Supply of Medulla

The medulla oblongata receives its blood supply from the following arteries.

1. Vertebral
2. Anterior spinal
3. Posterior spinal
4. Posterior inferior cerebellar

The vertebral artery supplies the medial and intermediate structures of the medulla, including the pyramids, hypoglossal nucleus, most of the inferior olive, olivocerebellar fibers, dorsal motor nucleus of the vagus, and the solitary nucleus and its tract. The anterior spinal artery supplies the medial structures of the medulla, including the pyramids, medial lemniscus, medial longitudinal fasciculus, and hypoglossal nucleus and nerve. The posterior spinal artery supplies the posterior (dorsal) structures of the medulla, including the posterior column nuclei and their tracts. The posterior inferior cerebellar artery supplies the dorsolateral part of the medulla, including the restiform body, the spinal trigeminal nucleus and its tract, the adjacent spinothalamic tract, nucleus ambiguus, dorsal motor nucleus of the vagus, and vestibular nuclei.

Applied Anatomy of Medulla Oblongata

Vascular lesions of the medulla oblongata lend themselves best to anatomicoclinical correlation; two syndromes are particularly illustrative.

Medial Medullary Syndrome

This syndrome (Fig. 5–26) is caused by occlusion of the anterior spinal artery or the paramedian branches of the vertebral artery. The affected area usually includes the following.

1. Medial lemniscus
2. Pyramid
3. Rootlets of the hypoglossal nerve or its nucleus within the medulla

Neurologic signs resulting from affection of these areas are the following.

1. Contralateral loss of kinesthesia and discriminative touch due to involvement of the medial lemniscus
2. Contralateral paralysis of the upper motor neuron type (weakness, hyperactive reflexes, Babinski sign, and spasticity) due to involvement of the pyramid
3. Lower motor neuron paralysis of the homolateral half of the tongue (weakness, atrophy, and fibrillation)

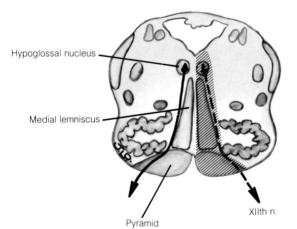

Hypoglossal nucleus

Medial lemniscus

Pyramid

XIIth n.

Medial Medullary Syndrome

Paralysis of homolateral half of tongue (lower motor neuron type)

Contralateral paralysis (upper motor neuron type)

Contralateral loss of kinesthesia and discriminative touch

5–26 Schematic diagram of the medullary areas involved in the medial medullary syndrome and the resulting clinical manifestations.

Lateral Medullary Syndrome

This syndrome (Fig. 5–27) is caused by occlusion of the vertebral artery or the posterior inferior cerebellar artery. It is also known as the posterior inferior cerebellar artery (PICA) syndrome or Wallenberg's syndrome. The affected area usually includes the following.

1. Spinal nucleus of the trigeminal nerve and its tract
2. Adjacent spinothalamic tract
3. Nucleus ambiguus or its axons
4. Base of the inferior cerebellar peduncle
5. Vestibular nuclei
6. Descending sympathetic fibers from the hypothalamus

Neurologic signs and symptoms resulting from affection of these areas are the following.

1. Loss of pain and temperature sensations from the ipsilateral face due to involvement of the spinal nucleus of the trigeminal and its tract
2. Loss of pain and temperature sensations over the contralateral half of the body due to involvement of the spinothalamic tract
3. Loss of gag reflex, difficulty in swallowing (dysphagia), hoarseness, and difficulty in articulation due to paralysis of pharyngeal muscles supplied by the nucleus ambiguus
4. Loss of coordination (ataxia) due to involvement of the base of the inferior cerebellar peduncle
5. Hallucination of turning (vertigo) due to involvement of the vestibular nuclei

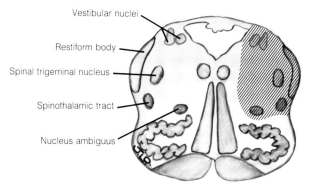

Vestibular nuclei

Restiform body

Spinal trigeminal nucleus

Spinothalamic tract

Nucleus ambiguus

Lateral Medullary Syndrome

Loss of pain and temperature sensations over the ipsilateral face and contralateral half of the body

Ataxia (loss of coordination)

Vertigo (hallucination of movement)

Loss of gag reflex, difficulty in swallowing, and difficulty in articulation

Ipsilateral Horner's syndrome

Vomiting

5–27 Schematic diagram of the medullary areas involved in the lateral medullary syndrome and the resulting clinical manifestations.

6. Horner's syndrome due to involvement of the descending sympathetic fibers from the hypothalamus. This syndrome consists of a small pupil (miosis), slight drooping of the upper eyelid (ptosis), and warm dry skin of the face (anhidrosis), all ipsilateral to the lesion
7. Vomiting, nystagmus, and nausea due to involvement of the vestibular nuclei
8. Hiccup of uncertain cause but usually attributed to involvement of the respiratory center in the reticular formation of the medulla

Pseudobulbar Palsy

Pseudobulbar palsy is a clinical syndrome caused by the interruption of the corticobulbar fibers to motor nuclei of cranial nerves. Most cranial nerve nuclei of the brain stem receive bilateral inputs from the cerebral cortex arising primarily from the precentral cortex. The majority of these fibers reach cranial nerve nuclei via the reticular formation (corticoreticulobulbar system). Some cranial nerve nuclei, however, receive direct corticobulbar fibers.

Bilateral interruption of the indirect corticoreticulobulbar or the direct corticobulbar fibers in the brain stem results in the syndrome of pseudobulbar palsy. The neurologic manifestations of this syndrome include the following.

1. Weakness (upper motor neuron variety) of muscles supplied by the corresponding cranial nerve nuclei
2. Inappropriate outbursts of laughing and crying

References

Beckstead, R.M.; Morse, J.R.; Norgren, R.: The Nucleus of the Solitary Tract in the Monkey: Projections to the Thalamus and Brain Stem Nuclei. J Comp Neurol 190 (1980) 259–282.

Ciriello, J.; Calaresu, F.R.: Vagal Bradycardia Elicited by Stimulation of the External Cuneate Nucleus in the Cat. Am J Physiol 235 (1978) R286–293.

Iwata, M.; Hirano, A.: Localization of Olivo-Cerebellar Fibers in Inferior Cerebellar Peduncle in Man. J Neurol Sci 38 (1978) 327–335.

Kalil, K.: Projections of the Cerebellar and Dorsal Column Nuclei upon the Inferior Olive in the Rhesus Monkey: An Autoradiographic Study. J Comp Neurol 188 (1979) 43–62.

Kawamura, K.; Hashikawa, T.: Olivocerebellar Projections in the Cat Studied by Means of Anterograde Axonal Transport of Labeled Amino Acids as Tracers. Neuroscience 4 (1979) 1615–1633.

Kotchabhakdi, N.; Rinvik, E.; Yingchareon, K.; Walberg, F.: Afferent Projections to the Thalamus from the Perihypoglossal Nuclei. Brain Res 187 (1980) 457–461.

Poulos, D.A.; Burton, H.; Molt, J.T.; Barron, K.D.: Localization of Specific Thermoreceptors in Spinal Trigeminal Nucleus of the Cat. Brain Res 165 (1979) 144–148.

Saint-Cyr, J.A.; Courville, J.: Projection from the Vestibular Nuclei to the Inferior Olive in the Cat: An Autoradiographic and Horseradish Peroxidase Study. Brain Res 165 (1979) 189–200.

Somana, R.; Walberg, F.: A Re-examination of the Cerebellar Projections from the Gracile, Main and External Cuneate Nuclei in the Cat. Brain Res 186 (1980) 33–42.

Uemura, M.; Matsuda, K.; Kume, M.; Takeuchi, Y.; Matsushima, R.; Mizuno, N.: Topographical Arrangement of Hypoglossal Motoneurons: An HRP Study in the Cat. Neurosci Lett 13 (1979) 99–104.

Weisberg, J.A.; Rustioni, A.: Differential Projections of Cortical Sensorimotor Areas upon the Dorsal Column Nuclei of Cats. J Comp Neurol 184 (1979) 401–422.

Zemlan, F.P.; Pfaff, D.W.: Topographical Organization in Medullary Reticulospinal Systems as Demonstrated by the Horseradish Peroxidase Technique. Brain Res 174 (1979) 161–166.

6

Pons

Gross Topography

The pons is that part of the brain stem between the medulla oblongata caudally and the midbrain rostrally. The cerebral peduncles mark its anterior boundary and the middle cerebellar peduncles (brachium pontis), which connect the pons and cerebellum, mark its lateral boundary. The dorsal surface is covered by the cerebellum.

Ventral Surface

The ventral surface (Fig. 6–1) of the pons forms a bulge, the pontine protuberance. In the middle of the protuberance is the pontine sulcus, which contains the basilar artery. Several cranial nerves leave the ventral surface of the pons. The abducens (CN VI) nerve emerges from the boundary between the pons and medulla oblongata (the inferior pontine sulcus). In the angle between the caudal pons, the rostral medulla, and the cerebellum (the cerebellopontine angle), the facial (CN VII) and cochleovestibular (CN VIII) nerves appear. From the lateral and rostral parts of the pons emerge the two components of the trigeminal (CN V) nerve, the larger sensory portion (portio major) and the smaller motor portion (portio minor). The crowding of the facial and cochleovestibular nerves in the cerebellopontine angle explains the early involvement of these two nerves in tumors (acoustic neuromas) arising in this angle.

Dorsal Surface

The dorsal surface (Fig. 6–2) of the pons forms the rostral portion of the floor of the fourth ventricle. This part of the floor features the facial colliculi; one is on each side of the midline sulcus (median sulcus). They represent the surface landmarks of the genu of the facial nerve and the underlying nucleus of the abducens nerve.

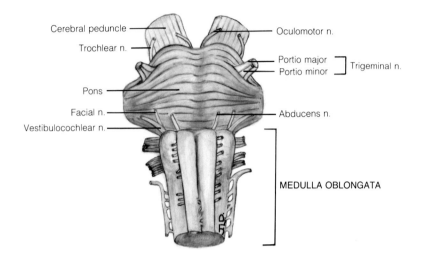

6-1 Schematic diagram of the ventral surface of the brain stem showing the major structures encountered on the ventral surface of the pons.

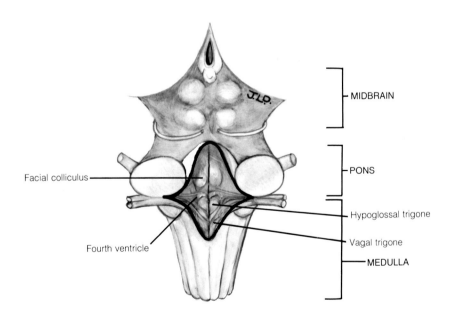

6-2 Schematic diagram of the dorsal surface of the brain stem showing the major structures encountered in the floor of the fourth ventricle at the medullary and pontine levels.

Microscopic Structure

Coronal sections of the pons reveal a basic organizational pattern of two parts; these are the basis pontis (ventral) and the tegmentum (dorsal).

Basis Pontis (Ventral)

The basis pontis (Fig. 6–3) corresponds to the pontine protuberance described under gross topography. It contains the pontine nuclei and multidirectional nerve fiber bundles.

The fibers in the basis pontis belong to three descending fiber systems.

1. Corticospinal fibers on their way from the cerebral cortex to the spinal cord pass through the basis pontis and continue caudally as the pyramids of the medulla oblongata.
2. Corticobulbar fibers descend from the cerebral cortex to cranial nerve nuclei of the brain stem. Some of these fibers project directly upon nuclei of cranial nerves; the majority, however, synapse on an intermediate reticular nucleus prior to reaching the cranial nerve nucleus. This latter indirect system is also known as corticoreticulobulbar. Corticobulbar and corticoreticulobulbar fibers projecting upon a cranial nerve nucleus usually arise from both cerebral hemispheres.

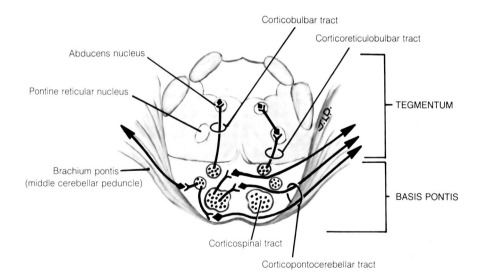

6–3 Schematic diagram of the pons showing its major divisions into tegmentum and basis pontis and types of fiber bundles traversing the basis pontis.

3. The corticopontocerebellar tract is the largest group of fibers in the basis pontis. This fiber system originates from wide areas of the cerebral cortex, projects upon ipsilateral pontine nuclei, and crosses the midline on its way to the cerebellum via the middle cerebellar peduncle. It is estimated that this fiber system, in man, contains approximately 19 million fibers on each side. The number of pontine neurons, in man, is estimated to be approximately 23 million in each half of the pons. Thus, the ratio of corticopontine fibers to pontine neurons is approximately 1:1. Although the corticopontine projection is believed to arise from wide areas of the cortex, it has been shown that it arises principally from the pre- and postrolandic sensorimotor cortices with minor contributions from the association cortices. A moderate contribution from the cingulate cortex has been demonstrated recently. The fact that pontine nuclei receive cortical input chiefly from primary cortical areas suggests that the corticopontocerebellar fiber system is concerned with rapid correction of movements. The functional significance of the cingulopontine fiber connection is not yet known, but it may represent the anatomic substrate for the effect of emotion on motor function.

A cortical region usually projects to more than one cell column of pontine nuclei and some pontine columns receive from more than one cortical region. It has also been shown that the cortical projection to pontine nuclei is exclusively through axodendritic synapses. Like the cortico-olivocerebellar system, the corticopontocerebellar system is somatotopically organized in a precise fashion. Thus, the prerolandic cortex projects to medial pontine nuclei, the postrolandic cortex to lateral pontine nuclei, the arm area of the sensorimotor cortex to dorsal pontine nuclei, and the leg area to ventral pontine nuclei. The projection from the cingulate gyrus to pontine nuclei has also been shown to be somatotopically organized with the anterior cingulate cortex projecting to the medial part of the pontine gray matter and the posterior cingulate cortex projecting to the lateral part. In contrast to projections from the sensorimotor cortex, those from the cingulate cortex terminate in the peripheral zone of the pontine gray matter and only occasionally in the central core traversed by fascicles of the corticospinal tract. Thus the cingulopontine projections form a ring around the periphery of the pontine gray matter.

The pontocerebellar projection is primarily crossed; it is estimated that 30% of the projection to the vermis and 10% of the projection to the cerebellar hemisphere is ipsilateral. The density of projection to the cerebellar hemispheres is three times that to the vermis. Like the corticopontine projection, the pontocerebellar projection is somatotopically organized with the caudal half of the pons projecting to the anterior lobe of the cerebellum and the rostral half of the pons projecting to the posterior lobe.

The basilar portion of the pons is the phylogenetically newer part and is present only in animals with well-developed cerebellar hemispheres.

Tegmentum (Dorsal)

The tegmentum is the phylogenetically older part of the pons and is composed largely of reticular formation. Lesions that destroy more than 25% of the tegmentum will result in loss of consciousness. In the basal part of the tegmentum, the medial lemniscus (which maintains a vertical orientation on each side of the midline in the medulla) becomes flattened in a mediolateral direction (Fig. 6–4). Fibers originating from the cuneate nucleus are located medially; gracile fibers are laterally placed. Lateral to the medial lemniscus lies the trigeminal tract, conveying sensations of pain, temperature, touch, and proprioception from the face. The spinothalamic tract is located lateral to the trigeminal tract and carries pain and temperature sensations from the contralateral half of the body. Thus, in the basal part of the tegmentum, separating it from the basis pontis, lies the specific sensory lemniscal system, which includes the medial lemniscus, trigeminal lemniscus, and spinothalamic tract.

Intermingled with the ascending fibers of the lemniscal system are transverse fibers of the trapezoid body. These arise from the cochlear nuclei,

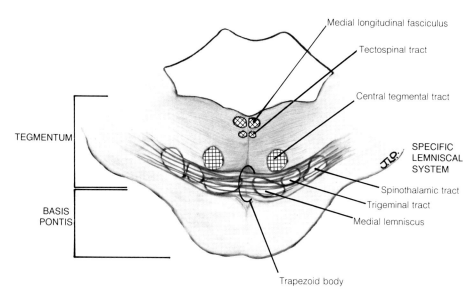

6–4 Schematic diagram of the pons showing the major tracts traversing the tegmentum.

course through the tegmentum and gather in the lateral portion of the pons to form the lateral lemniscus. This fiber system will be discussed later in connection with the cochlear division of the cochleovestibular (CN VIII) nerve.

Dorsal to the medial lemniscus is the central tegmental tract, which originates in the basal ganglia and midbrain and projects upon the inferior olive; it shifts positions in the tegmentum of the pons and lies dorsal to the lateral part of the medial lemniscus in the caudal pons (Fig. 6–4).

The medial longitudinal fasciculus and tectospinal tract retain the same dorsal and paramedian positions they occupied in the medulla just beneath the floor of the fourth ventricle (Fig. 6–4).

Other tracts coursing through the tegmentum of the pons include the rubrospinal tract located medial to the spinal trigeminal nucleus and the ventral spinocerebellar tract located medial to the restiform body. The ventral spinocerebellar tract enters the superior cerebellar peduncle to reach the cerebellum. The tegmentum of the pons also contains descending sympathetic fibers from the hypothalamus; these are located in the lateral part of the tegmentum. Interruption of these fibers will produce Horner's syndrome (see Chapter 5 on the medulla oblongata). Corticobulbar fibers and corticoreticulobulbar fibers on their way from the basis pontis to cranial nerve nuclei also pass through the tegmentum (Fig. 6–3).

Pontine Reticular Formation

The pontine reticular formation constitutes the major part of the tegmental portion of the pons and is a rostral continuation of the medullary reticular formation. As in the medulla, the pontine reticular nuclei are located medially and laterally (Fig. 6–5).

The medial pontine reticular nuclei include the nucleus reticularis pontis caudalis, which is a continuation of the gigantocellular reticular nucleus of the medulla. The rostral extension of this nucleus in the pons (nucleus reticularis pontis oralis) does not have large neurons.

From the reticularis pontis caudalis and oralis arise the pontine reticulospinal tract, which facilitates extensor motor neurons and inhibits flexor motor neurons, and the ascending reticular activating fiber system. The nucleus reticularis pontis caudalis has been associated with paradoxical sleep. Bilateral lesions in this nucleus result in complete elimination of paradoxical sleep.

Paramedian reticular nuclei (also known as raphe nuclei) occupy a position on each side of the central raphe. They contain small neurons and produce the transmitter substance serotonin.

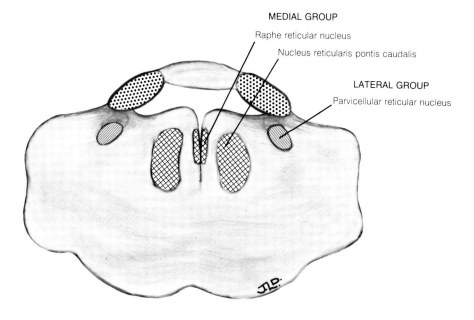

MEDIAL GROUP
Raphe reticular nucleus
Nucleus reticularis pontis caudalis

LATERAL GROUP
Parvicellular reticular nucleus

6–5 Schematic diagram of the pons showing the major divisions of pontine reticular nuclei.

The lateral pontine reticular nuclei consist primarily of the parvicellular reticular nucleus, which is an association center relating ascending and descending fiber systems to the medial group of reticular nuclei. In the rostral and dorsolateral part of the pontine tegmentum is the nucleus tegmentalis dorsolateralis, the pontine micturition center. Stimulation of this nucleus results in bladder contraction and micturition. Fiber connections have been shown between this nucleus and the intermediolateral autonomic cell column in the sacral spinal cord.

Cranial Nerve Nuclei

Cochleovestibular (CN VIII) Nerve

The cochleovestibular nerve has two divisions, the cochlear and the vestibular. The two divisions travel together from the peripheral end organs in the inner ear to the pons, where they separate; each then establishes its own distinct connections.

Cochlear Nerve The cochlear division (Fig. 6–6) of the cochleovestibular nerve is the larger of the two divisions. Nerve fibers in the cochlear nerve are central processes of bipolar neurons in the spiral ganglion located in the modiolus of the inner ear. The peripheral processes are linked to the hair cells of the auditory end organ in the organ of Corti. As fibers of the cochlear nerve reach the caudal part of the pons, they enter its lateral surface caudal and lateral to the vestibular division and project upon the dorsal and ventral cochlear nuclei. The dorsal cochlear nucleus, located on the dorsolateral surface of the restiform body, receives fibers originating in the basal turns of the cochlea (mediating high frequency sound), whereas the ventral cochlear nucleus, located on the ventrolateral aspect of the restiform body, receives fibers from the apical turns of the cochlea (mediating low frequency sound). It is estimated that the total number of

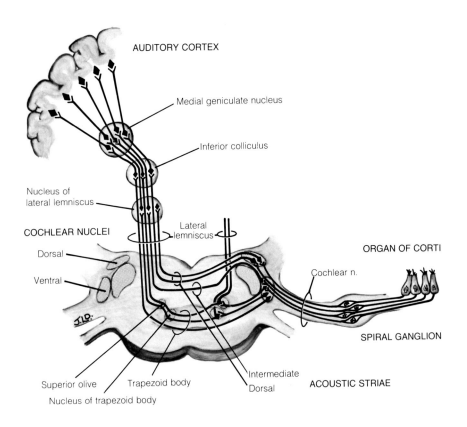

6–6 Schematic diagram of the auditory pathways.

neurons in the cochlear nuclei far exceeds the total number of cochlear nerve fibers, so that each fiber is believed to project upon several neurons.

Second order neurons from the cochlear nuclei course through the tegmentum of the pons forming the acoustic striae. The dorsal acoustic stria is formed by axons of neurons in the dorsal cochlear nucleus, whereas the intermediate and ventral acoustic striae originate in the inferior cochlear nucleus. The ventral acoustic stria (the trapezoid body) is the largest of the three striae. Fibers in this stria project upon neurons in the superior olivary nucleus and the nucleus of the trapezoid body. Third order neurons from these two nuclei contribute mainly to the contralateral lateral lemniscus, with some projection to the homolateral lateral lemniscus. The lateral lemniscus also receives fibers from both the dorsal and intermediate acoustic striae. Fibers in the lateral lemniscus project upon the nucleus of the lateral lemniscus. Subsequent stations in the auditory system include synapses in the inferior colliculus and medial geniculate body. The final station is the primary auditory cortex (transverse gyri of Heschl) in the temporal lobe. Tonotopic localization is believed to exist throughout the auditory system. In addition to this "classic" auditory pathway, there is evidence to suggest the existence of another multisynaptic auditory pathway through the reticular formation.

The auditory system is characterized by the presence of several inhibitory feedback mechanisms. However, the most important feedback mechanism is served by the olivocochlear bundle, also known as Rasmussen's efferent bundle (Fig. 6–7). This bundle has both crossed and uncrossed components. The crossed component arises from the accessory superior olive, courses dorsally in the pontine tegmentum, bypasses the nucleus of the abducens nerve, and crosses to the contralateral side. The uncrossed com-

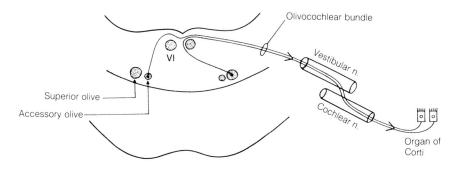

6–7 Schematic diagram showing the origin and course of the olivocochlear bundle.

ponent is smaller and originates in the main superior olive. Both components initially join the vestibular division of the cochleovestibular (CN VIII)
nerve but, at the vestibulocochlear anastomosis, leave it and travel with
the cochlear division as far as the hair cells of the organ of Corti. Stimulation
of the olivocochlear bundle suppresses the receptivity of the organ of Corti
and hence activity in the auditory nerve.

The hair cells of the organ of Corti transduce mechanical energy into
nerve impulses and exhibit a graded generator potential. Spike potentials
appear in the cochlear nerve.

Cochlear nerve fibers respond to both displacement and velocity of the
basilar membrane of the organ of Corti. Displacement of the basilar membrane toward the scala vestibuli produces inhibition, whereas displacement
toward the scala tympani produces excitation. A single fiber in the cochlear
nerve may respond to both displacement and velocity.

Reflex movements of eyes and neck toward a sound source are mediated
via two reflex pathways. The first is from the inferior colliculus to the
superior colliculus and from there via tectobulbar and tectospinal pathways
to the nuclei of the eye muscles and cervical musculature. The other pathway is from the superior olive to the abducens (CN VI) nerve nucleus and
then via the medial longitudinal fasciculus to the nuclei of cranial nerves
of extraocular muscles.

Vestibular Nerve Vestibular nerve fibers are central processes of bipolar cells in the ganglion of Scarpa. Peripheral processes of these bipolar
cells are distributed to the vestibular end organ in the three semicircular
canals, the utricle, and saccule. The semicircular canals are concerned with
angular acceleration; the utricle and saccule are concerned with linear
acceleration (gravity). The superior portion of the ganglion of Scarpa receives fibers from the anterior and horizontal canals, utricle and saccule. The
inferior portion of the ganglion receives fibers from the posterior semicircular canal and the saccule (Fig. 6–8). The vestibular nerve accompanies the cochlear nerve from the internal auditory meatus to the pons, where it enters the
lateral surface at the pontomedullary junction medial to the cochlear nerve.

Within the pons, vestibular nerve fibers course in the tegmentum between the restiform body and the spinal trigeminal complex. The major
portion of these fibers projects upon the four vestibular nuclei; a smaller
portion goes directly to the cerebellum via the juxtarestiform body. In the
cerebellum, they terminate as mossy fibers upon neurons in the flocculonodular lobe and the uvula. There are four vestibular nuclei: the medial,
inferior, lateral, and superior. The medial nucleus (principal nucleus or
nucleus of Schwalbe) appears in the medulla oblongata at the rostral end
of the inferior olive and extends to the caudal part of the pons. The inferior
nucleus (spinal nucleus) lies between the medial nucleus and the restiform

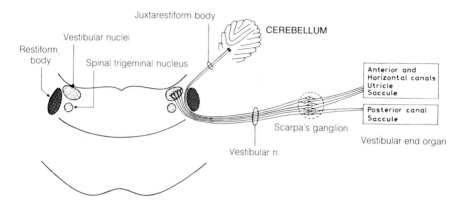

6–8 Schematic diagram showing the origin and termination of the vestibular nerve fibers.

body. The inferior nucleus, characterized in histologic sections by myelinated fibers traversing it from the vestibular nerve, extends from the rostral extremity of the gracile nucleus to the pontomedullary junction. The lateral nucleus (nucleus of Deiters), characterized in histologic sections by the presence of large multipolar neurons, extends from the pontomedullary junction to the level of the abducens (CN VI) nerve nucleus. The superior nucleus, or nucleus of von Bechterew, is smaller than the other nuclei and lies dorsal and medial to the medial and lateral nuclei. The number of neurons in the vestibular nuclei far exceeds the number of vestibular nerve fibers. Vestibular nerve fibers project only to limited regions within each vestibular nucleus. In addition to the input from the vestibular nerve, the vestibular nuclei receive fibers from 1) the spinal cord, 2) the cerebellum, and 3) the vestibular cortex (Fig. 6–9). The output from the vestibular nuclei is to 1) the spinal cord, 2) the cerebellum, 3) the thalamus, and 4) the nuclei of extraocular muscles.

The vestibular projection to the spinal cord (Fig. 6–10) is through the lateral vestibulospinal tract (from the lateral vestibular nucleus) and the medial vestibulospinal tract (from the medial vestibular nucleus) via the descending component of the medial longitudinal fasciculus. The lateral vestibulospinal tract facilitates extensor motor neurons, whereas the medial vestibulospinal tract facilitates flexor motor neurons. The medial vestibulospinal tract sends fibers to the dorsal motor nucleus of the vagus, which explains the nausea, sweating, and vomiting that occurs with stimulation of the vestibular end organ.

Projections from the vestibular nuclei to the cerebellum (Fig. 6–11) travel via the juxtarestiform body along with the primary vestibulocerebellar fibers. These projections arise from the superior, inferior, and medial

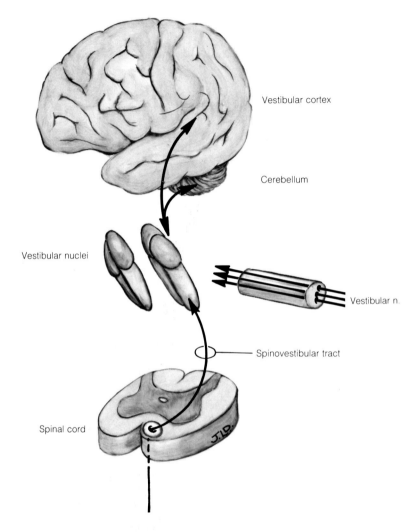

Vestibular cortex

Cerebellum

Vestibular nuclei

Vestibular n.

Spinovestibular tract

Spinal cord

6–9 Schematic diagram showing the major inputs to the vestibular nuclei.

vestibular nuclei and terminate mainly ipsilaterally (but also bilaterally) upon neurons in the flocculonodular lobe, the uvula, and the nucleus fastigi. Cerebellovestibular connections are much more abundant than vestibulocerebellar connections.

Vestibulothalamic projections have recently been described using autoradiography and retrograde axonal transport of horseradish peroxidase. These projections arise from the medial, lateral, and superior vestibular nuclei and project bilaterally upon several thalamic nuclei (ventral posterolateral, centrolateral, lateral geniculate, and posterior group). They

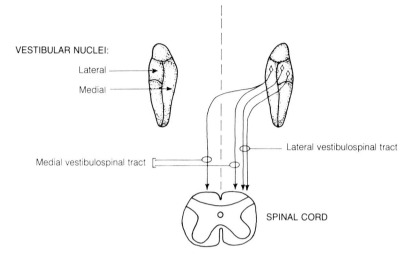

6–10 Schematic diagram showing the origin, course, and destination of the vestibulospinal pathways.

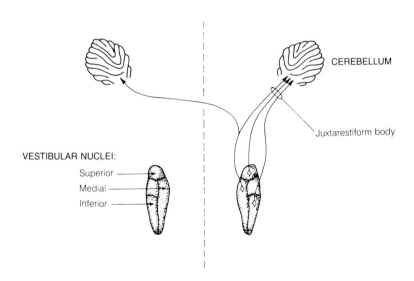

6–11 Schematic diagram showing the origin, course, and destination of the vestibulocerebellar pathways.

reach their destination via several pathways (lateral lemniscus, brachium conjunctivum, reticular formation), with a few traveling via the medial longitudinal fasciculus.

Vestibular projections to the nuclei of extraocular muscles travel via the ascending component of the medial longitudinal fasciculus. They arise from all four vestibular nuclei and project upon nuclei of the oculomotor (CN III), trochlear (CN IV), and abducens (CN VI) nerves.

A projection from the vestibular nuclei to the primary vestibular cortex in the temporal lobe is believed to exist; although the exact pathway of this projection is not well defined, it most likely reaches the vestibular cortex via relays in the thalamus.

The vestibular output to nuclei of extraocular muscles plays an important role in the control of conjugate eye movements. This control is mediated via two pathways (Fig. 6–12); these are the ascending component of the medial longitudinal fasciculus and the reticular formation. Reflex conjugate deviation of the eyes in a specific direction, known as nystagmus, has two components; these are a slow component away from the stimulated vestibular system and a fast component toward the stimulated side. In clinical medicine, nystagmus refers to the fast component. Although the mecha-

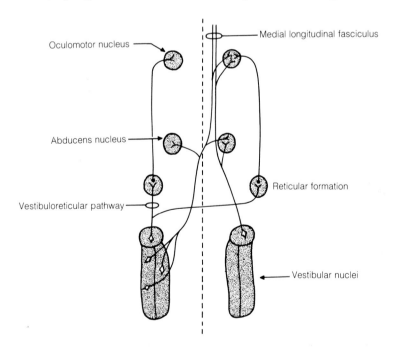

6–12 Schematic diagram showing the pathways by which the vestibular nuclei control conjugate eye movements.

nism of the slow component is fairly well understood in terms of neuronal connections, the same cannot be said of the fast component, which is believed to be a corrective attempt to return the eyes to a neutral position. Stimulation of the right horizontal semicircular canal (turning to the right in a Barani chair or pouring warm water in the right ear) or of the right medial, lateral, or inferior vestibular nuclei will result in a reflex conjugate horizontal deviation of the eyes (horizontal nystagmus) with a slow component to the left and a fast component to the right. Stimulation of the superior vestibular nucleus produces vertical nystagmus.

Lesions of the medial longitudinal fasciculus (MLF) rostral to the abducens nucleus will interfere with normal conjugate eye movements. In this condition, known as internuclear ophthalmoplegia or the MLF syndrome, there is paralysis of adduction ipsilateral to the lesion and horizontal monocular nystagmus of the abducting eye (Fig. 6–13). Such a condition is known to occur in the disease multiple sclerosis and in vascular disorders of the pons. Experimental evidence shows that such a lesion will interrupt MLF fibers destined for that part of the oculomotor nuclear complex which innervates the medial rectus, hence the loss of adduction. There is still no satisfactory explanation for the monocular horizontal nystagmus of the

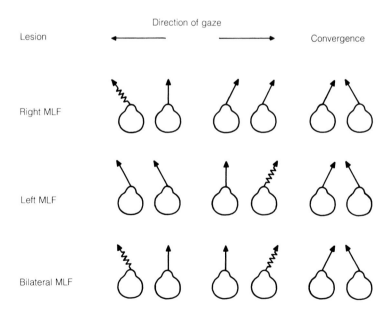

6–13   Schematic diagram showing the effects of lesions in the medial longitudinal fasciculus (MLF) on conjugate eye movements. *Zigzag arrows* indicate nystagmus.

abducting eye. Two theories have been proposed to explain this phenomenon. The first theory suggests that nystagmus is due to the utilization of convergence mechanisms to adduct the ipsilateral eye. This would induce adduction of the contralateral eye which will then jerk back to the position of fixation. The second theory suggests that the medial longitudinal fasciculus carries facilitatory fibers to the ipsilateral medial rectus neurons and inhibitory fibers to the contralateral medial rectus neurons. In lesions of the medial longitudinal fasciculus, failure of inhibition of adduction in the contralateral eye thus causes an abducting (corrective) nystagmus in that eye.

Facial (CN VII) Nerve

The facial nerve (Fig. 6–14) is a mixed nerve with both sensory and motor components.

Sensory Components   The facial nerve carries two types of sensory afferents. These are exteroceptive fibers from the external ear and taste fibers from the anterior two-thirds of the tongue.

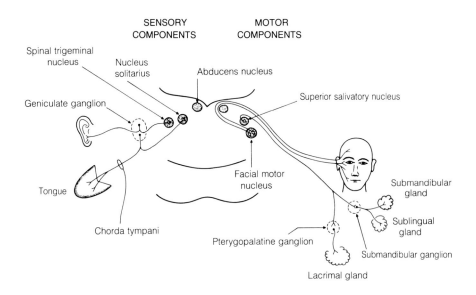

6–14   Schematic diagram showing the nuclei of origin, course, and areas of supply of the facial (CN VII) nerve.

The exteroceptive fibers from the external ear are peripheral processes of neurons in the geniculate ganglion. Central processes project upon neurons in the spinal trigeminal nucleus [similar to fibers from the same area carried by the glossopharyngeal (CN IX) and vagus (CN X) nerves].

The taste fibers have their neurons of origin in the geniculate ganglion. Peripheral processes of these neurons reach the taste buds in the anterior two-thirds of the tongue; central processes enter the brain stem with the nervus intermedius and project upon neurons in the gustatory part of the nucleus solitarius, along with fibers carried by the glossopharyngeal (from the posterior third of the tongue) and vagus nerves (from the epiglottic region).

Motor Components   The facial nerve carries two types of motor fibers.

Somatic Motor Fibers   These fibers supply the muscles of facial expression and the stapedius, stylohyoid, and posterior belly of the digastric. These fibers arise from the facial motor nucleus in the pontine tegmentum. From their neurons of origin, fibers course dorsomedially, then rostrally in the tegmentum, and form a compact bundle near the abducens (CN VI) nerve nucleus, in the floor of the fourth ventricle (the facial colliculus). They bend (genu) laterally over the abducens nucleus and turn ventrolaterally to emerge at the lateral border of the pons. This peculiar course of the facial nerve fibers in the tegmentum is the result of the migration of the facial motor nucleus from a position in the floor of the fourth ventricle caudally and ventrally, pulling its axons with it. The migration of the facial motor nucleus is explained by neurobiotaxis, in which neurons tend to migrate toward major sources of stimuli. In the case of the facial motor nucleus, this migration brings it closer to the trigeminal spinal nucleus and its tract.

The motor nucleus of the facial nerve receives fibers from the following sources.

Cerebral cortex   These fibers travel as direct corticobulbar or as corticoreticulobulbar fibers. The cortical input to the facial nucleus is bilateral to the part of the nucleus which supplies the upper facial muscles and only contralateral to the part of the nucleus that innervates the perioral musculature. In lesions affecting one hemisphere, only the lower facial muscles contralateral to the lesion are affected (Fig. 6–15). This is referred to as central facial paresis, in contradistinction to peripheral facial paralysis or paresis (resulting from lesions of the facial motor nucleus or the facial nerve), in which all of the muscles of facial expression ipsilateral to the lesion are affected.

Basal ganglia   This input to the facial motor nucleus explains the movement of paretic facial muscles in response to emotional stimulation. Patients with central facial paralysis who are unable to move the lower facial muscles

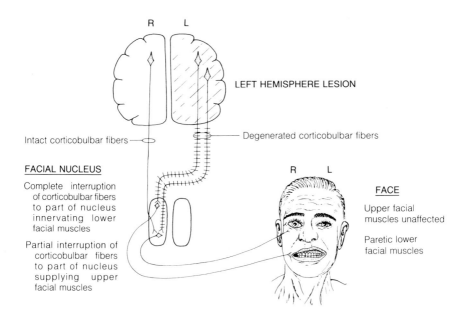

6–15 Schematic diagram illustrating the concept of central facial paresis.

voluntarily may be able to do so reflexly in response to emotional stimulation.

Superior olive This input is part of a reflex involving the facial and auditory nerves and explains the grimacing of facial muscles that occurs in response to loud noise.

Trigeminal system This input is also reflex in nature, linking the trigeminal and facial nerves, and underlies the blinking of the eyelids in response to corneal stimulation.

Superior colliculus This input via tectobulbar fibers is reflex in nature and provides for closure of the eyelids in response to intense light or a rapidly approaching object.

Secretomotor Fibers These fibers arise from the superior salivatory nucleus in the tegmentum of the pons. They are preganglionic fibers that synapse in collateral ganglia. They leave the brain stem with the nervus intermedius. Fibers destined for the lacrimal gland travel in the greater superficial petrosal nerve and synapse in the pterygopalatine ganglion from which postganglionic fibers reach the lacrimal gland. Fibers destined for the submandibular and sublingual glands join the chorda tympani and lingual nerves and synapse in the submandibular ganglion from which postganglionic fibers arise. Because fibers for the lacrimal, submandibular and sublingual glands leave the brain stem together, lesions of the facial nerve proximal to the geniculate ganglion may result in aberrant growth of regenerating fibers so that fibers destined to innervate the lacrimal glands reach the submandibular and sublingual salivary glands. Such an aberrant growth is responsible for the phenomenon of "crocodile tears," in which the patient lacrimates while chewing food.

Facial Nerve Lesions   Signs of facial nerve paralysis (Bell's palsy) vary with the location of the lesion (Fig. 6–16).

Proximal to Geniculate Ganglion   Lesions of the facial nerve proximal to the geniculate ganglion will result in the following signs.

1. Paralysis of all muscles of facial expression
2. Loss of taste in the anterior two-thirds of the ipsilateral half of the tongue

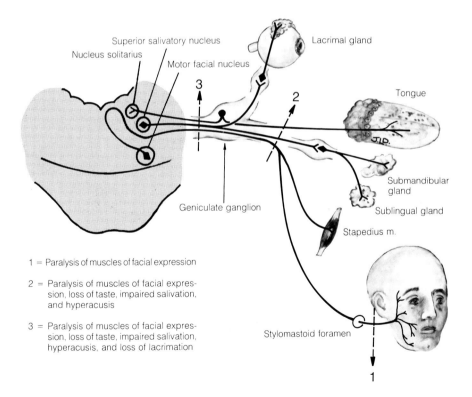

1 = Paralysis of muscles of facial expression

2 = Paralysis of muscles of facial expression, loss of taste, impaired salivation, and hyperacusis

3 = Paralysis of muscles of facial expression, loss of taste, impaired salivation, hyperacusis, and loss of lacrimation

6–16   Schematic diagram showing lesions in the facial nerve at different sites and the resulting clinical manifestations of each.

3. Impaired salivary secretion
4. Impaired lacrimation
5. Hyperacusis (hypersensitivity to sounds due to paralysis of the stapedius muscle)
6. Crocodile tears in some patients with aberrant growth of regenerating fibers

Distal to Geniculate Ganglion   Lesions of the facial nerve distal to the geniculate ganglion but proximal to the chorda tympani will result in the following ipsilateral signs.

1. Paralysis of all muscles of facial expression
2. Loss of taste in the anterior two-thirds of the tongue
3. Impaired salivary secretion
4. Hyperacusis

Lacrimation will not be affected by such a lesion, since the fibers destined for the lacrimal gland leave the nerve proximal to the level of the lesion.

Stylomastoid Foramen   Lesions of the facial nerve at the stylomastoid foramen (where the motor fibers destined for the muscles of facial expression leave the cranium) will result only in paralysis of muscles of facial expression ipsilateral to the lesion.

Abducens (CN VI) Nerve

The abducens nerve (Fig. 6–17) is a purely motor nerve that innervates the lateral rectus muscle. The abducens nucleus is located in a paramedian site in the tegmentum of the pons, in the floor of the fourth ventricle. It has recently been shown that the abducens nucleus has two populations of neurons, large and small (interneurons). Axons of the large neurons form the abducens nerve and supply the lateral rectus muscles. Axons of the small neurons join the contralateral medial longitudinal fasciculus and terminate upon those neurons in the oculomotor nucleus that supply the medial rectus muscle. Axons of the abducens nerve course in a ventral direction through the tegmentum and basis pontis and exit on the ventral surface of the pons in the groove between the pons and medulla oblongata (Fig. 6–1). The abducens nucleus (Fig. 6–17) receives fibers from the cerebral cortex (corticoreticulobulbar fibers) and from the vestibular nuclei via the medial longitudinal fasciculus. Direct afferent fibers from the ganglion of Scarpa to the abducens nucleus have been described recently. Lesions of the abducens nerve result in paralysis of the ipsilateral lateral rectus muscle and diplopia (double vision) on attempted horizontal gaze toward the side of the paralyzed muscle (Fig. 6–18, *A*); the two images are horizontal and the distance between them increases as the eyes move in the direction of action of the paralyzed muscle. The abducens nerve has

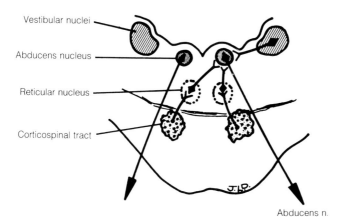

Vestibular nuclei

Abducens nucleus

Reticular nucleus

Corticospinal tract

Abducens n.

6–17 Schematic diagram showing the nuclei of origin, intrapontine course, and modulating inputs of the abducens (CN VI) nerve.

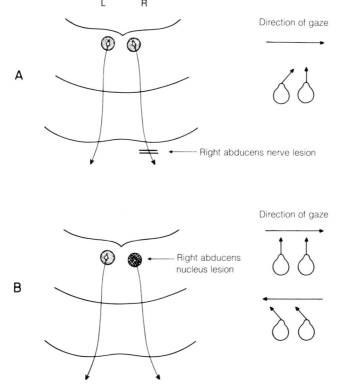

L   R

Direction of gaze

A

Right abducens nerve lesion

Direction of gaze

Right abducens nucleus lesion

B

6–18 Schematic diagram showing the clinical manifestations resulting from lesions in the abducens nucleus and nerve.

a long intracranial course and is therefore commonly affected in intracranial diseases of varying etiologies and sites. In contrast to lesions of the abducens nerve, lesions of the abducens nucleus do not result in paralysis of abduction, but in paralysis of horizontal gaze ipsilateral to the lesion; this is manifested by failure of both eyes to move on attempted ipsilateral horizontal gaze (Fig. 6–18, *B*). Paralysis of lateral gaze after abducens nucleus lesions was previously attributed to either the involvement of a hypothetic para-abducens nucleus in close proximity to the abducens nucleus or the interruption of two fiber systems (Fig. 6–19); these are 1) interruption of nerve fibers which originate from the abducens nucleus and supply the lateral rectus muscle, resulting in ipsilateral paralysis, and 2) interruption of reticular fibers of passage (from pontine reticular formation) through the abducens nucleus on their way to the contralateral oculomotor nucleus (the part of the nucleus that innervates the medial rectus muscle). With the recent discovery of the large and small neuronal populations within the abducens nucleus, paralysis of lateral gaze after abducens nu-

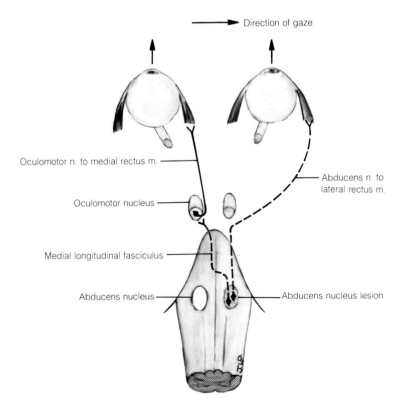

6–19 Schematic diagram illustrating the basis of lateral gaze paralysis in abducens nucleus lesions.

cleus lesions is now explained by involvement of the large neurons which results in paralysis of the ipsilateral lateral rectus and involvement of the small neurons (interneurons) which results in affection of the contralateral medial rectus neurons within the oculomotor nucleus. The previous notion that pontine reticular neurons are responsible for paralysis of adduction no longer appears tenable. Tritiated amino acids injected into the paramedian pontine reticular formation do not reveal terminations in the oculomotor nucleus, but rather in the interstitial nucleus of the medial longitudinal fasciculus, believed to be involved in vertical (downward) gaze.

Abducens nerve rootlets may also be involved in a variety of intra-axial vascular lesions within the pons. 1) Lesions in the basis pontis involving the corticospinal fibers and the rootlets of the abducens nerve will result in alternating hemiplegia manifested by ipsilateral lateral rectus paralysis and diplopia, as well as an upper motor neuron paralysis of the contralateral half of the body (Fig. 6–20, *A*). 2) Lesions of the pontine tegmentum involving the abducens rootlets and medial lemniscus will result in ipsilat-

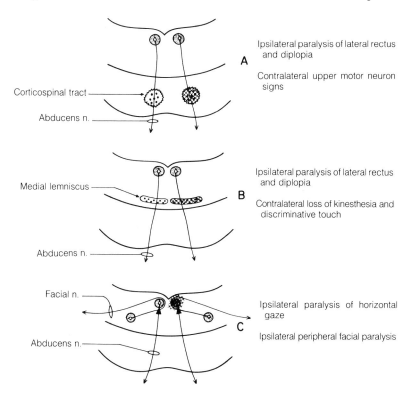

6–20   Schematic diagram of lesions of the abducens (CN VI) nerve and nucleus and the resulting clinical manifestations.

eral lateral rectus paralysis and contralateral loss of kinesthesia and discriminative touch (Fig. 6–20, *B*). 3) More dorsal lesions involving the abducens nucleus, the medial longitudinal fasciculus, and the curving rootlets of the facial nerve will produce paralysis of horizontal gaze and peripheral type facial paralysis both ipsilateral to the lesion (Fig. 6–20, *C*).

Trigeminal (CN V) Nerve

The trigeminal nerve has two roots, a smaller efferent (portio minor) and a larger afferent root (portio major).

Efferent Root   The efferent root (Fig. 6–21) of the trigeminal nerve arises from the motor nucleus of the trigeminal nerve located in the tegmentum of the pons. The efferent root supplies the muscles of mastication and the tensor tympani, tensor palati, mylohyoid, and anterior belly of the digastric. The motor nucleus receives fibers from the contralateral cerebral cortex (corticobulbar) and the sensory nuclei of the trigeminal nerve. Lesions affecting the motor nucleus or the efferent root will result in lower motor neuron type paralysis of the muscles supplied by this root.

Afferent Root   The afferent root (Fig. 6–22) of the trigeminal nerve contains two types of afferent fibers.

Proprioceptive Fibers   Proprioceptive fibers from deep structures of the face travel via the efferent and afferent roots. They are peripheral processes of unipolar neurons in the mesencephalic nucleus of the trigeminal located

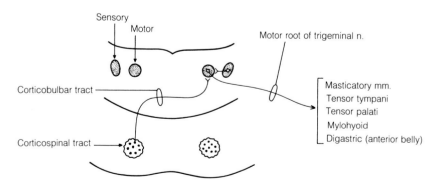

6–21 Schematic diagram showing the origin, intrapontine course and muscles supplied by the motor division of the trigeminal (CN V) nerve.

at rostral pontine and caudal mesencephalic levels. This nucleus is unique in that it is homologous to the dorsal root ganglion, yet is centrally placed. The output from the mesencephalic nucleus is destined for the cerebellum, thalamus, motor nuclei of the brain stem, and the reticular formation.

Exteroceptive Fibers　These are general somatic sensory fibers that convey pain, temperature, and touch sensations from the face and anterior aspect of the head. Neurons of origin of these fibers are located in the semilunar ganglion. Peripheral processes of neurons in the ganglion are distributed in the three divisions of the trigeminal nerve: the ophthalmic, maxillary, and mandibular. Central processes of these unipolar neurons enter the lateral aspect of the pons and distribute themselves as follows.

Some of these fibers descend in the pons, medulla and down to the level of the second or third cervical spinal segment as the descending (spinal) tract of the trigeminal nerve. They convey pain and temperature sensations. Throughout their caudal course, these fibers project upon neurons in the adjacent nucleus of the descending tract of the trigeminal (spinal trigeminal nucleus). The spinal trigeminal nucleus is divided into three parts on the

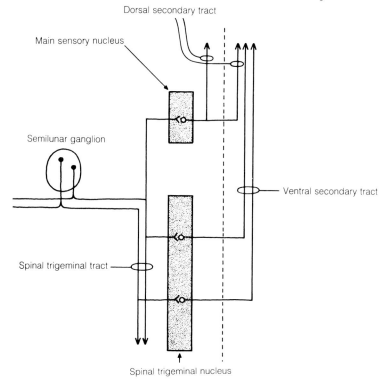

6–22　Schematic diagram showing the cells of origin and course of the sensory root of the trigeminal (CN V) nerve.

basis of its cytoarchitecture. These are 1) an oral part, which extends from the entry zone of the trigeminal nerve in the pons to the level of the rostral third of the inferior olivary nucleus in the medulla oblongata, 2) an interpolar part, which extends from the caudal extent of the oral part to just rostral to the pyramidal decussation in the medulla oblongata, and 3) a caudal part, which extends from the pyramidal decussation down to the second or third cervical spinal segments. Axons of neurons in the spinal trigeminal nucleus cross in the midline and form the ventral secondary ascending trigeminal tract which courses rostrally to terminate in the thalamus. During their rostral course, these second order fibers send collateral branches to several motor nuclei of the brain stem [hypoglossal (CN XII), facial (CN VII), and trigeminal (CN V)] to establish reflexes. Thus, the spinal tract of the trigeminal nerve is concerned mainly with transmission of pain and temperature sensations. It is sometimes cut surgically at a low level (trigeminal tractotomy) for the relief of intractable pain. Such operations may relieve pain but leave touch sensations intact. The spinal tract of the trigeminal nerve also carries somatic afferent fibers traveling with other cranial nerves [facial (CN VII), glossopharyngeal (CN IX), and vagus (CN X)] as outlined previously.

Other incoming fibers of the trigeminal nerve bifurcate upon entry to the pons into ascending and descending branches. These fibers convey touch sensation. The descending branches join the spinal tract of the trigeminal nerve and follow the course outlined above. The shorter ascending branches project upon the main sensory nucleus of the trigeminal. From the main sensory nucleus, second order fibers ascend ipsilaterally and contralaterally as the dorsal ascending trigeminal tract to the thalamus. Once formed, both secondary trigeminal tracts (the dorsal and ventral) lie lateral to the medial lemniscus between it and the spinothalamic tract. Since fibers that convey touch sensations bifurcate upon entry to the pons and terminate upon both the spinal and main sensory trigeminal nuclei, touch sensations are not abolished when the the spinal trigeminal tract is cut (trigeminal tractotomy). A schematic summary of the afferent and efferent trigeminal roots and their nuclei is shown in Figure 6–23. Recent studies on trigeminothalamic fibers have revealed that the bulk of these fibers arise from the main sensory nucleus and the interpolaris segment of the spinal nucleus. The majority of these fibers terminate in the contralateral thalamus with few terminations ipsilaterally.

Trigeminal neuralgia (tic douloureux) is a disabling painful sensation in the distribution of the branches of the trigeminal nerve. The pain is paroxysmal, stabbing, or lightning in nature and is usually triggered by eating, talking, or brushing the teeth. Several methods of treatment, including drugs, alcohol injection of the nerve, electrocoagulation of the ganglion, and surgical interruption of the nerve or the spinal tract in the medulla oblongata (tractotomy), have been tried with variable degrees of success.

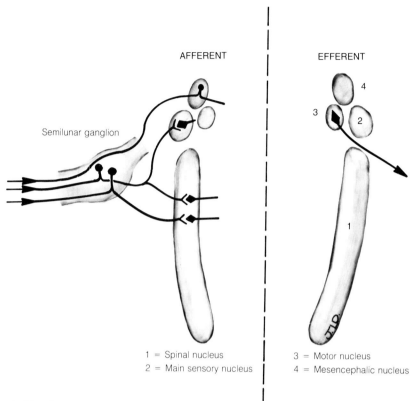

AFFERENT

EFFERENT

Semilunar ganglion

1 = Spinal nucleus
2 = Main sensory nucleus

3 = Motor nucleus
4 = Mesencephalic nucleus

6–23 Composite schematic diagram of the afferent and efferent roots of the trigeminal (CN V) nerve and their nuclei.

Applied Anatomy of the Pons

Vascular lesions of the pons lend themselves best to anatomicoclinical correlations; the following syndromes are particularly illustrative.

Basal Pontine Syndrome

This syndrome is caused by a lesion in the basal part of the pons affecting the rootlets of the facial nerve and the corticospinal tract bundles in the basis pontis (Fig. 6–24). The manifestations of this lesion include ipsilateral facial paralysis of the peripheral type and contralateral hemiplegia of the upper motor neuron type. This syndrome is known as the Millard-Gubler syndrome. Frequently, the lesion may extend medially and rostrally to include the rootlets of the sixth nerve (Fig. 6–25). In this situation, the patient will in addition manifest signs of ipsilateral sixth nerve paralysis.

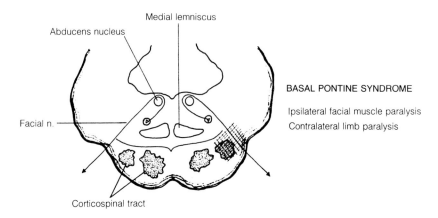

6-24 Schematic diagram of the structures involved in the caudal basal pontine syndrome (Millard-Gubler) and the resulting clinical manifestations.

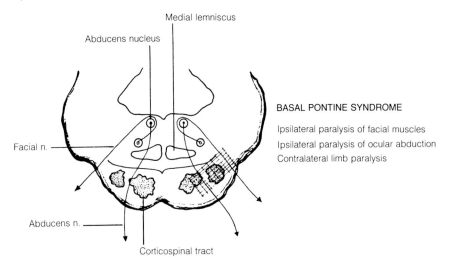

6-25 Schematic diagram of the structures involved in the medial basal pontine syndrome and the resulting clinical manifestations.

If the basal pontine lesion occurs more rostrally, at the level of the trigeminal nerve (Fig. 6-26), the manifestations will include ipsilateral trigeminal signs (sensory and motor) and a contralateral hemiplegia of the upper motor neuron variety.

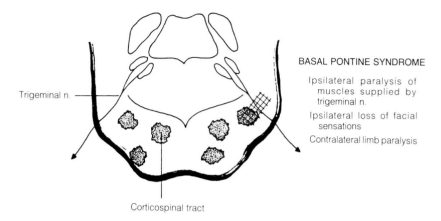

6–26 Schematic diagram showing structures involved in the rostral basal pontine syndrome and the resulting clinical manifestations.

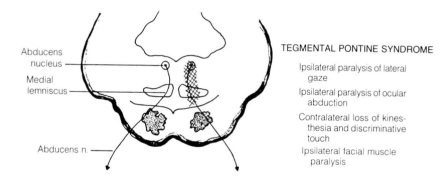

6–27 Schematic diagram showing structures involved in the tegmental pontine syndrome and the resulting clinical manifestations.

Tegmental Pontine Syndrome

This syndrome is caused by a lesion in the tegmentum of the pons affecting the nucleus of the sixth nerve and its rootlets, the genu of the facial nerve, and the medial lemniscus (Fig. 6–27). The manifestations of the lesion therefore include ipsilateral sixth nerve paralysis and a lateral gaze paralysis, ipsilateral facial paralysis of the peripheral variety, and contralateral loss of kinesthesia and discriminative touch.

References

Ash, P.R.; Keltner, J.L.: Neuro-ophthalmic Signs in Pontine Lesions. Medicine 58 (1979) 304–320.

Brodal, P.: The Pontocerebellar Projection in the Rhesus Monkey: An Experimental Study with Retrograde Axonal Transport of Horseradish Peroxidase. Neuroscience 4 (1979) 193–208.

Burton, H.; Craig, A.D.: Distribution of Trigeminothalamic Projection Cells in Cat and Monkey. Brain Res 161 (1979) 515–521.

Carpenter, M.B.; Batton, R.R.: Abducens Internuclear Neurons and Their Role in Conjugate Horizontal Gaze. J Comp Neurol 189 (1980) 191–209.

Gacek, R.R.: Location of Abducens Afferent Neurons in the Cat. Exp Neurol 64 (1979) 342–353.

Hu, J.W.; Sessle, B.J.: Trigeminal Nociceptive and Non-Nociceptive Neurons. Brain Stem Intranuclear Projections and Modulation by Orofacial, Periaqueductal Gray and Nucleus Raphe Magnus Stimuli. Brain Res 170 (1979) 547–552.

Jones, B.E.: Elimination of Paradoxical Sleep by Lesions of the Pontine Gigantocellular Tegmental Field in the Cat. Neurosci Lett 13 (1979) 285–293.

Korte, G.E.; Mugnaini, E.: The Cerebellar Projection of the Vestibular Nerve in the Cat. J Comp Neurol 184 (1979) 265–278.

Kotchabhakdi, N.; Rinvik, E.; Walberg, F.; Yingchareon, K.: The Vestibulothalamic Projections in the Cat Studied by Retrograde Axonal Transport of Horseradish Peroxidase. Exp Brain Res 40 (1980) 405–418.

Lang, W.; Büttner-Ennever, J.A.; Büttner, U.: Vestibular Projections to the Monkey Thalamus: An Autoradiographic Study. Brain Res 177 (1979) 3–17.

Loewy, A.D.; Saper, C.B.; Baker, R.P.: Descending Projection from the Pontine Micturition Center. Brain Res 172 (1979) 533–538.

Nakao, S.; Sasaki, S.: Excitatory Input from Interneurons in the Abducens Nucleus to Medial Rectus Motoneurons Mediating Conjugate Horizontal Nystagmus in the Cat. Exp Brain Res 39 (1980) 23–32.

Vilensky, J.A.; Van Hoesen, G.W.: Corticopontine Projections from the Cingulate Cortex in the Rhesus Monkey. Brain Res 205 (1981) 391–395.

Wiesendanger, R.; Wiesendanger, M; Rüegg, D.G.: An Anatomical Investigation of the Corticopontine Projection in the Primate (*Macaca Fascicularis and Saimiri Sciureus*). II. The Projection from Frontal and Parietal Association Areas. Neuroscience 4 (1979) 747–765.

7

Mesencephalon

Gross Topography

Ventral View (Fig. 7–1)

The inferior surface of the mesencephalon (midbrain) is marked by the divergence of two massive bundles of fibers, the cerebral peduncles, which carry corticofugal fibers to lower levels. Caudally, the cerebral peduncles pass into the basis pontis; rostrally, they continue into the internal capsule. Between the cerebral peduncles is the interpeduncular fossa, from which exit the oculomotor (CN III) nerves. The trochlear (CN IV) nerves emerge from the dorsal aspect of the mesencephalon, curve around and appear at the lateral borders of the cerebral peduncles. The optic tract passes under the cerebral peduncles before the latter disappear into the substance of the cerebral hemispheres.

Dorsal View (Fig. 7–2)

The dorsal surface of the mesencephalon features four elevations (corpora quadrigemina). The rostral and larger two are the superior colliculi; the caudal and smaller two are the inferior colliculi. The trochlear nerves emerge just caudal to the inferior colliculi.

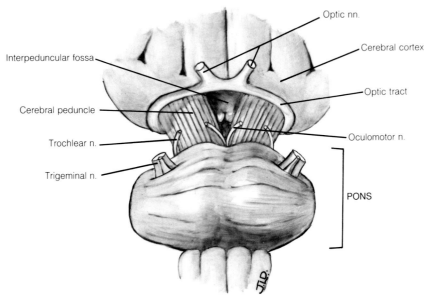

7-1 Schematic diagram of the ventral surface of the midbrain and pons, showing major midbrain structures encountered on this surface.

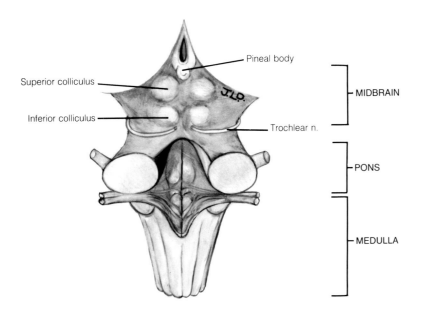

7-2 Schematic diagram of the dorsal surface of the midbrain, showing major structures encountered on this surface.

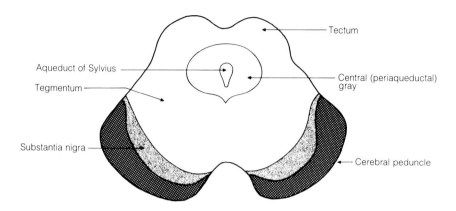

7–3 Cross-sectional diagram of the midbrain showing its major subdivisions.

Microscopic Structure

General Organization (Fig. 7–3)

Three subdivisions are generally recognized in sections of the mesencephalon.

1. The tectum is a mixture of gray and white matter dorsal to the central gray. It includes the superior and inferior colliculi.
2. The tegmentum, the main portion of the mesencephalon, lies inferior to the central gray and contains ascending and descending tracts, reticular nuclei, and well-delineated nuclear masses.
3. The basal portion includes the cerebral peduncles, a massive bundle of corticofugal fibers on the ventral aspect of the mesencephalon, and the substantia nigra, a pigmented nuclear mass between the dorsal surface of the cerebral peduncle and the tegmentum.

The components of each of these subdivisions will be discussed under two characteristic levels of the mesencephalon, the inferior colliculus and superior colliculus.

Inferior Colliculus Level

Tectum   The nucleus of the inferior colliculus occupies the tectum at this level. The nucleus is an oval mass of small and medium-sized neurons that have the following afferent and efferent connections.

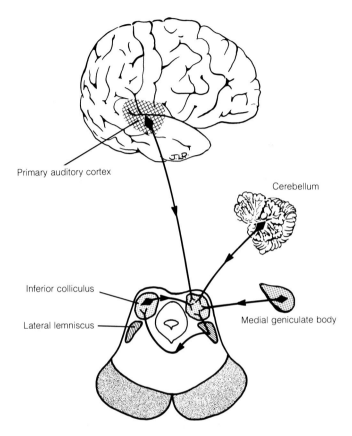

7–4 Schematic diagram showing the major afferent connections of the inferior colliculus.

Afferent Connections (Fig. 7–4)   Fibers come from the following sources.
Lateral lemniscus   These fibers terminate upon the ipsi- and contralateral inferior colliculi. Some lateral lemniscus fibers bypass the inferior colliculus to reach the medial geniculate body.
Contralateral inferior colliculus
Ipsilateral medial geniculate body   This connection serves as a feedback mechanism in the auditory pathway.
Cerebral cortex (primary auditory cortex)
Cerebellar cortex via the anterior medullary velum
Efferent Connections (Fig. 7–5)   The inferior colliculus projects to the following areas.
Medial geniculate body via the brachium of the inferior colliculus   This pathway is concerned with audition.
Contralateral inferior colliculus

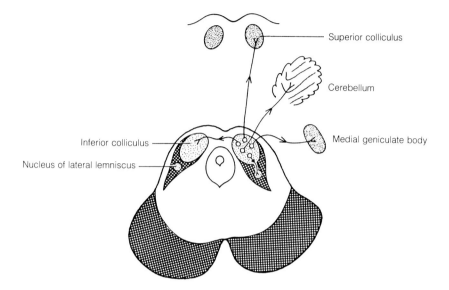

Superior colliculus

Cerebellum

Inferior colliculus

Medial geniculate body

Nucleus of lateral lemniscus

7–5 Schematic diagram showing the major efferent connections of the inferior colliculus.

Superior colliculus This establishes reflexes for turning the neck and eyes in response to sound.

Nucleus of the lateral lemniscus and other relay nuclei of the auditory system for feedback

Cerebellum via the anterior medullary velum The inferior colliculus is a major center for transmission of auditory impulses to the cerebellum. The inferior colliculus, thus, is a relay nucleus in the auditory pathway to the cerebral cortex and cerebellum. Physiologic studies suggest that the inferior colliculus plays a role in localization of source of sound.

Tegmentum At the level of the inferior colliculus, the tegmentum of the mesencephalon contains fibers of passage (ascending and descending tracts) and nuclear groups.

Fibers of Passage (Fig. 7–6) The following fiber tracts pass through the mesencephalon.

Brachium conjunctivum (superior cerebellar peduncle) The brachium conjunctivum is a massive bundle of fibers arising in the deep cerebellar nuclei. These fibers decussate in the tegmentum of the midbrain at this level; some proceed rostrally to terminate upon the red nucleus and others form the capsule of the red nucleus and continue rostrally to terminate upon the ventrolateral nucleus of the thalamus.

Medial lemniscus The medial lemniscus is located lateral to the decussating brachium conjunctivum and above the substantia nigra. This fiber

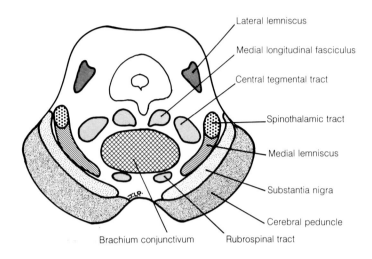

Lateral lemniscus

Medial longitudinal fasciculus

Central tegmental tract

Spinothalamic tract

Medial lemniscus

Substantia nigra

Cerebral peduncle

Brachium conjunctivum   Rubrospinal tract

7–6   Cross-sectional diagram of the midbrain at the inferior colliculus level, showing its major fibers of passage.

system, conveying kinesthesia and discriminative touch from more caudal levels, continues its course toward the thalamus.

Trigeminal lemniscus   The trigeminal lemniscus is composed of the ventral secondary trigeminal tracts and travels with the medial lemniscus on its way to the thalamus.

Spinothalamic tract   The spinothalamic tract conveys pain and temperature sensations from the contralateral half of the body and is located lateral to the medial lemniscus. Mingled with the spinothalamic fibers are the spinotectal fibers on their way to the tectum.

Lateral lemniscus   The lateral lemniscus conveys auditory fibers and occupies a position lateral and dorsal to the spinothalamic tract.

Medial longitudinal fasciculus   The medial longitudinal fasciculus maintains its position dorsally in the tegmentum in a paramedian position.

Central tegmental tract   The central tegmental tract conveys fibers from the basal ganglia and midbrain to the inferior olive and occupies a dorsal position in the tegmentum, ventrolateral to the medial longitudinal fasciculus.

Rubrospinal tract   The rubrospinal tract conveys fibers from the red nucleus to the spinal cord and is located dorsal to the medial lemniscus.

Nuclear Groups (Fig. 7–7)   The following nuclei are seen at the level of the inferior colliculus.

Mesencephalic nucleus   The mesencephalic nucleus of the trigeminal nerve is homologous to the dorsal root ganglion but is uniquely placed within the central nervous system. It contains unipolar neurons with axons

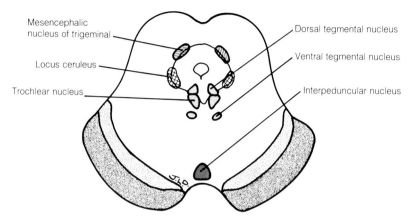

7–7 Schematic diagram of the midbrain at the inferior colliculus level, showing its major nuclear groups.

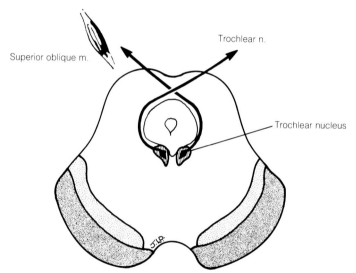

7–8 Schematic diagram of the midbrain showing origin, course, and area of supply (superior oblique muscle) of the trochlear (CN IV) nerve.

(the mesencephalic root of the trigeminal) which convey proprioceptive impulses from the muscles of mastication and the periodontal membranes. As these fibers approach the nucleus, they gather in a bundle close to the nucleus.

Nucleus of the trochlear (CN IV) nerve The nucleus of the trochlear nerve lies in the V-shaped ventral part of the central gray. Axons of this nerve arch around the central gray, cross in the anterior medullary velum, and emerge from the dorsal aspect of the mesencephalon (Fig. 7–8). These axons supply the superior oblique eye muscle. The trochlear nerve is thus unique in two respects. 1) It is the only cranial nerve that crosses before emerging from the brain stem and 2) it is the only cranial nerve that emerges on the dorsal aspect of the brain stem. Because of decussation, lesions of the trochlear nucleus result in paralysis of the contralateral superior oblique muscle, whereas lesions of the nerve after it emerges from the brain stem result in paralysis of the ipsilateral superior oblique. The superior oblique acts by intorsion of the abducted eye and depression of the adducted eye. Patients with trochlear nerve lesions complain of vertical diplopia, especially marked when looking contralaterally downward while descending stairs and usually corrected by head tilt (toward the normal nerve) to compensate for the action of the paralyzed muscle. The trochlear nucleus receives 1) contralateral and probably some ipsilateral corticobulbar fibers and 2) vestibular fibers from the medial longitudinal fasciculus concerned with coordination of eye movements. Vestibular fibers to the trochlear nucleus originate from the superior and medial vestibular nuclei. The fibers from the superior vestibular nucleus are ipsilateral and inhibitory; those from the medial vestibular nucleus are contralateral and excitatory.

Interpeduncular nucleus   The interpeduncular nucleus, indistinct in man, is a poorly understood nuclear group located in the base of the tegmentum between the cerebral peduncles. It receives fibers mainly from the habenular nuclei through the habenulopeduncular tract and sends fibers to the dorsal tegmental nucleus through the pedunculotegmental tract.

Dorsal tegmental nucleus   The dorsal tegmental nucleus is located dorsal to the medial longitudinal fasciculus in the central gray. It is made up of conspicuously small cells. It receives fibers from the interpeduncular nucleus and projects upon autonomic nuclei of the brain stem and the reticular formation.

Ventral tegmental nucleus   The ventral tegmental nucleus is located ventral to the dorsal tegmental nucleus in the midbrain tegmentum. It receives fibers from the mamillary bodies. The dorsal and ventral tegmental nuclei are part of the circuit that is concerned with emotion and behavior.

Nucleus pigmentosus (locus ceruleus)   The nucleus pigmentosus is seen in the rostral pons and caudal mesencephalon. At the level of the inferior colliculus, it is located at the edge of the central gray, between the mesencephalic nucleus of the trigeminal and the dorsal tegmental nucleus. Its pigmented cells contain melanin granules which are lost in the disease parkinsonism. The neurons of the locus ceruleus produce norepinephrine. Axons of neurons of the locus ceruleus are elaborately branched and ramify throughout practically the entire brain. These axons reach their destinations via three major ascending tracts: the central tegmental tract, the dorsal longitudinal fasciculus, and the medial forebrain bundle. Through these tracts, the locus ceruleus innervates the thalamus, hypothalamus, and basal telencephalon. In addition, the locus ceruleus projects to the cerebellum

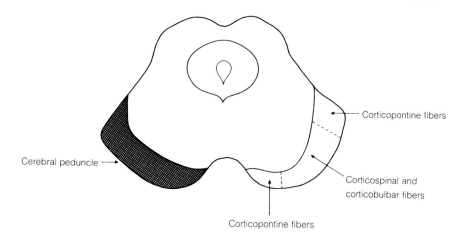

Corticopontine fibers

Cerebral peduncle →

Corticospinal and
corticobulbar fibers

Corticopontine fibers

7–9 Schematic diagram of the midbrain showing the major subdivisions of the cerebral peduncle.

via the brachium conjunctivum, to the spinal cord and to sensory nuclei of the brain stem. The nucleus is believed to play a role in regulation of respiration as well as in the rapid eye movement (REM) stage of sleep.

Basal Portion   At the level of the inferior colliculus, the basal portion of the mesencephalon includes the cerebral peduncle and substantia nigra.

Cerebral Peduncle   The cerebral peduncle (Fig. 7–9) is the massive fiber bundle occupying the most ventral part of the mesencephalon. It is continuous with the internal capsule rostrally and merges caudally into the basis pontis. This massive fiber bundle conveys corticofugal fibers from the cerebral cortex to several subcortical centers. The middle three-fifths of the cerebral peduncle is occupied by the corticospinal tract, which is continuous caudally with the pyramids. The corticopontine fibers occupy the areas of the cerebral peduncle on each side of the corticospinal tract. These fibers originate in wide areas of the cerebral cortex, synapse on pontine nuclei and enter the contralateral cerebellar hemisphere via the middle cerebellar peduncle (brachium pontis). The corticobulbar fibers destined for cranial nerve nuclei accompany the corticospinal fibers.

Substantia Nigra   The substantia nigra is a pigmented mass of neurons sandwiched between the cerebral peduncles and the tegmentum. It is made of two zones, a dorsal zona compacta containing melanin pigment and a ventral zona reticulata containing iron compounds. It has been observed that dendrites of neurons in the zona compacta arborize in the zona reticulata. The zona reticulata represents the receptive zone of the substantia nigra, whereas the zona compacta is the effector zone. The pars lateralis represents the oldest part of this nucleus. The neural connectivity of the substantia nigra is not fully elucidated; it no doubt plays an important role in the regulation of motor activity. Lesions of the substantia nigra are almost always seen in the disease parkinsonism, characterized by tremor, rigidity, and slowness of motor activity. The known afferent and efferent connections of the substantia nigra are outlined below.

Afferent connections
Caudate and Putamen Nuclei
Cerebral Cortex —The corticonigral projection is not as massive as previously believed. Most of the fibers are fibers of passage and relatively few of them terminate on nigral neurons.
Globus Pallidus
Efferent connections
Nigrostriate Fibers—Nigrostriate fibers project to the caudate and putamen. It is generally recognized that two types of fibers connect the nigra with the caudate nucleus. The first is a cholinergic system of very small caliber fibers which facilitates caudate activity. The second is a dopaminergic fiber system which is inhibitory to caudate activity. Interruption of the nigrostriate fibers results in the accumulation of catecholamines such as dopamine in the substantia nigra and their depletion in the caudate. This fiber system is believed to be affected in parkinsonism. The latter condition is treated by replacement of depleted dopamine.

Nigrocortical Tract—The nigrocortical fibers originate in the zona compacta, course through the medial forebrain bundle and terminate in the anterior part of the cingulate gyrus. Affection of this pathway in parkinsonism may explain the akinesia of this disease.
Nigropallidal Tract
Nigrorubral Tract
Nigrosubthalamic Tract
Nigrothalamic Tract—The nigrothalamic tract is mainly to the ventral anterior nucleus of the thalamus.
Nigrotegmental Tract
Nigrocollicular Tract
Nigroamygdaloid Tract—The nigroamygdaloid tract originates from dopaminergic neurons of the zona compacta and pars lateralis of the substantia nigra and projects upon the lateral and central amygdaloid nuclei.

The nigral origin of many of these efferent fiber systems remains in doubt and needs further exploration. Many of these systems may represent fibers of passage interrupted by nigral lesions and may not be originating in nigral neurons.

Superior Colliculus Level

Tectum The nucleus of the superior colliculus occupies the tectum at this level. The superior colliculus is a laminated mass of gray matter that

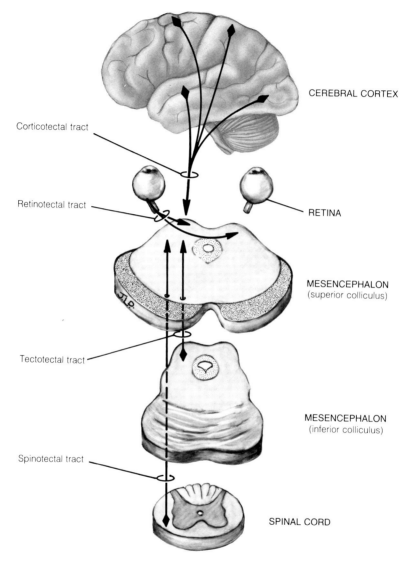

7-10 Schematic diagram showing the major afferent connections of the superior colliculus.

plays a role in visual reflexes. The laminated appearance is the result of alternating strata of white and gray matter.

Afferent connections to the superior colliculus (Fig. 7-10) come from the following sources.

Cerebral Cortex Corticocollicular fibers arise from all over the cerebral cortex but most abundantly from the occipital (visual) cortex. Those fibers originating from the frontal lobe are concerned with conjugate eye movements. Occipitotectal fibers are concerned with reflex scanning eye movements in pursuit of a passing object. Corticotectal fibers are ipsilateral.

Retina   Retinal fibers project upon the same layer of the superior colliculus as those of the cerebral cortex. In contrast to cortical fibers, those from the retina are bilateral, with a preponderance of contralateral input.

Spinal Cord   Spinotectal fibers arise in the spinal cord and ascend in the anterolateral part of the cord to the superior colliculus. They may belong to a multisynaptic system conveying pain sensation.

Inferior Colliculus   This input is part of a reflex arc which turns the neck and eyes toward the source of sound.

Efferent connections (Fig. 7–11) leave the superior colliculus via three main tracts.

Tectospinal Tract   From their neurons of origin in the superior colliculus, fibers of this system cross in the dorsal tegmental decussation in the midbrain tegmentum and descend as part of or in close proximity to the medial longitudinal fasciculus to reach the cervical spinal cord. They are concerned with reflex neck movement in response to visual stimuli.

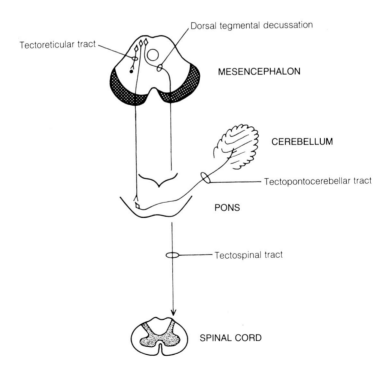

7–11   Schematic diagram showing the major efferent connections of the superior colliculus.

Tectopontocerebellar Tract   This tract descends to the ipsilateral pontine nuclei and is believed to convey visual impulses from the superior colliculus to the cerebellum via the pontine nuclei.

Tectoreticular Tract   This tract projects upon reticular nuclei of the midbrain as well as on the accessory oculomotor nuclei.

Rostral to the superior colliculus at the mesencephalic-diencephalic junction is the pretectal area (pretectal nucleus). This area is an important station in the reflex pathway for pupillary reflexes. It receives fibers from the retina and projects fibers bilaterally to both oculomotor nuclei.

Experiments in which the pretectal area and/or the posterior commissure were ablated suggest strongly that these structures are essential for vertical gaze. This may explain the paralysis of vertical gaze in pineal tumors, which compress these structures.

Tegmentum   At the level of the superior colliculus, the tegmentum contains fibers of passage and nuclear groups.

Fibers of Passage   These include all the fiber tracts encountered at the inferior colliculus level except the lateral lemniscus, which terminates upon inferior colliculus neurons and is not seen at superior colliculus levels. The brachium conjunctivum fibers, which decussate at inferior colliculus levels, terminate in the red nucleus at this level or else form the capsule of the red nucleus on their way to the thalamus. The other tracts discussed under the inferior colliculus level maintain approximately the same positions at this level.

Nuclear Groups (Fig. 7–12)   These include the red nucleus, oculomotor nucleus, and accessory oculomotor nuclei.

Red nucleus   This nucleus, so named because in fresh preparations its

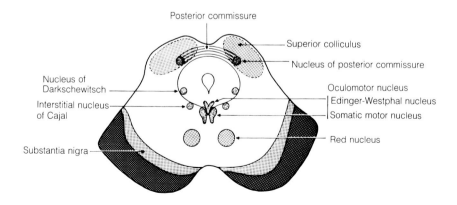

7–12   Schematic diagram of the midbrain at the superior colliculus level, showing its major nuclear groups.

rich vascularity gives it a pinkish hue, is a prominent feature of the tegmentum at this level. It is composed of a rostral, phylogenetically recent small cell part (parvicellular) and a caudal, phylogenetically older large cell part (magnocellular). The rostral part is well developed in man. The nucleus is traversed by the following fiber systems: 1) superior cerebellar peduncle (brachium conjunctivum), 2) oculomotor (CN III) root fibers, and 3) habenulopeduncular tract. Of the three, only the brachium conjunctivum projects upon this nucleus; the other two are related to the nucleus only by proximity. The nucleus has the following afferent and efferent connections.

Afferent connections are most documented from two sources (Fig. 7–13).

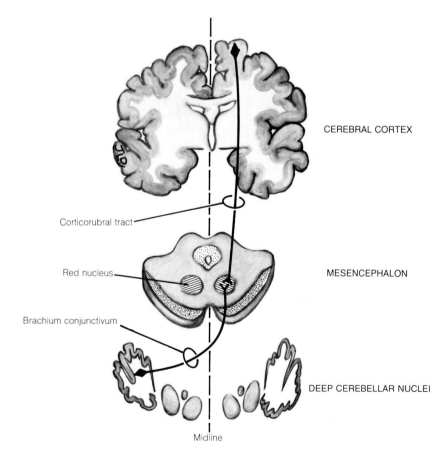

CEREBRAL CORTEX

Corticorubral tract

Red nucleus

MESENCEPHALON

Brachium conjunctivum

DEEP CEREBELLAR NUCLEI

Midline

7–13 Schematic diagram showing the major afferent connections of the red nucleus.

Deep Cerebellar Nuclei—The cerebellorubral fibers arise from the dentate, globose and emboliform nuclei of the cerebellum. They travel via the brachium conjunctivum, decussate in the tegmentum of the inferior colliculus, and project partly to the contralateral red nucleus. Interruption of this fiber system results in a volitional type tremor manifested when the extremity is in motion (*e.g.*, attempting to reach for an object). Electron microscopic studies have shown that the cerebellorubral input establishes mainly axosomatic synapses in the red nucleus.

Cerebral Cortex—Corticorubral fibers arise mainly from the motor and premotor cortices and project mainly to the ipsilateral red nucleus. This projection is somatotopically organized. The corticorubral and rubrospinal tracts are considered an indirect corticospinal fiber system. The corticorubral input to the red nucleus establishes mainly axodendritic synapses. Deafferentation experiments have shown that following cerebellar ablation the cerebral input to the red nucleus establishes axosomatic synapses to replace the deafferented cerebellar input.

The above two afferent connections are the most well established. Other possible afferent tracts include tectorubral from the superior colliculus and pallidorubral from the globus pallidus.

Efferent connections project to the following areas (Fig. 7–14).

Spinal Cord—Rubrospinal fibers arise from the caudal part of the nucleus, cross in the ventral tegmental decussation, and descend to the spinal cord. They project upon the same spinal cord laminae as the corticospinal tract. Like the corticospinal tract, the rubrospinal tract facilitates flexor motor neurons and inhibits extensor motor neurons. Because of their common termination, and the fact that the red nucleus receives cortical input, the rubrospinal tract has been considered an indirect corticospinal tract.

Cerebellum—The rubrocerebellar fibers are from the rubrospinal tract. In the upper pons, some rubrospinal fibers leave the descending tract and accompany the superior cerebellar peduncle to the cerebellum. In the cerebellum, these fibers terminate upon the same nuclei from which the cerebellorubral fibers arise.

Reticular Formation—Rubroreticular fibers are also offshoots from the rubrospinal tract. They separate from the descending tract in the medulla oblongata and terminate upon the ipsilateral lateral reticular nucleus. The lateral reticular nucleus, as described in the chapter on the medulla oblongata, in turn projects to the cerebellum. Thus, a feedback circuit is established between the cerebellum, red nucleus, lateral reticular nucleus, and back to the cerebellum.

Inferior Olive—The rubro-olivary tract is a fiber system which arises in the rostral small cell part of the nucleus and projects to the ipsilateral inferior olive via the central tegmental tract. The inferior olive in turn projects to the cerebellum, thus establishing another feedback circuit be-

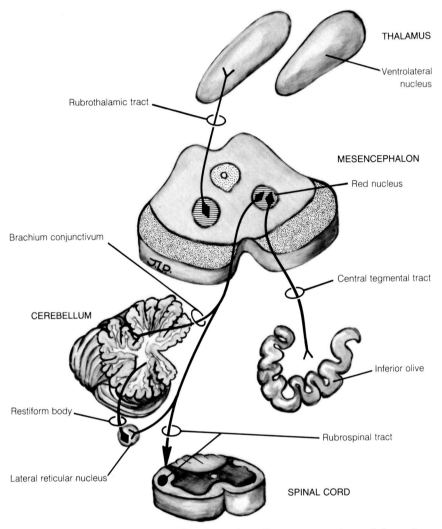

THALAMUS

Ventrolateral
nucleus

Rubrothalamic tract

MESENCEPHALON

Red nucleus

Brachium conjunctivum

Central tegmental tract

CEREBELLUM

Inferior olive

Restiform body

Rubrospinal tract

Lateral reticular nucleus

SPINAL CORD

7–14 Schematic diagram showing the major efferent connections of the red nucleus.

tween the cerebellum, red nucleus, inferior olive, and back to the cerebellum.

Thalamus—Rubrothalamic fibers to the ventrolateral nucleus of the thalamus accompany fibers of the superior cerebellar peduncle to the same nucleus. Recent work using autoradiographic tracer methods has questioned the existence of such a tract.

Other Projections—Recently described efferent projections include fibers to the nucleus of Darkschewitsch, Edinger-Westphal nucleus, mesencephalic reticular formation, tectum, and pretectum.

Thus, the red nucleus is a synaptic station in the following systems concerned with movement.

1. Cerebellothalamic system (deep cerebellar nuclei to red nucleus to ventrolateral nucleus of the thalamus)
2. Corticospinal system (cerebral cortex to red nucleus to spinal cord)
3. Cerebellospinal system (deep cerebellar nuclei to red nucleus to spinal cord)

Lesions of the red nucleus result in contralateral tremor.

Oculomotor nucleus   The oculomotor nucleus is located dorsal to the medial longitudinal fasciculus at the level of the superior colliculus. It is composed of a lateral somatic motor cell column and a medial visceral cell column.

The oculomotor nucleus receives fibers from the following sources.

Cerebral Cortex—Corticoreticulobulbar fibers are mainly from the contralateral hemisphere.

Mesencephalon—Mesencephalic projections to the oculomotor nucleus originate from the interstitial nucleus of Cajal, interstitial nucleus of the medial longitudinal fasciculus, and the pretectal nucleus. The fibers from the interstitial nucleus of Cajal course in the posterior commissure and project mainly upon the contralateral oculomotor nucleus. Interruption of these fibers results in paralysis of upward gaze. The interstitial nucleus of the medial longitudinal fasciculus is a recently described nucleus located just rostral to the interstitial nucleus of Cajal. The projection from the interstitial nucleus of the medial longitudinal fasciculus to the oculomotor nucleus is mainly ipsilateral. Lesions of the interstitial nucleus of the medial longitudinal fasciculus lead to paralysis of downward gaze. Physiologic studies have shown that neurons in the interstitial nucleus of Cajal and the interstitial nucleus of the medial longitudinal fasciculus are active just prior to vertical eye movements. The interstitial nucleus of Cajal and the interstitial nucleus of the medial longitudinal fasciculus project fibers to the somatic motor cell column of the oculomotor nucleus, whereas the pretectal area projects mainly to the Edinger-Westphal nucleus of the visceral cell column. The pretectal area receives fibers from both retinae and projects to both oculomotor nuclei. This connection plays a role in the pupillary light reflex.

Pons and Medulla—Pontine and medullary projections to the oculomotor nucleus arise from the vestibular nuclei and the abducens nucleus. The vestibular projections originate in the superior, medial, and inferior vestibular nuclei. The projection from the abducens nucleus is crossed and reaches the oculomotor nucleus via the medial longitudinal fasciculus along with vestibular fibers. The connection between the abducens and oculomotor nuclei provides the anatomic substrate for the coordination between the lateral rectus and medial rectus muscles in conjugate horizontal gaze.

Cerebellum—Cerebello-oculomotor fibers arise from the contralateral dentate nucleus and are concerned with regulation of eye movements. In addition, physiologic studies have shown that the cerebellum exerts an influence on autonomic neurons of the oculomotor nucleus. Short latency (direct), as well as long latency (indirect), responses have been elicited in the Edinger-Westphal nucleus following stimulation of the interposed and fastigial cerebellar nuclei. This connection is believed to course in the brachium conjunctivum and plays a role in both pupillary constriction and accommodation. The short latency connection is facilitatory, whereas the long latency connection is inhibitory.

The somatic motor cell column is organized into subgroups for each of the eye muscles supplied by the oculomotor nerve. Axons of neurons in the somatic motor column course through the tegmentum of the mesencephalon, pass near or through the red nucleus and emerge through the interpeduncular fossa medial to the cerebral peduncle. The axons leave the brain stem between the superior cerebellar artery and posterior cerebral artery and supply the superior rectus, inferior rectus, medial rectus, and inferior oblique, all of which are extraocular muscles, and the levator palpebrae superioris of the eyelid. Lesions of this component of the nerve result in paralysis of the above muscles that is manifested by downward and outward deviation of the eye and drooping of the upper lid.

The visceral cell column includes the Edinger-Westphal nucleus and the nucleus of Perlia.

The Edinger-Westphal nucleus is concerned with the light reflex. The nucleus of Perlia is probably concerned with accommodation, but has not been identified in man.

The axons of neurons in the visceral cell column accompany those of the somatic motor column as far as the orbit. In the orbit they part company and project to the ciliary ganglion. Postganglionic fibers from the ciliary ganglion innervate the sphincter pupillae and ciliaris muscles. Lesions of this component of the oculomotor nerve result in a dilated pupil that is unresponsive to light or accommodation.

Lesions of the oculomotor nerve outside the brain stem (Fig. 7–15, *A*) result in 1) paralysis of muscles supplied by the nerve, manifested by drooping of the ipsilateral eyelid and deviation of the ipsilateral eye downward and outward; 2) diplopia; and 3) paralysis of sphincter pupillae and ciliaris muscles, manifested by ipsilateral dilated pupil unresponsive to light and accommodation. Lesions at the interpeduncular fossa of the mesencephalon (Fig. 7–15, *B*) involving the cerebral peduncle and the rootlets of the oculomotor nerve result in 1) deviation of the ipsilateral eye downward and outward, with drooping of the eyelid; 2) diplopia; 3) ipsilateral loss of light and accommodation reflexes; 4) dilatation of the ipsilateral pupil; and 5) contralateral upper motor neuron paralysis.

Lesions in the mesencephalon involving the red nucleus and rootlets of the oculomotor nerve (7–15, C) are manifested by 1) deviation of the ipsilateral eye downward and outward, with drooping of the eyelid; 2) diplopia; 3) ipsilateral loss of light and accommodation reflexes; 4) dilatation of the ipsilateral pupil; and 5) contralateral tremor.

The relationship of the oculomotor nerve to the posterior cerebral and superior cerebellar arteries makes it vulnerable to aneurysms of these vessels. Rupture of these aneurysms is usually manifested by sudden onset of signs of oculomotor nerve lesion.

It is worth noting that the parasympathetic fibers concerned with the pupillary light reflex are located in the outer part of the oculomotor nerve and are therefore relatively unaffected in vascular ischemic diseases of the nerve such as in diabetes mellitus. The blood supply of the oculomotor nerve dips deep into the nerve and hence interruption of blood supply will adversely affect deeper fibers and spare more superficial fibers.

Accessory oculomotor nuclei (Fig. 7–12) The nuclei include the following.

Interstitial Nucleus of Cajal—The nucleus is composed of a mass of small cells located lateral to the medial longitudinal fasciculus.

Interstitial Nucleus of the Medial Longitudinal Fasciculus—The nucleus (also known as the nucleus of the prerubral field) is composed of a mass of small cells located just rostral to the interstitial nucleus of Cajal.

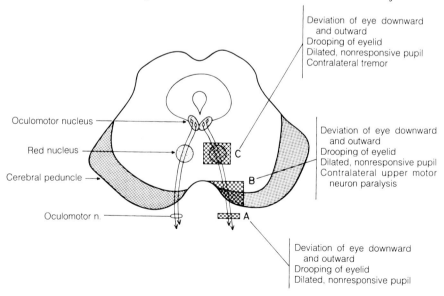

7–15 Schematic diagram showing lesions of the oculomotor nerve in its intra- and extra-axial course and their respective clinical manifestations.

Nucleus of Darkschewitsch—The nucleus is located lateral to the somatic motor cell column of the oculomotor nerve.

Nucleus of the Posterior Commissure—The nucleus is located within the posterior commissure.

The accessory oculomotor nuclei are directly or indirectly connected with the oculomotor complex. The interstitial nucleus of Cajal, in addition, sends fibers to the spinal cord via the medial longitudinal fasciculus.

Central (Periaqueductal) Gray—This region of the mesencephalon surrounds the aqueduct of Sylvius and contains scattered neurons, several nuclei and some fine myelinated and unmyelinated fibers. The accessory oculomotor, oculomotor, and trochlear nuclei, as well as the mesencephalic nucleus of the trigeminal nerve, are located at the edge of this region. The dorsal longitudinal fasciculus (of Schütz) courses in the central gray. It arises in part from the hypothalamus and contains autonomic fibers. Its projections are not well delineated but probably include cranial nerve nuclei. Recent interest in the central gray has focused on its role in pain. The neuropeptide enkephalin has been identified in the central gray. Stimulation of certain sites within the central gray releases enkephalins which act on serotonergic neurons in the medulla oblongata, which in turn project on primary afferent axons (concerned with pain conduction) in the dorsal horn of the spinal cord to produce analgesia. Stimulus-produced analgesia has been achieved by stimulation of the caudal and medial region of the central gray. In contrast, stimulation of the rostral and lateral central gray facilitates pain sensation.

Light Reflex

Stimulation of the retina by light will set off a reflex with the following afferent and efferent pathways (Fig. 7–16).

Afferent Pathway

From the retina the impulse will travel via the optic nerve and optic tract to the pretectal area. After synapsing on neurons of the pretectal area, the impulse will travel via the posterior commissure to both Edinger-Westphal nuclei of the oculomotor complex.

Efferent Pathway

From the Edinger-Westphal nucleus, parasympathetic preganglionic fibers travel with the somatic motor component of the oculomotor nerve as far as the orbit. In the orbit, the parasympathetic fibers project upon neurons

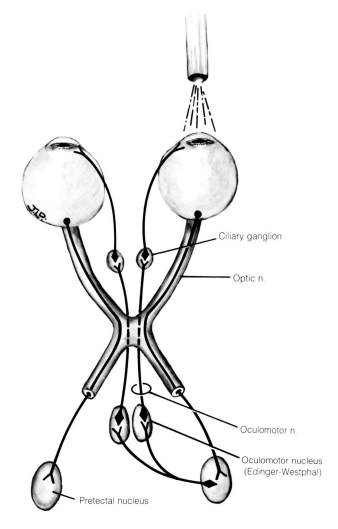

7–16 Schematic diagram showing the afferent and efferent pathways of the light reflex.

in the ciliary ganglion. Postganglionic fibers arise from the ciliary ganglion (short ciliary nerves) and innervate the sphincter pupillae and ciliaris muscles.

Thus, when light is thrown on one retina, both pupils respond by constriction. The response of the ipsilateral pupil is the direct light reflex, whereas that of the contralateral pupil is the consensual light reflex. A consensual light reflex is possible because of the projection of the pretectal area to both oculomotor nuclei.

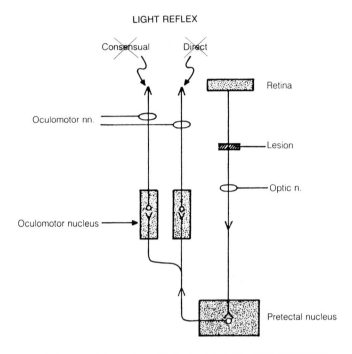

LIGHT REFLEX

Optic nerve lesion --→ loss of both direct and consensual light reflexes

7-17 Schematic diagram showing the effects of optic nerve lesions on the direct and consensual light reflexes.

Lesions of the optic nerve (Fig. 7–17) abolish both the direct and consensual light reflexes in response to light stimulation of the ipsilateral retina.

Lesions of the oculomotor nerve (Fig. 7–18) abolish the direct light reflex, but not the consensual light reflex, in response to light stimulation of the ipsilateral retina.

Accommodation-Convergence Reflex

This reflex involves the following processes.

1. Assumption of convex shape by the lens is secondary to contraction of the ciliary muscle and relaxation of the suspensory ligament. This is a process of accommodation of the lens, which thickens to maintain the image in sharp focus.
2. Contraction of the medial rectus muscles (convergence) brings the eyes into alignment.

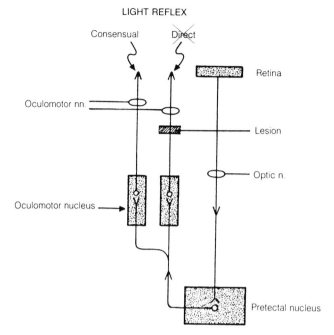

7–18   Schematic diagram showing the effects of oculomotor nerve lesions on the direct and consensual light reflexes.

3. Pupillary constriction occurs as an aid in regulating the depth of focus for sharper images.

The accommodation-convergence reflex occurs when the eyes converge voluntarily to look at a near object or when the eyes make a reflex response to an object approaching the eye.

The pathway of the accommodation-convergence reflex is not well delineated. It is believed, however, that afferent impulses from the retina reach the occipital cortex and that the efferent pathway from the occipital cortex reaches the oculomotor complex after synapsing in the pretectal nucleus and/or the superior colliculus. In the oculomotor complex, the nucleus of Perlia has been assumed to play a role in convergence. The pathway for the accommodation-convergence reflex is thus different from that of the light reflex. This is supported clinically by a condition known as the Argyll Robertson pupil, in which the light reflex is lost while the accommodation-convergence reflex persists. The site of the lesion in this condition has not been established with certainty, but its etiology is known to be syphilis of the nervous system.

Mesencephalic Reticular Formation

This structure is a continuation of the medial pontine reticular nuclei and merges rostrally with the zona incerta. It receives fibers from most of the ascending fiber pathways (except the medial lemniscus) and from the limbic lobe. Although the mesencephalic reticular formation does not send direct reticulospinal fibers, it does influence spinal activity indirectly through the reticular nuclei of the pons and medulla. The major output from the mesencephalic reticular formation ascends to the diencephalon and cerebral cortex and is involved in behavior mechanisms as well as in sleep mechanisms. Unilateral lesions in the mesencephalic reticular formation in monkeys result in profound neglect of tactile, auditory, and visual sensations in the contralateral half of the body. This neglect is believed to be due to interruption of the corticolimbic reticular alerting system which includes the mesencephalic reticular formation.

Applied Anatomy of the Mesencephalon

The clinical syndromes associated with mesencephalic dysfunction fall into one of the following categories: alternating hemiplegia, disorders of ocular motility, disturbances of consciousness, and decerebrate rigidity. These result from occlusion of branches of the basilar or, rarely, the posterior cerebral artery.

Alternating Hemiplegia

The most common syndromes are the Moritz-Benedikt and the Weber. In the former syndrome, the patient presents with signs of ipsilateral oculomotor nerve paralysis and contralateral tremor. The vascular lesion affects rootlets of the oculomotor nerve within the tegmentum of the mesencephalon and the underlying red nucleus (Fig. 7–15, C). In Weber's syndrome, the patient presents with signs of ipsilateral oculomotor nerve paralysis and contralateral upper motor neuron paralysis. The vascular lesion affects rootlets of the oculomotor nerve and the underlying cerebral peduncle (Fig. 7–15, B).

Disorders of Ocular Motility

In addition to disturbances of ocular motility described in lesions of the oculomotor and trochlear cranial nerves, tectal lesions of the rostral mesencephalon (pretectal region) result in paralysis of upward gaze (Parinaud's syndrome). It is believed that such lesions interrupt fibers from the interstitial nucleus of Cajal coursing in the posterior commissure and destined for the contralateral oculomotor nucleus. Parinaud's syndrome is often encountered in pineal gland tumors which compress the pretectal-posterior commissure region.

Disturbances of Consciousness

Various levels of unconsciousness occur with lesions of the mesencephalic reticular formation. Evidence from experimental work points to a tonic role of the mesencephalic reticular formation in cortical excitability and the maintenance of awareness. Bilateral limited lesions of the mesencephalic reticular formation have been associated with akinetic mutism, a clinical condition characterized by absolute mutism and complete immobility except for the eyes, which are kept open and move in all directions. No communication with the patient through either painful or auditory stimuli can be established. This condition may result from injury to the mesencephalic reticular formation caused by transtentorial herniation with edema, hemorrhage, or occlusion of branches of the basilar artery.

Decerebrate Rigidity

Decerebrate rigidity in man occurs in lesions of the brain stem caudal to the red nucleus and rostral to the vestibular nuclei. The body is forced backward with the head bent extremely dorsally. The shoulders are internally rotated, the elbows are extended, and the distal parts of the upper limbs are hyperpronated with finger extension at the metacarpophalangeal joints and flexion at the interphalangeal joints. The hips and knees are extended; the feet and toes are plantar flexed. This syndrome is associated with severe head trauma and compression of the brain stem by herniation.

References

Afifi, A.K.; Kaelber, W.W.: Efferent Connections of the Substantia Nigra: An Experimental Study in Cats. Exp Neurol 11 (1965) 474–482.

Anderson, M.E.; Yoshida, M.: Axonal Branching Patterns and Location of Nigrothalamic and Nigrocollicular Neurons in the Cat. J Neurophysiol 43 (1980) 883–895.

Fog, M.; Hein-Sørensen, O.: Mesencephalic Syndromes. In: Handbook of Clinical Neurology, Vol. 2, pp. 272–285. Ed. by P.J. Vinken and G.W. Bruyn. North-Holland Publishing Co., Amsterdam, 1969.

Gebhart, G.F.; Toleikis, J.R.: An Evaluation of Stimulation-Produced Analgesia in the Cat. Exp Neurol 62 (1980) 570–579.

Hartmann-von Monakow, K.; Akert, K.; Künzle, H.: Projections of Precentral and Premotor Cortex to the Red Nucleus and Other Midbrain Areas in *Macaca Fascicularis*. Exp Brain Res 34 (1979) 91–105.

Kaelber, W.W.; Afifi, A.K.: Nigroamygdaloid Fiber Connections in the Cat. Am J Anat 148 (1977) 129–135.

Meibach, R.C.; Katzman, R.: Origin, Course and Termination of Dopaminergic Substantia Nigra Neurons Projecting to the Amygdaloid Complex in the Cat. Neuroscience 6 (1981) 2159–2171.

Steiger, H.J.; Buttner-Ennever, J.A.: Oculomotor Nucleus Afferents in the Monkey Demonstrated with Horseradish Peroxidase. Brain Res 160 (1979) 1–15.

Trojanowski, J.Q.; Wray, S.H.: Vertical Gaze Ophthalmoplegia: Selective Paralysis of Downgaze. Neurology 30 (1980) 605–610.

Usunoff, K.G.; Romansky, K.V.; Malinov, G.B.; Ivanov, D.P.; Blagov, Z.A.; Galobov, G.P.: Electron Microscopic Evidence for the Existence of a Corticonigral Tract in the Cat. J Hirnforsch 23 (1982) 17–23.

Walberg, F.; Nordby, T.: A Re-examination of the Rubro-Olivary Tract in the Cat, Using Horseradish Peroxidase as a Retrograde and an Anterograde Neuronal Tracer. Neuroscience 6 (1981) 2379–2391.

Weber, J.T.; Martin, G.F.; Behan, M; Huerta, M.F.; Harting, J.K.: The Precise Origin of the Tectospinal Pathway in Three Common Laboratory Animals: A Study Using the Horseradish Peroxidase Method. Neurosci Lett 11 (1979) 121–127.

8

Diencephalon

Gross Topography (Figs. 8–1 and 8–2)

The diencephalon or "in-between brain" is completely surrounded by the cerebral hemispheres except at its ventral surface. It is limited posteriorly by the posterior commissure and anteriorly by the lamina terminalis and the foramen of Monro. The posterior limb of the internal capsule limits the diencephalon laterally. Medially, the diencephalon forms the lateral wall of the third ventricle. The dorsal surface forms the floor of the lateral ventricle and is marked medially by a band of nerve fibers, the stria medullaris thalami. The ventral surface is exposed and contains hypothalamic structures. A groove extending between the foramen of Monro and the aqueduct of Sylvius (the hypothalamic sulcus) divides the diencephalon into a dorsal portion, the thalamus, and a ventral portion, the hypothalamus. The two thalami are connected across the midline in about 70% of humans through the interthalamic adhesion (massa intermedia).

Divisions of Diencephalon

The diencephalon is divided into four major subdivisions. These are the epithalamus, the thalamus and metathalamus, the subthalamus, and the hypothalamus.

Epithalamus

The epithalamus occupies a position dorsal to the thalamus and includes the following structures (Fig. 8–1).

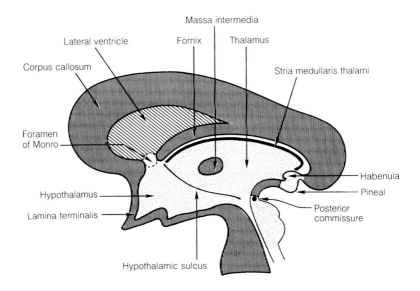

8–1 Schematic diagram showing the major subdivisions of the diencephalon as seen in a midsagittal view.

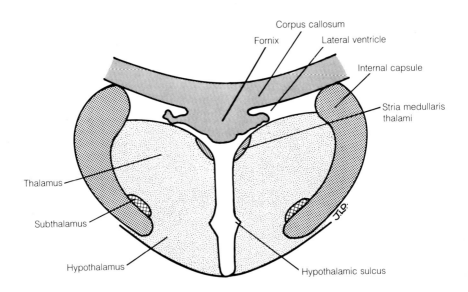

8–2 Schematic diagram showing the subdivisions of the diencephalon as seen in a composite coronal section.

Stria Medullaris Thalami   This band of nerve fibers courses dorsomedial to the thalamus and connects the septal (medial olfactory) area, located underneath the rostral end of the corpus callosum in the frontal lobe, with the habenular nuclei.

Habenular Nuclei   These nuclei are located in the caudal diencephalon; one is on each side, dorsomedial to the thalamus. They receive the stria medullaris and project via the habenulointerpeduncular tract (fasciculus retroflexus of Meynert) to the interpeduncular nucleus of the midbrain. The two habenular nuclei are connected by the habenular commissure. The habenular nuclei, part of a neural network that includes the limbic and olfactory systems, are concerned with mechanisms of emotion and behavior.

Pineal Gland   This endocrine gland is located just rostral to the superior colliculi in the roof of the third ventricle. The functions of the pineal gland are not well understood. It may have a role in gonadal function. The pineal gland calcifies after the age of 16 years. This fact is used in the detection of midline shifts in skull X-rays. In normal skull X-rays, pineal calcifications are seen in the midline. Shifts of pineal calcification away from the midline suggest the presence of space-occupying lesions displacing the pineal. Such a lesion could be blood in the subdural or epidural space, a hematoma within the brain or a brain tumor. Pineal gland tumors which develop around the age of puberty may interfere with the onset of puberty, causing either delayed or premature onset. Such tumors also interfere with vertical gaze. This loss of vertical gaze, known as Parinaud's syndrome, results from the pressure of the pineal lesion on the pretectal area and/or the posterior commissure.

Thalamus and Metathalamus

The thalamus is the largest component of the diencephalon and is subdivided into the following major nuclear groups (Fig. 8–3).

1. Anterior
2. Medial
3. Lateral
4. Intralaminar and reticular
5. Metathalamus
6. Posterior thalamus

The thalamus is traversed by a band of myelinated fibers, the internal medullary lamina, which runs along the rostral caudal extent of the thalamus. The internal medullary lamina separates the medial from the lateral group of nuclei. Rostrally and caudally, the internal medullary lamina splits

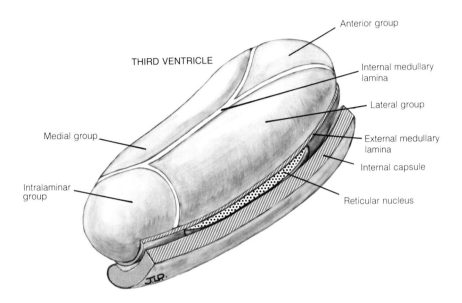

THIRD VENTRICLE

Anterior group

Internal medullary lamina

Lateral group

Medial group

External medullary lamina

Internal capsule

Intralaminar group

Reticular nucleus

8-3   Schematic diagram showing the major nuclear groups of the thalamus.

to enclose the anterior and intralaminar nuclear groups, respectively. The internal medullary lamina contains intrathalamic fibers connecting the different nuclei of the thalamus with each other. Another medullated band, the external medullary lamina, forms the lateral boundary of the thalamus medial to the internal capsule. Between the external medullary lamina and the internal capsule is the reticular nucleus of the thalamus. The external medullary lamina contains nerve fibers leaving or entering the thalamus on their way to or from the adjacent capsule.

Anterior Nuclear Group   The anterior tubercle of the thalamus is formed by the anterior nuclear group. It has reciprocal connections with the mamillary body and the cingulate gyrus (Fig. 8-4).

The reciprocal fibers between the anterior thalamic nucleus and the mamillary body travel via the mamillothalamic tract (tract of Vicq d'Azyr). The reciprocal connections between the anterior nucleus and the cingulate gyrus accompany the internal capsule. The anterior nucleus of the thalamus is part of the limbic system, which is concerned with emotional behavior and memory mechanisms. The anterior group of thalamic nuclei includes the anterior dorsal, anterior medial, and anterior ventral nuclei.

Medial Nuclear Group   Of the medial nuclear group, the dorsomedial nucleus is the most highly developed in man. The dorsomedial nucleus is

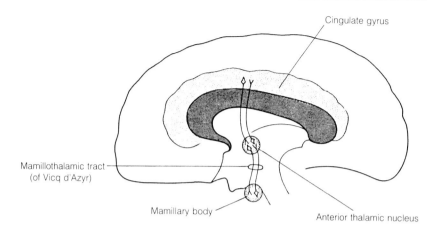

8-4 Schematic diagram showing the reciprocal connections among the anterior nucleus of the thalamus, mamillary body, and cingulate gyrus.

reciprocally connected with the prefrontal cortex and hypothalamus (Fig. 8-5). It also receives fibers from other thalamic nuclei, particularly the lateral and intralaminar groups.

With the radioactive amino acid technique, a projection was recently demonstrated from the precentral gyrus (primary motor area) to the dorsomedial nucleus. This connection suggests that the dorsomedial nucleus represents a link between the motor and prefrontal (association) cortex of the frontal lobe. Other reported connections include those with the amygdaloid nucleus and the corpus striatum. The dorsomedial nucleus belongs to a neural system concerned with affective behavior and memory. The reciprocal connections between the prefrontal cortex and dorsomedial nucleus can be interrupted surgically to relieve severe anxiety states and other psychiatric disorders. The operation known as prefrontal lobotomy (ablation of prefrontal cortex) or prefrontal leukotomy (severance of the prefrontal-dorsomedial nucleus pathway) is rarely practiced nowadays, having been largely replaced by medical treatment that achieves the same result without undesirable side effects.

Lateral Nuclear Group The lateral nuclear group of the thalamus is subdivided into two groups, dorsal and ventral.

Dorsal Subgroup This subgroup includes from rostral to caudal the lateral dorsal, lateral posterior, and pulvinar nuclei. The borderline between the lateral posterior nucleus and the pulvinar is vague and the term pulvinar-LP complex has been used to refer to this nuclear complex.

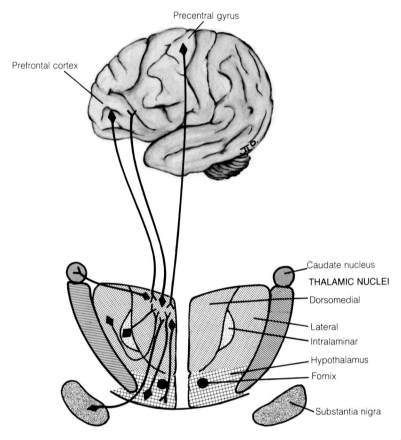

Precentral gyrus

Prefrontal cortex

Caudate nucleus

THALAMIC NUCLEI

Dorsomedial

Lateral

Intralaminar

Hypothalamus

Fornix

Substantia nigra

8–5   Schematic diagram showing the major afferent and efferent connections of the dorsomedial nucleus of the thalamus.

The connections of this subgroup are poorly understood; of the three nuclei, those of the pulvinar are most documented. The pulvinar has reciprocal connections caudally with the medial and lateral geniculate bodies and rostrally with the association areas of the parietal, temporal, and occipital cortices (Fig. 8–6). The pulvinar is thus a relay station between subcortical auditory and visual centers and their respective association cortices in the temporal and occipital lobes. There is evidence that the pulvinar plays a role in speech mechanisms. Stimulation of the pulvinar of the dominant hemisphere has produced anomia. The pulvinar has also been shown to play a role in pain mechanisms. Lesions in the pulvinar have been effective in the treatment of intractable pain. Experimental studies have demonstrated connections between the pulvinar and several cortical and subcortical areas concerned with pain mechanisms.

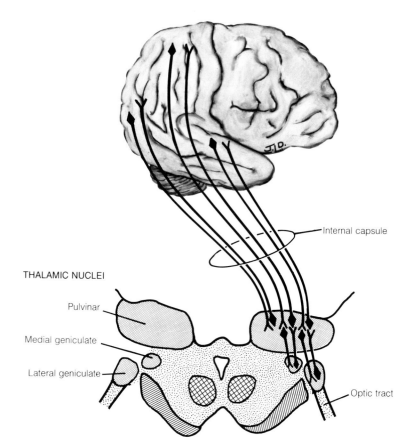

8–6 Schematic diagram showing the major afferent and efferent connections of the pulvinar.

The dorsal subgroup and the dorsomedial nucleus are known collectively as the association thalamic nuclei. They all have the following in common.

1. They do not receive a direct input from the long ascending tracts.
2. Their input is mainly from other thalamic nuclei.
3. They project mainly to the association areas of the cortex.

Ventral Subgroup This subgroup includes the ventral anterior, ventral lateral, and ventral posterior nuclei.

The neural connectivity and functions of this subgroup are much better understood than those of the dorsal subgroup. In contrast to the dorsal subgroup, which belongs to the association thalamic nuclei, the ventral subgroup belongs to the specific relay thalamic nuclei. These nuclei share the following characteristics.

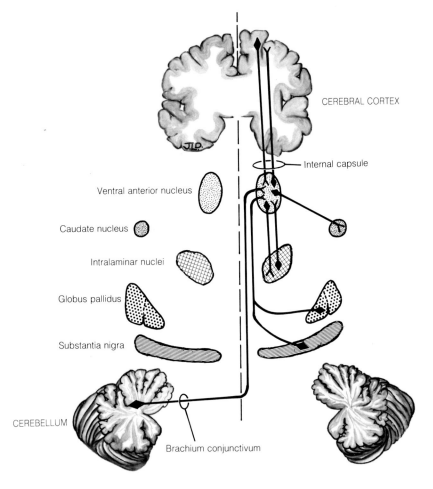

CEREBRAL CORTEX

Internal capsule

Ventral anterior nucleus

Caudate nucleus

Intralaminar nuclei

Globus pallidus

Substantia nigra

CEREBELLUM

Brachium conjunctivum

8–7 Schematic diagram showing the major connections of the ventral anterior nucleus of the thalamus.

1. They receive a direct input from the long ascending tracts.
2. They have reciprocal relationships with specific cortical areas.
3. They degenerate upon ablation of the specific cortical area to which they project.

Ventral Anterior Nucleus   This is the most rostrally placed of the ventral subgroup. It receives fibers from several sources (Fig. 8–7).

Globus Pallidus—A major input to this nucleus is from the globus pallidus. Fibers from the globus pallidus form the ansa and lenticular fasciculi and reach the nucleus via the thalamic fasciculus.

Deep Cerebellar Nuclei—Another input is from the deep cerebellar nuclei. Fibers from the cerebellum travel via the dentatorubrothalamic system. They project upon the ventral lateral nucleus but also contribute fibers to the ventral anterior nucleus.

Substantia Nigra
Intralaminar Thalamic Nuclei
Premotor, Motor and Association Frontal Cortices
The major output of the ventral anterior nucleus goes to the motor and premotor cortices and, possibly, to wide areas of the frontal cortex as well. It also has reciprocal connections with the intralaminar nuclei. The questionable projection from the ventral anterior nucleus to the caudate nucleus has recently been confirmed with the horseradish peroxidase technique. A cortical projection to the association parietal cortex (areas 5 and 7) has recently been described.

Thus, the ventral anterior nucleus is a major relay station in the motor pathways from the basal ganglia and cerebellum to the cerebral cortex. As such it is involved in the regulation of movement. Lesions in this nucleus and adjacent areas of the thalamus have been placed surgically (thalamotomy) to relieve disorders of movement, especially parkinsonism. Through its connection with the intralaminar nuclei of the thalamus, the ventral anterior nucleus seems to play a role in the ascending activating reticular system.

Ventral Lateral Nucleus   This nucleus is located caudal to the ventral anterior nucleus and plays a major role similar to the latter in motor integration. The afferent fibers to the ventral lateral nucleus come from the following sources (Fig. 8–8).

Deep Cerebellar Nuclei—The dentatorubrothalamic system constitutes the major input to the ventral lateral nucleus. As detailed elsewhere, this fiber system originates in the deep cerebellar nuclei (mainly dentate), leaves the cerebellum via the superior cerebellar peduncle and decussates in the mesencephalon. Some fibers synapse in the red nucleus, while others bypass it to reach the thalamus.

Globus Pallidus—Although the pallidothalamic fiber system projects primarily upon ventral anterior neurons, some fibers reach the ventral lateral nucleus.

Red Nucleus—The rubrothalamic fibers are part of the dentatorubrothalamic system. Some recent studies question the projection of fibers from the red nucleus to the thalamus.

Substantia Nigra
Primary Motor Cortex—There is a reciprocal relationship between the primary motor cortex and the ventral lateral nucleus. The efferent fibers of the ventral lateral nucleus go to the primary motor cortex in the precentral gyrus.

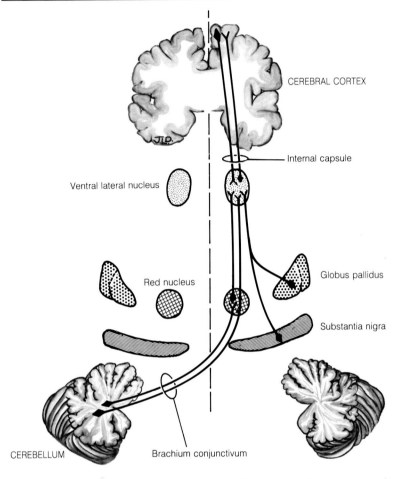

CEREBRAL CORTEX

Internal capsule

Ventral lateral nucleus

Red nucleus

Globus pallidus

Substantia nigra

CEREBELLUM

Brachium conjunctivum

8-8 Schematic diagram showing the major afferent and efferent connections of the nucleus ventralis lateralis of the thalamus.

Thus, the ventral lateral nucleus, like the ventral anterior nucleus, is a major relay station in the motor system linking the cerebellum, the basal ganglia, and the cerebral cortex. As in the case of the ventral anterior nucleus, lesions in the ventral lateral nucleus have been surgically produced to relieve disorders of movement manifested by tremor. Deep cerebellar nuclei have been shown to project equally to ventral anterior and ventral lateral thalamic nuclei, whereas the projections from the globus pallidus and substantia nigra project mainly to the ventral anterior nucleus with overflow to the ventral lateral nucleus. Physiologic studies have shown that the cerebellar and pallidonigral projection zones in the ventral anterior and ventral lateral nuclei are separate; very few cells have been identified that respond to both cerebellar and pallidonigral stimulation.

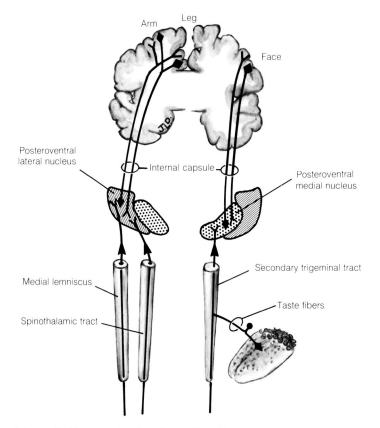

8–9 Schematic diagram showing the major afferent and efferent connections of the posteroventral lateral and posteroventral medial nuclei of the thalamus.

Ventral Posterior Nucleus This nucleus is located in the caudal part of the thalamus. It receives the long ascending tracts conveying sensory modalities (including taste) from the contralateral half of the body and face. These tracts (Fig. 8–9) include the medial lemniscus, trigeminal lemniscus (secondary trigeminal tracts), and spinothalamic tract.

Vestibular information is relayed to the cortex via the ventral posterior as well as the intralaminar and posterior group of thalamic nuclei.

The ventral posterior nucleus is made up of two parts; these are the posteroventral medial nucleus, which receives the trigeminal lemniscus and taste fibers, and the posteroventral lateral nucleus, which receives the medial lemniscus and spinothalamic tracts. Both nuclei receive reciprocal input from the primary sensory cortex.

The output from both nuclei is to the primary sensory cortex in the postcentral gyrus. The projection to the cortex is somatotopically organized in such a way that fibers from the posteroventral medial nucleus project to the face area, while different parts of the posteroventral lateral nucleus project to corresponding areas of body representation in the cortex. A cortical projection from the part of the posteroventral medial nucleus that receives taste fibers to the orbital gyrus has been demonstrated recently with the horseradish peroxidase technique.

The posteroventral lateral and posteroventral medial nuclei are collectively referred to as the ventrobasal complex.

Intralaminar and Reticular Nuclei   The intralaminar nuclei, as their name suggests, are enclosed within the internal medullary lamina in the caudal thalamus. The reticular nuclei occupy a position between the external medullary lamina and the internal capsule (Fig. 8–3).

The intralaminar nuclei include several nuclei, of which the most important functionally, in man, are the centromedian and parafascicular nuclei. The intralaminar nuclei have the following afferent and efferent connections.

Afferent Connections (Fig. 8–10)   Fibers projecting upon the intralaminar nuclei come from the following sources.

Reticular Formation   This constitutes the major input to the intralaminar nuclei.

Cerebellum   The dentatorubrothalamic system projects upon the ventral lateral and ventral anterior nuclei of the thalamus, but also contains fibers that project upon the intralaminar nuclei.

Red Nucleus   The rubrothalamic fiber system projects mainly upon the ventral lateral nucleus of the thalamus, but also projects upon the intralaminar nuclei.

Spinothalamic and Trigeminal Lemniscus   Afferent fibers from the ascending pain pathways project largely upon the ventral posterior nucleus, but also project upon the intralaminar nuclei.

Globus Pallidus   Pallidothalamic fibers project mainly upon the ventral anterior nucleus, but also project upon the intralaminar nuclei.

Cerebral Cortex   Cortical fibers arise primarily from the motor and premotor areas.

Other Connections   Retrograde transport studies of horseradish peroxidase have recently identified afferent connections to the intralaminar nuclei from the vestibular nuclei, periaqueductal gray matter, superior colliculus, and the locus ceruleus.

Efferent Connections   The intralaminar nuclei project to the following structures.

Other Thalamic Nuclei   The intralaminar nuclei influence cortical activity through other thalamic nuclei. There are no direct cortical connections for the intralaminar nuclei. One exception has been demonstrated recently with both the horseradish peroxidase technique and autoradiog-

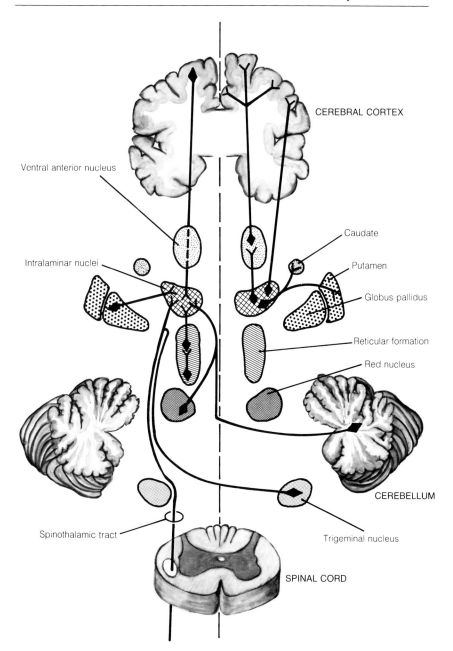

8–10 Schematic diagram showing the major afferent and efferent connections of the intralaminar nuclei of the thalamus.

raphy showing a direct projection from one of the intralaminar nuclei (centrolateral) to the primary visual cortex (area 17) in the cat. The significance of this finding is twofold. First, it shows that intralaminar nuclei, contrary to previous concepts, do project directly to cortical areas. Secondly, it explains the reported response of area 17 neurons to nonvisual stimuli (pinprick, sound, etc); such responses would be mediated through the intralaminar nuclei.

The Striatum (Caudate and Putamen)

The reticular nucleus is a continuation of the reticular formation of the brain stem into the diencephalon. It receives the multisynaptic ascending reticular fiber system and projects widely and diffusely to the cerebral cortex, from which it also receives reciprocal connections.

Thus, the intralaminar nuclei and reticular nucleus collectively receive fibers from several sources, motor and sensory, and project diffusely to the cerebral cortex either directly or indirectly through other thalamic nuclei. Their multisource input and diffuse cortical projection enable them to play a role in the cortical arousal response. The intralaminar nuclei are also involved in the awareness of painful sensory experience. The awareness of sensory experience in the intralaminar nuclei is poorly localized and has an emotional quality, in contrast to cortical awareness, which is well localized.

Metathalamus   The term metathalamus refers to two thalamic nuclei, the medial geniculate and lateral geniculate.

Medial Geniculate Nucleus   This is a relay thalamic nucleus in the auditory system. It receives fibers from the lateral lemniscus directly or, more frequently, after a synapse in the inferior colliculus. These auditory fibers reach the medial geniculate body via the brachium of the inferior colliculus (inferior quadrigeminal brachium). The medial geniculate nucleus also receives feedback fibers from the primary auditory cortex in the temporal lobe. The efferent outflow from the medial geniculate nucleus forms the auditory radiation of the internal capsule to the primary auditory cortex in the temporal lobe. Some of the efferent outflow projects upon neurons of the pulvinar.

Lateral Geniculate Nucleus   This is a relay thalamic nucleus in the visual system. It receives fibers from the optic tract conveying impulses from both retinae. The lateral geniculate nucleus is laminated and the inflow from each retina projects upon different laminae. Feedback fibers also reach the nucleus from the primary visual cortex in the occipital lobes. The efferent outflow from the lateral geniculate nucleus forms the optic radiation of the internal capsule to the primary visual cortex in the occipital lobe. Some of the efferent outflow projects to the pulvinar.

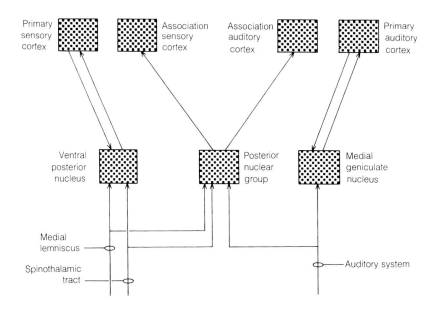

8-11 Schematic diagram comparing the afferent and efferent connections of the specific thalamic nuclei (ventral posterior and medial geniculate) with the posterior nuclear group of thalamic nuclei.

Posterior Thalamus   This group embraces the caudal pole of the ventral posterior group of thalamic nuclei and extends caudally to merge with the medial geniculate body and the gray matter medial to it. It receives from all somatic ascending tracts (medial lemniscus and spinothalamic), as well as from the auditory pathways and possibly the visual pathways. The outflow from the posterior group projects to the association cortices in the parietal, temporal, and occipital lobes. The posterior nuclear group is thus a convergence center for varied sensory modalities. It lacks the modal and spatial specificity of the classic ascending sensory systems, but allows for interaction among the divergent sensory systems that project upon it. Unlike the specific sensory thalamic nuclei, the posterior group does not receive reciprocal feedback connections from the cerebral cortex (Fig. 8–11).

The function of the thalamus is to integrate sensory and motor activities. In addition, it has roles to play in arousal and consciousness, as well as in affective behavior. In a sense it is the gateway to the cortex.

The thalamus receives two major inputs. These are a peripheral input conveying several types of sensory modalities and a central input arriving mainly from the cerebral cortex, but also from some brain stem nuclei (basal ganglia and reticular). There are also intrathalamic connections linking the different thalamic nuclei with each other. The interaction between the peripheral input and the thalamic neurons takes place in a synaptic island, the glomerulus, which is a cluster of terminals surrounded by glial membranes. Within the glomerulus, the afferent axon synapses with dendrites of both the principal and intrinsic neurons. In addition, the glomerulus contains dendrodendritic and axodendritic synapses between the principal and intrinsic neurons of a thalamic nucleus. Outside the glomerulus, the cortical input establishes axodendritic synapses with both the principal and intrinsic neurons. The principal neuron also projects upon the intrinsic neuron via axon collaterals. The interactions within the glomerulus and outside the glomerulus between principal and intrinsic neurons permit local feedback and feed forward circuits to modify the input from the periphery. On the other hand, the input from the cortex upon the dendrites of both principal and intrinsic neurons allows for long feedback loops. A characteristic of thalamic neurons is their tendency to rhythmic activity. In response to stimulation of an afferent input, principal thalamic neurons manifest a burst of excitatory postsynaptic potentials (EPSPs), followed by a prolonged inhibitory postsynaptic potential (IPSP). At the end of the IPSP, another burst of impulses occurs, followed by an IPSP, and so on. It is believed that the rhythmically generated IPSPs are responsible for the phasing of the bursts. The basis for the IPSP could be one of two mechanisms.

1. Axon collaterals from the principal neuron may project to the intrinsic neuron, which in turn inhibits not only the principal neuron of the axon collateral but neighboring principal neurons as well, thus allowing for rhythmic, synchronous excitations and inhibitions of a population of principal neurons.
2. The inhibition may be effected in addition by dendrodendritic connections between the principal and intrinsic neurons, with the latter in turn inhibiting a number of principal neurons. In view of the paucity of axon collaterals in principal thalamic neurons, this mechanism becomes the more likely one to effect inhibition.

Another hypothesis to explain rhythmic activity postulates that the principal neuron becomes hyperexcitable (postinhibitory exaltation) at the end of inhibition, resulting in a burst of EPSPs, followed by IPSP, and so on.

Nuclei of the thalamus are generally categorized into specific relay nuclei and nonspecific nuclei. This categorization is based upon both the anatomic and physiologic properties of the two groups.

The specific relay nuclei receive specific ascending systems and project to specific cortical areas from which they in turn receive a feedback loop. Low frequency stimulation of the specific relay nuclei or their peripheral afferents results in a characteristic physiologic cortical response known as the augmenting response. This response consists of a primary EPSP followed by augmentation of the amplitude and latency of the primary EPSP recorded from the specific cortical area to which the specific relay thalamic nucleus projects. The specific relay nuclei include the sensory relay nuclei (medial geniculate, lateral geniculate, and ventral posterior) and the cortical relay nuclei (anterior, ventral lateral, and ventral anterior).

The nonspecific nuclei of the thalamus include the intralaminar and reticular nuclei. They receive mainly from the reticular formation and project widely and diffusely to the cerebral cortex. Stimulation of the nonspecific nuclei gives rise to the characteristic recruiting response in the cortex. This is a bilateral generalized cortical response (in contrast to the localized augmenting response) characterized by a predominantly surface negative EPSP which increases in amplitude and with continued stimulation will wax and wane.

The thalamus plays a central role in sensory integration. All somatic and special senses, except olfaction, pass through the thalamus before reaching the cerebral cortex. Sensory activity within the thalamus is channeled in one of three routes.

The first route is through the specific sensory relay nuclei (medial geniculate, lateral geniculate, and ventral posterior). Sensations relayed in the specific sensory relay nuclei have direct access to the respective sensory cortical areas. They are strictly organized with regard to topographic and modal specificities and are discriminative and well localized.

The second route is through the nonspecific nuclei. With its many sources of input and diffuse projection to the cortex, this route serves the low extreme of the modality specificity gradient.

The third route is through the posterior nuclear group. This route receives from multiple sensory sources and projects to the association cortical areas. It plays an intermediate role between the specific and nonspecific routes described above.

Some sensory modalities are perceived at the thalamic level and are not affected by ablation of the sensory cortex. Following sensory cortical lesions, all sensory modalities are lost, but soon pain, thermal sense, and crude touch return. The sense of pain that returns is the aching, burning type of pain that is carried by C-fibers. It is this type of pain that is believed to terminate in the thalamus, whereas the pricking, well-localized pain carried by the A-fibers terminates in the sensory cortex and is lost with its ablation. In patients with intractable pain, placement of a surgical lesion in the ventral posterior and/or intralaminar nuclei (centromedian) may provide relief.

The role of the thalamus in motor control is evident from the input it receives from the cerebellum, basal ganglia, and the motor areas of the cortex. A tremorogenic center has been postulated for the ventral lateral nucleus. Lesions have been placed in the ventral lateral nucleus to relieve abnormal movement resulting from cerebellar and basal ganglia disorders.

The thalamus, as part of the ascending reticular activating system, has a central role in the conscious state and attention.

The connections of the medial thalamus with the prefrontal cortex reflect its role in affective behavior. Ablation of the prefrontal cortex or the dorsomedial nucleus causes changes in personality characterized by lack of drive, flat affect, and indifference to pain.

The connections of the anterior thalamic nuclei with the hypothalamus and cingulate gyrus enable them to play a role in memory, visceral function, and emotional behavior.

Vascular lesions of the thalamus result in a characteristic clinical syndrome known as the thalamic syndrome. Following an initial period of loss of all sensations contralateral to the thalamic lesion, pain, thermal sense, and some crude touch return. However, the threshold of stimulation which elicits these sensations is elevated and the sensations are exaggerated and unpleasant when perceived. The syndrome is usually associated with a marked affective response attributed to the intact dorsomedial nucleus, usually unaffected by the vascular lesion.

Subthalamus

The subthalamus is a mass of gray and white substance in the caudal diencephalon. It is bordered medially by the hypothalamus, laterally by the internal capsule, dorsally by the thalamus, and ventrally by the internal capsule.

The subthalamus consists of three main structures; these are the subthalamic nucleus, fields of Forel, and zona incerta.

Subthalamic Nucleus   The subthalamic nucleus (of Luys) is a biconvex gray mass which replaces the substantia nigra in caudal diencephalic levels. It has a major and reciprocal connection with the globus pallidus via the subthalamic fasciculus. The two subthalamic nuclei communicate via the supramamillary commissure. The subthalamic nucleus also receives a small input from the substantia nigra (Fig. 8–12). The subthalamic nucleus is important for the regulation of movement. Lesions in man and experimental animals produce involuntary, flinging, violent movements involving the proximal musculature of the contralateral upper and lower extremities. Facial and neck muscles may also be involved. This condition is known as hemiballismus and is relieved by lesions in the ventral lateral nucleus of the thalamus.

Fields of Forel (Fig. 8–12)   This term refers to fiber bundles containing pallidal and cerebellar efferents to the thalamus. Efferent pallidal fibers that course across the internal capsule gather dorsal to the subthalamic

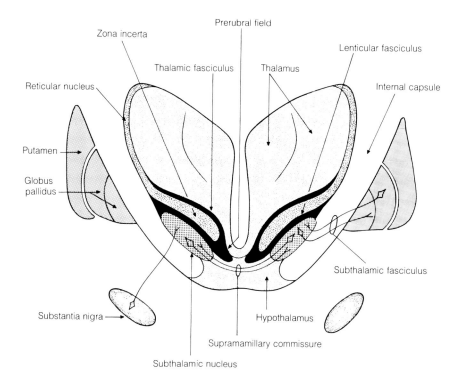

8–12 Schematic diagram of the subthalamic region showing its components and the major afferent and efferent connections of the subthalamic nucleus.

nucleus to form the lenticular fasciculus or H_2 field of Forel. Dentatoru-brothalamic fibers gather in the caudal diencephalon in a bundle known as the prerubral field or H field of Forel, which also contains pallidotha-lamic fibers. Both the prerubral field fibers and the lenticular fasciculus contribute to the thalamic fasciculus or H_1 field of Forel, which enters the ventral lateral and ventral anterior nuclei of the thalamus.

Zona Incerta   The zona incerta (Fig. 8–12) is the rostral continuation of the mesencephalic reticular formation and extends laterally into the reticular nucleus of the thalamus. It is sandwiched between the lenticular fasciculus and the thalamic fasciculus. The neural connectivity of the zona incerta is not well delineated. Lesions have been placed in the zona incerta to relieve abnormal movement.

Hypothalamus

The hypothalamus is the area of the diencephalon ventral to the hypothalamic sulcus (Fig. 8–1). It is limited anteriorly by the lamina terminalis and is continuous posteriorly with the mesencephalon. In coronal sections, the hypothalamus is seen to be bordered medially by the third ventricle and laterally by the subthalamus (Fig. 8–2). The fornix divides the hypothalamus into medial and lateral regions (Fig. 8–5). The lateral region contains mainly longitudinally oriented fiber bundles, among which are scattered neurons of the lateral hypothalamic nucleus. The medial region has a cluster of nuclei organized into four major groups. In a rostrocaudal orientation, these nuclear groups are as follows.

1. Preoptic
2. Suprachiasmatic (supraoptic)
3. Tuberal
4. Mamillary

Preoptic Region   The gray matter in the most rostral part of the hypothalamus, just caudal to the lamina terminalis, is the preoptic region and contains medial and lateral preoptic nuclei.

Suprachiasmatic (Supraoptic) Region   This nuclear group contains the supraoptic, paraventricular, and anterior hypothalamic nuclei.

The supraoptic nucleus is located above the optic tract, whereas the paraventricular nucleus is dorsal to it, lateral to the third ventricle (Fig. 8–13). Axons of both nuclei course in the pituitary stalk to reach the posterior lobe of the pituitary (hypothalamo-neurohypophyseal system), transporting neurosecretory material elaborated in these nuclei and stored in axonal swellings within the posterior lobe. The neurosecretory material consists of vasopressin, antidiuretic hormone (ADH), and oxytocin. There is evidence to suggest that the supraoptic nucleus elaborates ADH, whereas the paraventricular nucleus elaborates oxytocin. ADH acts on the distal convoluted tubules of the kidney to increase reabsorption of water. Lesions of the supraoptic nucleus, the hypothalamo-neurohypophyseal system, or the posterior lobe of the pituitary result in excessive excretion of urine (polyuria) of low specific gravity. This condition is known as diabetes insipidus. Another symptom of this condition is excessive intake of water (polydipsia). Unlike diabetes mellitus, diabetes insipidus is not associated with alterations in the sugar content of blood or of urine. Production of ADH is controlled by the osmolarity of the blood which bathes the supraoptic nucleus. An increase in blood osmolarity, as occurs in dehydration, increases ADH production, whereas the reverse occurs in states of lowered blood osmolarity, such as excessive hydration. Vasopressin secretion is increased by pain, stress, and drugs like morphine, nicotine, and barbiturates; it is decreased by alcohol intake.

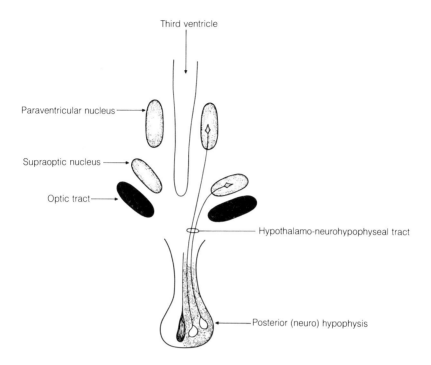

Third ventricle

Paraventricular nucleus

Supraoptic nucleus

Optic tract

Hypothalamo-neurohypophyseal tract

Posterior (neuro) hypophysis

8–13   Schematic diagram showing the hypothalamo-neurohypophyseal fiber system.

Oxytocin causes contraction of uterine musculature. Commercially produced oxytocin is used to induce labor.

The anterior nucleus merges with the preoptic region. Stimulation of the anterior part of the hypothalamus in animals results in excessive intake of water, suggesting that a center for thirst is located in this region. Tumors in this region in children are associated with refusal of patients to drink in spite of severe dehydration.

Tuberal Region   This is the widest region of the hypothalamus and the one in which the division of the hypothalamus into medial and lateral areas by the fornix is best illustrated. The tuberal region contains the ventromedial hypothalamic, dorsomedial hypothalamic, and arcuate nuclei.

The ventromedial nucleus, a poorly delineated area of small neurons, is concerned with satiety. Bilateral lesions in the ventromedial nucleus in animals produce a voracious appetite, obesity, and savage behavior. Lesions in the lateral hypothalamus at this level produce loss of appetite. Thus, a center for satiety is believed to be associated with the ventromedial nucleus and a feeding center with the lateral hypothalamus.

The dorsomedial nucleus is a poorly delineated mass of small neurons dorsal to the ventromedial nucleus.

The arcuate nucleus consists of small neurons located ventral to the third ventricle. It possibly may have an endocrine function.

The neural connectivity of the three nuclei mentioned above is not well defined; all probably have reciprocal connections with the midline thalamic nuclei.

Mamillary Region   The most caudal region of the hypothalamus is the mamillary region; it contains mamillary and posterior hypothalamic nuclei.

The mamillary nuclei (bodies) (Fig. 8–14) are two spherical masses protruding from the ventral surface of the hypothalamus in the interpeduncular fossa. They receive the following afferents.

1. The fornix comprises the major input to the mamillary body. Arising from the hippocampus, the fornix follows a C-shaped course underneath the corpus callosum as far forward as the interventricular foramen of Monro, where it disappears in the substance of the diencephalon to reach the mamillary bodies. Although the major component of the fornix comes from the hippocampus, it also carries fibers from the septal area to the mamillary bodies.
2. Fibers from the anterior thalamic nuclei reach the mamillary bodies via the mamillothalamic tract and provide a feedback mechanism to the mamillary bodies.
3. The mamillary peduncle, a bundle of fibers of diverse origin containing collaterals from most of the ascending sensory systems, projects upon the mamillary bodies.
4. The medial forebrain bundle is a pathway which brings afferents to the mamillary bodies from the premotor frontal cortex.

The efferent connections of the mamillary bodies are as follows.

1. The mamillothalamic tract (tract of Vicq d'Azyr) is a two-way system connecting the mamillary bodies with the anterior nucleus of the thalamus.
2. Fibers in the mamillotegmental tract course caudally to terminate upon reticular nuclei of the mesencephalon and secondarily upon autonomic cranial and spinal nuclei.

The posterior hypothalamic nucleus (Fig. 8–15) is a mass of large neurons located dorsal to the mamillary bodies. It is the main source of descending hypothalamic fibers to the brain stem. The posterior hypothalamic and

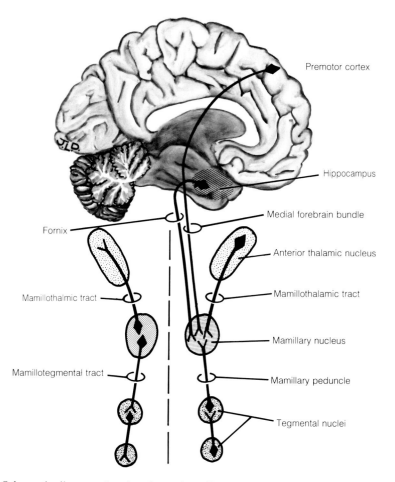

8-14 Schematic diagram showing the major afferent and efferent connections of the mamillary bodies.

lateral hypothalamic nuclei have common afferent and efferent connections.

Afferent connections include the following fiber systems.

1. The medial forebrain bundle contains fibers from the septal nuclei, the basal olfactory area, the periamygdaloid area, and the frontal cortex. These fibers project upon or pass through the lateral and posterior hypothalamic regions to reach the mesencephalic tegmentum.
2. Amygdalohypothalamic fibers.
3. Thalamohypothalamic fibers from the dorsomedial and midline thalamic nuclei reach the lateral and posterior hypothalamus.

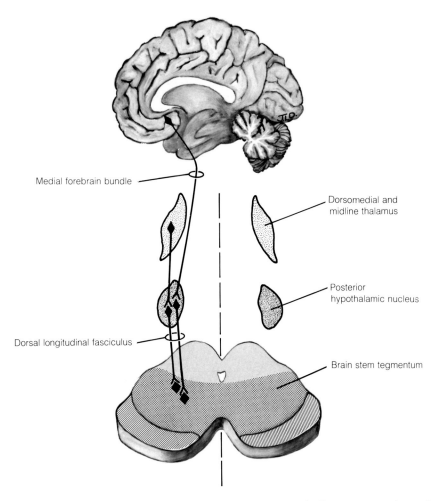

8-15 Schematic diagram showing the major afferent and efferent connections of the posterior nucleus of the hypothalamus.

The efferent connections of the lateral and posterior hypothalamic nuclei constitute the main source of hypothalamic fibers to lower brain stem regions. These fibers travel via the periventricular fiber system. The majority of these fibers arise in the posterior hypothalamic nucleus. Some of them course dorsally alongside the third ventricle to reach the dorsomedial and midline thalamic nuclei. The majority of these fibers, however, descend as the dorsal longitudinal fasciculus (dorsal bundle of Schütz), located in the periaqueductal gray, to project on autonomic and motor nuclei in the brain stem tegmentum.

Functions of Hypothalamus The functions of the hypothalamus, mediated through its varied and complex connections, involve several important bodily activities. The following is a listing of some of the most important and best known.

Control of Posterior Pituitary (Neurohypophysis) This is served through the hypothalamo-neurohypophyseal system discussed above.

Control of Anterior Pituitary Several trophic factors are produced in the hypothalamus and influence production of hormones in the anterior pituitary. Trophic factors are released into capillaries of the median eminence from which they reach the anterior pituitary via the hypophyseal portal circulation. In the anterior lobe, trophic factors act upon the appropriate chromophil cell to release or inhibit the appropriate trophic hormone. The anterior pituitary trophic hormones then act upon the appropriate target gland. The serum hormone level of the target gland has a feedback effect on hypothalamic trophic factors. The known hypothalamic trophic factors include corticotropin-releasing factor, which influences production of adrenocorticotropic hormone (ACTH) by the pituitary basophils; thyrotropin-releasing factor, which influences secretion of thyroid-stimulating hormone (TSH) from the basophils; gonadotropin-releasing factor, which influences production of follicle-stimulating and luteinizing hormones (LH) from the basophils; growth hormone-releasing factor, which influences growth hormone (GH) secretion from the acidophils; and prolactin-inhibiting factor, which inhibits production of prolactin from the acidophils.

Autonomic Regulation The hypothalamus is known to control brain stem autonomic centers. Stimulation or ablation of the hypothalamus influences cardiovascular, respiratory, and gastrointestinal functions. Autonomic influences are mediated via the dorsal longitudinal fasciculus and the mamillotegmental tract. Although definite delineation within the hypothalamus of sympathetic and parasympathetic centers is not feasible, it is generally held that the rostral hypothalamus is concerned with parasympathetic control, whereas the caudal hypothalamus is concerned with sympathetic control mechanisms.

Temperature Regulation Some regions of the hypothalamus are sensitive to changes in the temperature of blood perfusing these regions. Anterior regions of the hypothalamus are sensitive to a rise in blood temperature and trigger the mechanism for heat dissipation, which includes sweating and cutaneous vascular dilatation in man. Damage to this region, through surgery or by tumors or vascular lesions, results in elevation of body temperature (hyperthermia). In contrast, the posterior hypothalamic region is sensitive to the lowering of blood temperature and triggers the mechanism for heat conservation, which includes cessation of sweating, shivering, and vascular constriction.

Emotional Behavior The hypothalamus is a major component of the central compartment of the autonomic nervous system and as such plays a role in emotional behavior. Lesions of the ventromedial hypothalamic nuclei in animals are associated with a rage reaction characterized by hissing, snarling, biting, piloerection, arching of the back, and pupillary dilatation. Stimulation of some hypothalamic regions elicits a pleasurable response. Stimulation of other regions produces unpleasant responses, as evidenced by the attempts of such animals to avoid repetitive stimulation of these regions. The role of the hypothalamus in behavior and emotion is intimately related to that of the limbic system.

Feeding Behavior As detailed above, lesions in the ventromedial nucleus elicit hyperphagia (excessive feeding), whereas lesions in the lateral hypothalamus produce loss of hunger, suggesting the presence of a satiety center and feeding center, respectively, in these regions.

Drinking and Thirst In addition to the control of body water by ADH, stimulation of the lateral region of the hypothalamus elicits drinking behavior which persists in spite of overhydration. Lesions of the same area abolish thirst.

Sleep and Wakefulness The hypothalamus is believed to play a role in the daily sleep-wakefulness cycle. Such cycles are disturbed by lesions of the anterior hypothalamus.

Internal Capsule (Fig. 8–16)

The internal capsule is a broad compact band of nerve fibers that are continuous rostrally with the corona radiata and caudally with the cerebral peduncles. It contains afferent and efferent nerve fibers passing to and from the brain stem to the cerebral cortex. In horizontal sections of the cerebral hemispheres, the internal capsule is bent with a lateral concavity to fit the wedge-shaped lentiform nucleus. It is divided into an anterior limb, genu, posterior limb, retrolenticular part, and sublenticular part.

The anterior limb is sandwiched between the head of the caudate nucleus medially and the lentiform nucleus (putamen and globus pallidus) laterally. It contains frontopontine, thalamocortical, and corticothalamic bundles; the latter two bundles reciprocally connect the dorsomedial and anterior thalamic nuclei with the prefrontal cortex and cingulate gyrus. Some investigators add the caudatoputamenal interconnections to components of the anterior limb.

The genu of the internal capsule contains corticobulbar fibers which terminate upon motor nuclei of the brain stem. Evidence obtained from stimulation of the internal capsule during stereotaxic surgery and from vascular lesions of the internal capsule suggest, however, that corticobulbar fibers are located in the posterior third of the posterior limb rather than in the genu.

ANTERIOR LIMB
Frontopontine fibers
Thalamocortical fibers
Corticothalamic fibers
Caudatoputamenal fibers

CAUDATE

GENU
Corticobulbar fibers

PUTAMEN

GLOBUS PALLIDUS

THALAMUS

SUBLENTICULAR PART
Auditory radiation
Corticopontine
Visual radiation

MEDIAL GENICULATE

RETROLENTICULAR PART
Visual radiation
Corticotectal
Corticonigral
Corticotegmental

LATERAL GENICULATE

POSTERIOR LIMB
Corticospinal fibers
Corticorubral fibers
Corticothalamic fibers
Thalamocortical fibers

8–16 Schematic diagram showing component parts of the internal capsule and the fiber bundles within each component.

The posterior limb is bounded medially by the thalamus and laterally by the lentiform nucleus. It contains corticospinal and corticorubral fibers, as well as fibers that reciprocally connect the lateral group of thalamic nuclei (ventral lateral and ventral posterior) with the cerebral cortex. The corticospinal bundle is somatotopically organized in such a way that the fibers to the upper extremity are located more anteriorly, followed by fibers to the trunk and the lower extremity.

The retrolenticular part of the internal capsule contains corticotectal, corticonigral, and corticotegmental fibers, as well as part of the visual radiation.

The sublenticular part of the internal capsule contains corticopontine fibers, the auditory radiation, and part of the visual radiation.

References

Akert, K; Hartman-Von Monakow, K.; Künzle, H.: Projection of Precentral Motor Cortex upon Nucleus Medialis Dorsalis Thalami in Monkey. Neurosci Lett 11 (1979) 103–106.

Bertrand, G.: Stimulation during Stereotactic Operation for Dyskinesia. J Neurosurg 24 (1966) 419–423.

Blum, P.S.; Day, M.J.; Carpenter, M.B.; Gilman, S.: Thalamic Components of the Ascending Vestibular System. Exp Neurol 64 (1979) 587–603.

Donnan, G.A.; Tress, B.M.; Bladin, P.F.: A Prospective Study of Lacunar Infarction Using Computerized Tomography. Neurology 32 (1982) 49–56.

Groothuis, D.R.; Duncan, G.W.; Fisher, C. M.: The Human Thalamocortical Sensory Path in the Internal Capsule: Evidence from a Small Capsular Hemorrhage Causing a Pure Sensory Stroke. Ann Neurol 2 (1977) 328–331.

Hanaway, J.; Young, R.; Netsky, M., Adelman, L.: Localization of the Pyramidal Tract in the Internal Capsule. Neurology 31 (1981) 365–366.

Hendry, S.H.C.; Jones, E.G.; Graham, J.: Thalamic Relay Nuclei for Cerebellar and Certain Related Fiber Systems in the Cat. J Comp Neurol 185 (1979) 679–714.

Hirayama, K.; Tsubaki, T.; Toyokura, Y., Okinaka, S.: The Representation of the Pyramidal Tract in the Internal Capsule and Basis Pedunculi. A Study Based on Three Cases of Amyotrophic Lateral Sclerosis. Neurology 12 (1962) 337–342.

Madarasz, M.; Tömböl T.; Hajdu, F.; Somogyi, G.: A Combined Horseradish Peroxidase and Golgi Study on the Afferent Connections of the Ventrobasal Complex of the Thalamus in the Cat. Cell Tiss Res 199 (1979) 529–538.

McGuinness, C.M.; Krauthamer, G.M.: The Afferent Projections to the Centrum Medianum of the Cat as Demonstrated by Retrograde Transport of Horseradish Peroxidase. Brain Res 184 (1980) 255–269.

Miller, J.W.; Benevento, L.A.: Demonstration of a Direct Projection from the Intralaminar Central Lateral Nucleus to the Primary Visual Cortex. Neurosci Lett 14 (1979) 229–234.

Nomura, S.; Itoh, K.; Mizuno, N.: Topographical Arrangement of Thalamic Neurons Projecting to the Orbital Gyrus in the Cat. Exp Neurol 67 (1980) 601–610.

Royce, G.J.: Cells of Origin of Subcortical Afferents to the Caudate Nucleus: A Horseradish Peroxidase Study in the Cat. Brain Res 153 (1978) 465–475.

Goldman, P. S.: Contralateral Projections to the Dorsal Thalamus from Frontal Association Cortex in the Rhesus Monkey. Brain Res 166 (1979) 166–171.

Tekian, A.; Afifi, A.K.: Efferent Connections of the Pulvinar Nucleus in the Cat. J Anat 132 (1981) 249–265.

9

Basal Ganglia

Terminology

The term basal ganglia has carried varying connotations from time to time. Early anatomists used it to refer to all of the nuclear masses in the interior of the brain, including the thalamus. Currently, the term is used to refer to the following nuclei.

1. Caudate
2. Putamen
3. Globus pallidus
4. Amygdaloid nucleus
5. Claustrum

Functionally, the caudate, putamen, and globus pallidus are more closely related, whereas the amygdaloid nucleus is functionally a part of the limbic system. The function and connections of the claustrum, a gray mass located lateral to the putamen, are not well understood.

The term extrapyramidal system is used to refer to the basal ganglia and their associated brain stem nuclei. It includes, in addition to the basal ganglia, the following nuclei.

1. Red nucleus
2. Subthalamic nucleus
3. Substantia nigra
4. Reticular formation

The extrapyramidal system plays an important role in motor control.

The term corpus striatum refers to the caudate, putamen, and globus pallidus, which appear striated in myelin preparations because of the myelinated fibers traversing these gray masses. The term striatum or neostriatum refers to the caudate and putamen nuclei. The term lenticular nucleus refers to the putamen and globus pallidus. The term pallidum refers to the globus pallidus. The terms neostriatum, paleostriatum, and archistriatum refer to the caudate-putamen, globus pallidus, and amygdaloid nucleus, respectively.

Neostriatum

Caudate Nucleus

The caudate nucleus is a C-shaped structure with an expanded rostral extremity, the head, which tapers down in size to form a body and a tail. The head of the caudate bears a constant and characteristic relationship to the anterior horn of the lateral ventricle. This part of the caudate characteristically bulges into the ventricle. In degenerative central nervous diseases involving the caudate nucleus, such as chorea, this bulge is lost and the lateral surface of the ventricle becomes flat or even slightly concave. While the head of the caudate is related to the lateral wall of the anterior horn of the lateral ventricle, the tail of the caudate occupies a position in the roof of the inferior horn of the lateral ventricle.

Putamen

The putamen is located lateral to the globus pallidus and medial to the external capsule. It is separated from the caudate nucleus by the internal capsule, except rostrally, where the head of the caudate and the putamen are continuous around the anterior limb of the internal capsule.

Histologically, the structures of the caudate and putamen are similar. The majority of neurons are small (10 to 15 μm); some large neurons, however, are present. Nerve fibers traversing both nuclei are small in diameter and are either thinly myelinated or nonmyelinated. The latter observation explains the difficulties encountered by early investigators using myelin degeneration techiques in studying the fiber connections of these nuclei. Small neurons are primarily receptive and associative in function, although some contribute to the outflow from the neostriatum. Most of the outflow fibers from the neostriatum, however, arise from the large neurons. Recent studies in the cat have challenged the proposed role of small and large neurons by suggesting that the small neurons, rather than the large ones, are the major source of outflow projections from the neostriatum. Synaptic terminals within the caudate nucleus have been demonstrated with either clear acetylcholine-containing vesicles or dense catecholamine-containing vesicles.

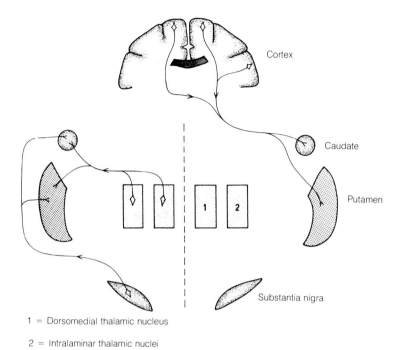

Cortex

Caudate

Putamen

1

2

Substantia nigra

1 = Dorsomedial thalamic nucleus

2 = Intralaminar thalamic nuclei

9-1 Schematic diagram showing the major afferent connections of the neostriatum.

Neostriatal Connections

Afferent connections to the neostriatum (Fig. 9–1) arise from the following sources.

Cerebral Cortex Wide areas of the cerebral cortex project in axodendritic and axosomatic terminals upon neostriate neurons in a topographic manner. Most of these cortical fibers arise from the sensory motor cortex in the frontal and parietal lobes, but other cortical areas also contribute to this system. Corticostriate fibers reach the neostriatum via the external and internal capsules as well as via the subcallosal fasciculus. Corticostriate connections are ipsilateral, except those from the sensorimotor and supplementary motor cortices, which are bilateral.

Much overlap has been demonstrated in corticostriate connections so that no part of the neostriatum is under the sole control of one cortical area. Some of the corticostriate connections are short latency direct pro-

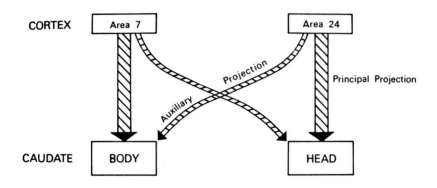

9-2 Schematic diagram showing the two types of corticostriate projections: principal and auxiliary.

jections to the neostriatum; others are long latency indirect projections via the thalamus. The latter are considered of importance in coordinating basal ganglia and cerebellar activities. Collateral projections to the neostriatum have been demonstrated to arise from cortico-olivary and corticopontine projections.

Recent anatomic studies on corticostriate projections, using axonal transport methods, have suggested the existence of two types of projections: principal and auxiliary. A cortical area, area 7, has been shown to send a principal projection to the body of the caudate and an auxiliary projection to the head of the caudate. Another cortical area, area 24, has been shown to send a principal projection to the head of the caudate and an auxiliary connection to the body of the caudate. These cortical areas (7 and 24) are known to be interconnected via corticocortical association fibers. Thus, cortical areas related via reciprocal corticocortical connections project, in part, to similar areas within the caudate nucleus (Fig. 9–2).

Thalamus Thalamostriate fibers arise primarily from the intralaminar and dorsomedial nuclei of the thalamus.

Substantia Nigra Nigrostriate connections are now well established by anatomic and physiologic techniques. These connections play an important role in motor control and their interruption contributes to the genesis of parkinsonism. The nigrostriate connections to the caudate nucleus are of two varieties. These are a classic cholinergic fiber system in which the neurotransmitter is acetylcholine and a dopaminergic system in which the neurotransmitter is dopamine. A disturbance in the balance between these two systems contributes to parkinsonism.

Efferent connections from the neostriatum project upon the following areas.

Globus Pallidus   The neostriatum projects to the pallidum via the stria-
topallidal tract.

Substantia Nigra (Striatonigral Tract)   The substantia nigra is an intermediate station in a system through which caudate neurons influence the
thalamus.

Globus Pallidus

The globus pallidus is a wedge-shaped nuclear mass located between the
putamen and internal capsule. A lamina of fibers (external pallidal lamina)
separates the globus pallidus from the putamen. Another lamina (internal
pallidal lamina) divides the globus pallidus into a larger lateral and a smaller
medial segment. Neurons of the globus pallidus are of the large multipolar
variety. The entopeduncular nucleus of nonprimate mammals is part of
the medial pallidal segment in primate mammals.

Afferent Connections

Afferent connections (Fig. 9–3) to pallidum are mainly from three sources.

Subthalamic Nucleus   Rich reciprocal connections exist between the
subthalamic nucleus and the globus pallidus via the subthalamic fasciculus.

Neostriatum   Fibers from both the caudate and putamen terminate upon
the globus pallidus.

Substantia Nigra   Nigropallidal fibers have been described by some investigators.

Efferent Connections

Efferent connections (Fig. 9–3) of the globus pallidus project to the following areas.

Subthalamic Nucleus   The globus pallidus projects via the subthalamic
fasciculus which traverses the internal capsule.

Thalamus   Pallidothalamic fibers project via the ansa and fasciculus
lenticularis. The globus pallidus is the source of the efferent outflow of the
basal ganglia. Pallidothalamic fibers follow one of two routes. Some traverse the internal capsule and gather dorsal to the subthalamic nucleus as
the lenticular fasciculus (H_2 field of Forel); others pass around the internal
capsule (ansa lenticularis). Both groups of fibers gather together to form

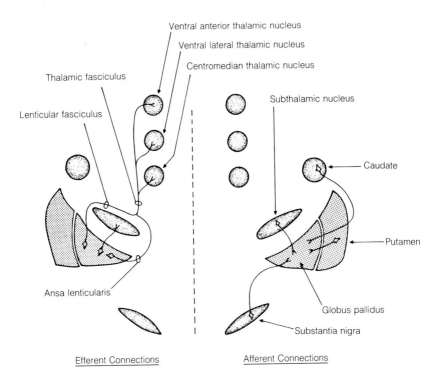

Ventral anterior thalamic nucleus

Ventral lateral thalamic nucleus

Centromedian thalamic nucleus

Thalamic fasciculus

Lenticular fasciculus

Subthalamic nucleus

Caudate

Putamen

Ansa lenticularis

Globus pallidus

Substantia nigra

Efferent Connections

Afferent Connections

9-3   Schematic diagram showing the major afferent and efferent connections of the globus pallidus.

the prerubral field (H field of Forel) and then join the thalamic fasciculus (H_1 field of Forel) to reach the ventral anterior nucleus of the thalamus, with some going to the ventrolateral nucleus, reticular nucleus, and centromedian nucleus of the thalamus. Pallidal projections to the thalamus are somatotopically organized so that the rostral pallidum projects to the ventral anterior nucleus, while the caudal pallidum projects to the ventral lateral thalamic nucleus.

Other Pallidal Efferents   These include projections to the inferior olive via the central tegmental tract and to the reticular nuclei of the brain stem via pallidoreticular fibers. Pallidal efferents have also been described projecting to the neostriatum, substantia nigra (pars compacta), habenular nucleus, and cortex.

Recent evidence suggests that while the two pallidal segments have similar inputs, their outputs are distinctively different. The lateral pallidal segment projects to the subthalamic nucleus, reticular nucleus of the thalamus, neostriatum, substantia nigra (pars compacta), and cortex. The medial pallidal segment projects to the ventral anterior, ventral lateral, and intralaminar nuclei of the thalamus, habenular nucleus, and mesencephalic tegmentum.

Telencephalic-Striatal Organization

Based on such criteria as common internal histology, similar input-output patterns, and characteristic neurotransmitters, the telencephalic-striatal complex has been organized into three concentric tiers. The outermost tier (tier I or cortex) includes the neo- and allocortices. The second tier (tier II or neostriatum) includes the caudate nucleus, putamen, and nucleus accumbens septi (a nuclear group separated from the caudate nucleus by the frontal horn of the lateral ventricle). The third tier (tier III or pallidum) is composed of the lateral and medial segments of the globus pallidus, substantia innominata (a nuclear group separated from the globus pallidus by the anterior commissure), and the substantia nigra (pars reticulata). The components of each tier share common histologic characteristics, common diencephalic input, and a characteristic pattern of monoaminergic innervation.

Tier I receives a major diencephalic input from the dorsomedial and ventrolateral thalamic nuclei and a monoamine input which is noradrenergic. Tier II receives a diencephalic input from the intralaminar thalamic nuclei and a monoamine input which is dopaminergic from the midbrain. Tier III receives a diencephalic input from the subthalamic nucleus and a serotonergic monoamine input from the midbrain raphe nuclei. The three tiers are interconnected through their projection fiber system. Practically every area of tier I projects to tier II. Similarly, every area of tier II projects to tier III. The volume and number of neurons in each tier diminish from tier I to tier III; thus the whole system resembles a funnel. Although there is considerable circumferential interaction within tier I (corticocortical association fiber system), the same is not true of tiers II and III.

In contrast to the converging projections from tier I to II and from tier II to III, the projections from tier III are divergent and widespread, reaching the epithalamus, thalamus, subthalamus, superior colliculus, midbrain tegmentum, substantia nigra, caudate nucleus, putamen, and, possibly, cortex. This divergent and extensive output is in marked contrast to the classic concept of the corpus striatum with output solely directed at the

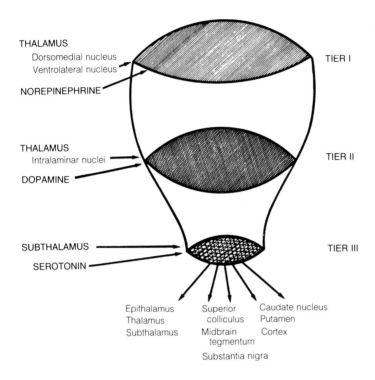

THALAMUS
Dorsomedial nucleus
Ventrolateral nucleus

NOREPINEPHRINE

TIER I

THALAMUS
Intralaminar nuclei

DOPAMINE

TIER II

SUBTHALAMUS

SEROTONIN

TIER III

Epithalamus   Superior   Caudate nucleus
Thalamus   colliculus   Putamen
Subthalamus   Midbrain   Cortex
             tegmentum
          Substantia nigra

9–4 Schematic diagram illustrating the concept of telencephalic-striatal organization.

motor cortex via thalamic nuclei. Figure 9–4 is a diagrammatic representation of the concepts presented above.

Functional Considerations

In spite of the voluminous neuroanatomic and neurophysiologic data available on the basal ganglia, knowledge of their function remains elementary and full of discrepancies. From the available data, however, the following statements summarize the major functional aspects of the corpus striatum.

Caudate Nucleus

Rapid stimulation of the caudate nucleus in experimental unanesthetized animals elicits turning movements of the head and circling of the animal away from the direction of the stimulus. On the other hand, low frequency stimulation or chronic stimulation results in cessation of ongoing motor activity and sleep.

Unilateral ablation of the caudate nucleus in animals coupled with administration of L-dopa elicits circling movements toward the ablated side. Bilateral ablation results in the phenomenon of "forced progression," in which the animal has an irresistible tendency to move straight ahead.

In general, the caudate seems to have an inhibitory function on cortically induced motor activity.

Putamen

Stimulation and ablation experiments on the putamen result in manifestations indistinguishable from those observed after similar procedures on the caudate.

Globus Pallidus

Stimulation of the globus pallidus produces contraversive running movement. Prolonged stimulation produces contralateral tremor.

Unilateral ablation of the globus pallidus produces little or no effect. Bilateral ablation, however, produces a hypoactive sleepy animal which seldom moves around or even changes position.

Clinical Correlation

Basal ganglia disorders in man are categorized as hyperkinetic and hypokinetic. The hyperkinetic category includes such clinical entities as chorea, athetosis, and ballism. The hypokinetic variety occurs in parkinsonism.

Chorea

Chorea is a disorder of movement characterized by sudden, involuntary, purposeless, and quick jerks of the extremities and head associated with facial grimaces. The lesion producing chorea is believed to be in the caudate nucleus. Two varieties of chorea are known to occur. These are a benign, reversible variety (Sydenham's chorea) occurring in children as a complication of rheumatic fever and a malignant variety (Huntington's chorea) which is a hereditary disorder associated with mental deficiency and progressive deterioration.

Athetosis

Athetosis is a disorder of movement characterized by slow, writhing, worm-like movements of the distal parts of the extremities, chiefly in the fingers, which show bizarre posturing. The lesion producing athetosis is probably in the putamen.

Ballism

Ballism is a disorder of movement caused by a lesion in the subthalamic nucleus. The movements of the limbs in this disorder may be unusually violent and are flinging in nature.

Parkinsonism

Parkinson's disease is a disorder characterized by tremor, rigidity, and hypo- or akinesia.

The tremor of Parkinson's disease is rhythmic fine tremor recurring at the rate of 3 to 6 cps and is best seen when the extremity is in a fixed posture rather than in motion.

The rigidity is characterized by resistance to passive movement of a joint throughout the range of motion (cogwheel rigidity), resulting from an increase in tone of muscles with opposing action (agonists and antagonists).

Hypokinesia or akinesia is manifested by a diminution or loss of associated movements, slow movement, and expressionless facies.

The lesion producing Parkinson's disease is widespread in the central nervous system but affects the substantia nigra most consistently. The lesion affects the dopaminergic nigrocaudate fiber system and depletes the nigrocaudate dopamine stores. The disease can be ameliorated by administration of L-dopa. Extensive studies on the genesis of parkinsonism have elucidated the existence of two fiber systems between the substantia nigra and striatum; these are an inhibitory dopaminergic system and excitatory cholinergic system.

Reduced activity of the dopaminergic system releases the globus pallidus and sets in motion a series of events in the ventrolateral nucleus of the thalamus and the motor cortex culminating in the genesis of the rhythmic tremor of parkinsonism.

Prior to the discovery of the significance of L-dopa in parkinsonism, the tremor and rigidity of parkinsonism were treated by surgical lesions either in the globus pallidus or the ventrolateral nucleus of the thalamus. The former was more effective in the relief of rigidity and the latter in the relief of tremor. These surgical procedures are still used as an adjunct mode of therapy to L-dopa.

The abnormal movements of basal ganglia disorders all disappear during sleep and are best seen when the extremities are in static posture rather than in motion. This is in contrast to cerebellar tremor which is best seen when the extremity is in motion.

It is evident from the above that the basal ganglia play an important role in motor control. They exert this control via two systems, the thalamo-cortical and corticospinal pathways and the nigroreticular and reticulospinal pathways. Thus, there is no direct connection from the basal ganglia onto the final common path in the spinal cord.

Pharmacology

Many neurotransmitters have been demonstrated in the basal ganglia: dopamine, acetylcholine, serotonin, substance P, enkephalins, L-glutamic acid, and gamma-aminobutyric acid (GABA). Dopamine, stored in neurons of the substantia nigra (zona compacta), is the inhibitory neurotransmitter in the nigrostriatal system and exerts its influence on cholinergic interneurons of the neostriatum. Two types of interneurons have been identified in the neostriatum: cholinergic and enkephalinergic. Glutamic acid is believed to be the neurotransmitter in the corticostriatal projection system. Serotonin has been demonstrated in the projection of the raphe nuclei of the brain stem upon the substantia nigra and striatum. Substance P and GABA have been identified as neurotransmitters in the striatopallidonigral system. The highest levels of GABA in mammalian brains have been shown in the neostriatum, pallidum, and substantia nigra. Within the neostriatum, most GABA is located within inhibitory interneurons, although some is present in output (principal) neurons, with terminals which synapse in the pallidum and substantia nigra. Some studies suggest the presence of a major GABA pathway arising in the pallidum and terminating upon dopaminergic neurons in the substantia nigra. The striatopallidonigral GABA pathway exerts an inhibitory influence on target dopaminergic cells. Figure 9–5 is a proposed schema of neurotransmitter pathways in the basal ganglia. The noradrenergic input shown in the diagram arises from cell bodies in the hindbrain, the largest group of which is the locus ceruleus.

Parkinsonism

The pharmacology of parkinsonism consists of selective depletion of dopaminergic neurons in the substantia nigra (zona compacta). As a result of this, two events occur. The first is a loss of tonic inhibitory dopaminergic influence on striatal cholinergic interneurons (Fig. 9–5), resulting in increased release of acetylcholine and excessive stimulation of postsynaptic

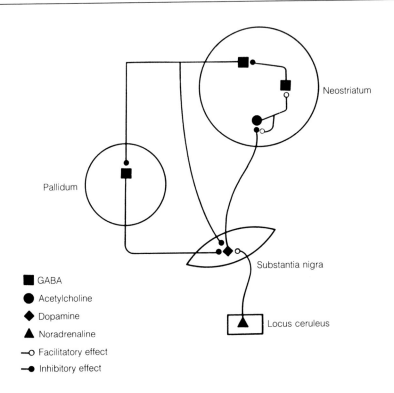

9–5 Schematic diagram showing neurotransmitter pathways in the basal ganglia.

muscarinic receptors. The second event consists of an increase in density and in sensitivity of dopamine receptors due to depletion of dopamine (denervation supersensitivity).

Huntington's Chorea

In Huntington's chorea, there is a progressive degeneration of striatal neurons. As a result of this, three events occur. The first is a loss of cholinergic interneurons in the striatum, resulting in decreased postsynaptic activation of muscarinic receptors. The second is a loss of the striatonigral GABA-ergic inhibitory feedback pathway (Fig. 9–5), resulting in disinhibition of GABA-ergic neurons. The third event consists of a relative enrichment of dopaminergic terminals with resultant functional hyperinnervation by dopaminergic pathways.

References

Cherubini, E.; Novak, G.; Hull, C.D.; Buchwald, N.A.; Levine, M.S.: Caudate Neuronal Responses Evoked by Cortical Stimulation: Contribution of an Indirect Corticothalamic Pathway. Brain Res 173 (1979) 331–336.

Divac, I.; Diemer, N.H.: Prefrontal System in the Rat Visualized by Means of Labelled Deoxyglucose. Further Evidence for Functional Heterogeneity of the Neostriatum. J Comp Neurol 190 (1980) 1–13.

Fallon, J.H.; Ziegler, B.T.S.: The Crossed Cortico-Caudate Projection in the Rhesus Monkey. Neurosci Lett 15 (1979) 29–32.

Filion, M.; Harnois, C.: A Comparison of Projections of Entopeduncular Neurons to the Thalamus, the Midbrain and the Habenula in the Cat. J Comp Neurol 181 (1978) 763–780.

Graybiel, A.M.; Ragsdale, C.W., Jr.; Moon Edley, S.: Compartments in the Striatum of the Cat Observed by Retrograde Cell Labeling. Exp Brain Res 34 (1979) 189–195.

Jinnai, K.; Matsuda, Y.: Neurons of the Motor Cortex Projecting Commonly on the Caudate Nucleus and the Lower Brain Stem in the Cat. Neurosci Lett 13 (1979) 121–126.

Kemp, J.M.; Powell, T.P.S.: The Cortico-Striate Projection in the Monkey. Brain 93 (1970) 525–546.

Nauta, H.J.W.: A Proposed Conceptual Reorganization of the Basal Ganglia and Telencephalon. Neuroscience 4 (1979) 1875–1881.

Spokes, E.G.S.: Neurochemical Alterations in Huntington's Chorea. A Study of Post-Mortem Brain Tissue. Brain 103 (1980) 179–210.

Yeterian, E.H.; Van Hoesen, G.W.: Corticostriate Projections in the Rhesus Monkey: The Organization of Certain Cortico-Caudate Connections. Brain Res 139 (1978) 43–63.

10

Cerebellum

Gross Features

The cerebellum or "small brain" is a development of the rhombic lip, a zone of cells between the alar and roof plates at the level of the pontine flexure. Although it develops from a "sensory" region, the cerebellum is concerned primarily (but not exclusively) with motor function.

The cerebellum is located in the posterior fossa of the skull, separated from the occipital lobes by a dural fold, the tentorium cerebelli. It overlies the dorsal portions of the pons and medulla and contributes to the formation of the roof of the fourth ventricle.

The cerebellum consists of a midline vermis and two laterally placed hemispheres. The parts of the hemispheres adjacent to the vermis are known as the paravermal or intermediate zones. (Fig. 10–1).

The dorsal cerebellar surface is rather flat, with a midline elevation; the demarcation of vermis and hemispheres is not evident on this surface. The inferior surface is convex with a deep groove (vallecula) in the midline through which the inferior vermis is apparent.

In midsagittal sections, the cerebellum is divided by two fissures into three lobes (Fig. 10–2). The most rostrally placed lobe is the anterior lobe. This lobe is separated from the posterior lobe by the primary fissure. The posterior lobe is separated from the most caudally placed lobe, the flocculonodular lobe, by the posterolateral (prenodular) fissure. Each of these lobes is divided into lobules which are in turn subdivided into folia. The different lobules and folia are separated by fissures or sulci that have no functional significance. The posterior lobe contains the cerebellar tonsils.

Tonsillar herniation through the foramen magnum resulting from an increase in intracranial pressure is a neurosurgical emergency, a life-threatening situation due to compromise of vital centers in the brain stem.

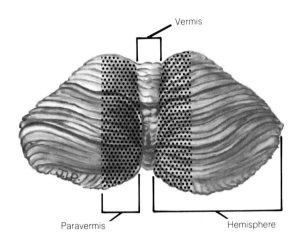

10–1   Schematic diagram showing the subdivisions of the cerebellum.

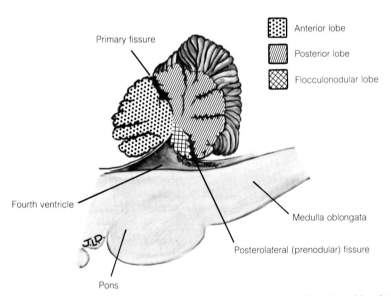

10–2   Schematic diagram showing the three lobes of the cerebellum in midsagittal section.

Phylogenetically, the cerebellum is divided into three zones. The archicerebellum, the oldest zone, corresponds to the flocculonodular lobe and is related functionally to the vestibular system. The paleocerebellum, of more recent phylogenetic development than the archicerebellum, corresponds to the anterior lobe and a small part of the posterior lobe. This

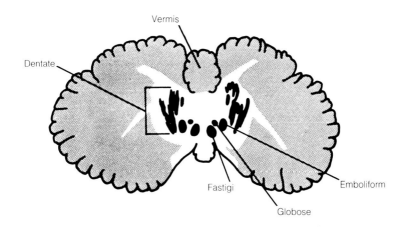

Vermis

Dentate

Fastigi

Globose

Emboliform

10–3 Schematic diagram showing the spatial arrangement of the deep cerebellar nuclei.

zone is functionally related to the spinal cord and is concerned with posture, muscle tone, and gait. The neocerebellum, the most recent phylogenetically, corresponds to the posterior lobe. This zone is functionally related to the corticopontocerebellar system and through this system it exerts a regulating effect on the discrete movement of limbs.

The adult human cerebellum weighs approximately 150 gm (10% of brain weight) and has a surface area of approximately 1000 cm² (40% of that of the cerebral cortex).

The cerebellum is connected to the midbrain, pons, and medulla oblongata by three pairs of peduncles.

1. The superior cerebellar peduncle (brachium conjunctivum) connects the cerebellum with the midbrain.
2. The middle cerebellar peduncle (brachium pontis) connects the cerebellum with the pons.
3. The inferior cerebellar peduncle (restiform and juxtarestiform bodies) connects the cerebellum with the medulla oblongata.

The contents of each of these peduncles are discussed in the chapters on the mesencephalon, pons, and medulla oblongata.

The cerebellum consists of a highly convoluted layer of gray matter, the cerebellar cortex, surrounding a core of white matter which contains the afferent and efferent tracts. Embedded in the white matter core are four pairs of deep cerebellar nuclei (Fig. 10–3).

1. Fastigial nucleus
2. Globose nucleus
3. Emboliform nucleus
4. Dentate nucleus

The globose and emboliform nuclei are referred to collectively as the interposed nucleus.

Unlike the cerebral cortex, body representation in the cerebellum is patchy. In the anterior lobe, the body appears inverted with the hindlimbs represented rostral to the forelimbs. In the posterior lobe, the body appears noninverted and dually represented on each side of the midline.

Microscopic Structure

The cerebellar cortex is made up of the following three layers.

1. Outermost molecular layer (about 300 μm in thickness)
2. Middle Purkinje cell layer (about 100 μm in thickness)
3. Innermost granule cell layer (about 200 μm in thickness)

The cerebellar cortex contains five cell types distributed in the different cortical layers. Basket and stellate cells are in the molecular layer, Purkinje cells are in the Purkinje cell layer, and granule and Golgi cells are in the granule cell layer.

Of these five cell types, the Purkinje cell constitutes the principal neuron of the cerebellum, since it is the only cerebellar neuron that sends its axons outside the cerebellum. All of the other cells of the cerebellum are therefore intrinsic neurons and establish connections within the cerebellum.

Principal Neuron

Cell bodies of Purkinje cells (Fig. 10–4) are arranged in a single sheet at the border zone between the molecular and granule cell layers. The cell is flask-shaped when viewed in the transverse plane and is narrow and vertical when viewed in longitudinal sections. The Purkinje cell measures approximately 30 to 35 μm in tranverse diameter. Adjacent Purkinje cells are separated by 50 μm in the transverse plane and by 50 to 100 μm in the longitudinal plane. Each Purkinje cell has an elaborate dendritic tree that stretches throughout the extent of the molecular layer and is arranged at right angles to the long axis of the folium. The dendritic tree is made up of a sequence of primary, secondary, and tertiary branches, with the smaller dendritic branches profusely covered with dendritic spines or gemmules. It is estimated that each Purkinje cell has over 150,000 spines on its dendritic tree.

Each Purkinje cell has a single axon that courses through the granule cell layer and deep white matter to project upon deep cerebellar nuclei. Some Purkinje cell axons (from the vermis) bypass the deep cerebellar nuclei to reach the lateral vestibular nucleus. Recurrent collateral axonal branches arise from Purkinje cell axons and project upon adjacent Purkinje

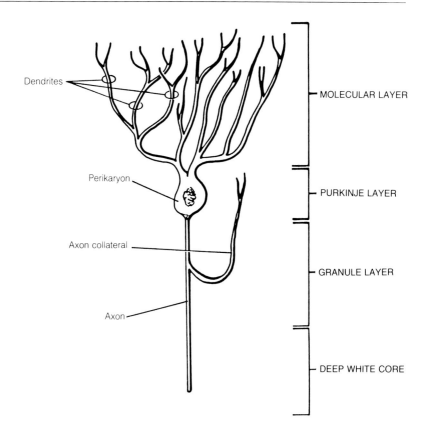

Dendrites

MOLECULAR LAYER

Perikaryon

PURKINJE LAYER

Axon collateral

GRANULE LAYER

Axon

DEEP WHITE CORE

10–4 Schematic diagram of the components of a Purkinje cell and their spatial relationships to cerebellar layers.

cells as well as upon basket, stellate and Golgi cells in neighboring or even distant folia. It is estimated that there are about 15 million Purkinje cells in the human cerebellum.

Intrinsic Neurons

Basket Cell Basket cells (Fig. 10–5) are situated in deeper parts of the molecular layer in close proximity to Purkinje cells. Dendritic arborizations of basket cells are disposed in the transverse plane of the folium in a manner similar to but less elaborate than the Purkinje cells. The axon courses in the molecular layer in the transverse plane of the folium just above the cell bodies of Purkinje cells. Each axon gives rise to several descending branches that surround Purkinje cell perikarya and initial segments of their axons in the form of a basket, hence their name. Each basket cell axon

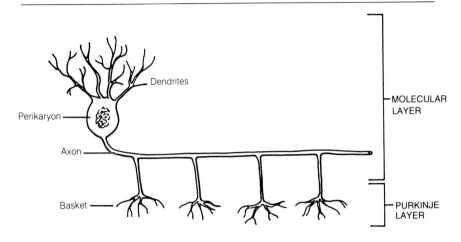

10–5 Schematic diagram of the components of a basket cell and their spatial relationships to cerebellar layers.

covers the territory of about 10 Purkinje cells. Basket formation, however, skips the Purkinje cell immediately adjacent to the basket cell and descends upon the second Purkinje cell and onward in the row. In addition, axonal branches extend in the longitudinal plane of the folium to reach an additional three to six rows of Purkinje cells on both sides of the main axons. As a result of this, a single basket cell may reach as many as 200 Purkinje cells. More than one basket cell may contribute to a single basket formation around one Purkinje cell. While the descending branches of basket cell axons establish contact with Purkinje cell perikarya and initial segments of their axons, ascending branches of basket cell axons ascend in the molecular layer to reach the proximal dendrites of Purkinje cells. It is estimated that there are about seven million basket cells in the human cerebellum.

Stellate Cell Stellate cells (Fig 10–6) are located in the superficial and deeper parts of the molecular layer. Dendrites of stellate cells are also disposed transversely in the folium and terminate upon Purkinje cell dendrites. It is estimated that there are 12 million stellate cells in the human cerebellum.

The basket and stellate cells can be considered as belonging to the same class. Both receive the same input and both act upon Purkinje cells. The difference lies in the fact that stellate cells establish contact with the dendrites of Purkinje cells, whereas basket cells establish contact with dendrites, perikarya, and axons of Purkinje cells.

Granule Cell Granule cells (Fig 10–7) are among the smallest cells in the brain (6 to 9 μm) and fill the granule cell layer. Each cell gives rise to about three to five dendrites that establish synaptic contacts with axons in

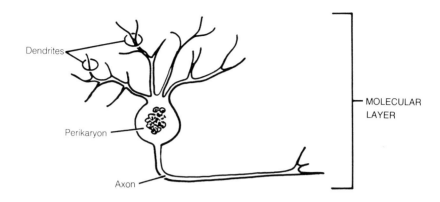

10–6 Schematic diagram of the components of a stellate cell and their orientation in the molecular layer.

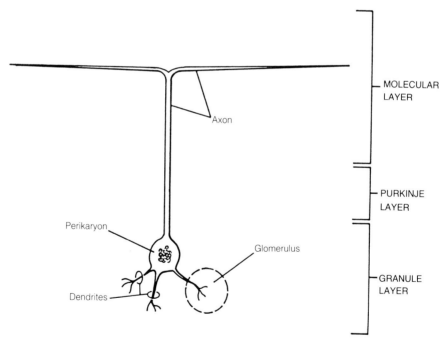

10–7 Schematic diagram of the components of a granule cell and their spatial relationships to cerebellar layers.

a synaptic zone within the granule cell layer, the glomerulus. Axons of granule cells ascend in the granule cell layer, the Purkinje layer, and the molecular layer, where they bifurcate in a T fashion to form the parallel fiber system, which runs horizontally in the molecular layer perpendicular to the plane of the Purkinje dendrites. Each parallel fiber branch is 1 to 1.5 mm in length; thus, the axon of a single granule cell spans an area of

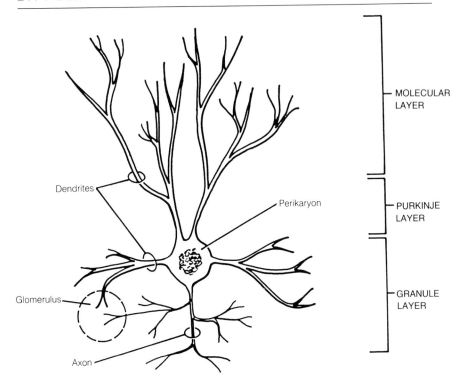

10–8 Schematic diagram of the components of a Golgi cell and their spatial relationships to cerebellar layers.

approximately 3 mm. The parallel fibers establish contact with dendrites of Purkinje cells, Golgi cells, stellate cells, and basket cells. Generally, a parallel fiber comes in contact with a Purkinje cell only once or, rarely, twice. A single Purkinje cell, however, can receive up to 100,000 parallel fibers. The total number of granule cells is estimated to be in the order of 2.2 billion.

Golgi Type II Cell Golgi neurons (Fig. 10–8) occupy the superficial part of the granule cell layer adjacent to the Purkinje cells. They are large neurons, about the same size as the Purkinje cell bodies. Dendrites of Golgi neurons arborize either in the molecular or granule cell layer. Those that remain in the granule cell layer contribute to the glomerulus of that layer. Those that reach the molecular layer arborize widely and overlap the territories of three Purkinje cells in both the transverse and longitudinal planes. The Golgi neuron dendritic arborization is thus three times that of the Purkinje cell.

Axons of Golgi cells take part in the formation of the glomerulus. They are characterized by a dense arborization of short axonal branches that

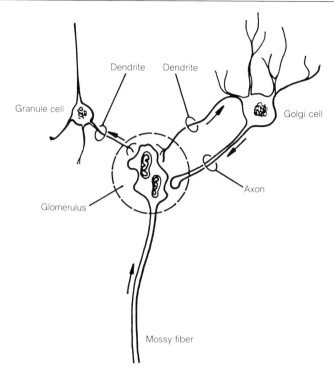

10–9 Schematic diagram of a cerebellar glomerulus showing the different sources of converging fibers.

span the entire granule cell layer. The field of axonal arborization approaches that of dendritic arborization. The axonal arborization of the Golgi neurons is among the most unique in the brain. It is estimated that there are four million Golgi cells. The Golgi neuron forms the central point of a functional hexagon within the cerebellar cortex. The hexagon includes about 10 Purkinje cells.

Cerebellar Glomerulus

In histologic sections of the cerebellar cortex, there are islands between granule cells which stain lighter than the rest of the granule cell layer. These are the cerebellar glomeruli (Fig. 10–9). Such islands are the sites of synaptic contact between the incoming cerebellar fibers (mossy fiber system) and processes of neurons within the granule cell layer. The elements that form a cerebellar glomerulus are the following.

1. Cerebellar input via the mossy fiber system (origins of this system will be discussed later)
2. Dendrites of granule cells

3. Axon terminals of Golgi neurons
4. Proximal parts of Golgi dendrites

Electron micrographs have shown that the mossy fiber axonal terminal is the central element in the glomerulus around which are clustered dendrites of granule cells and axons of Golgi neurons. Both mossy fiber axons and Golgi axons act upon the dendrites of granule cells. In addition, mossy fiber axons project upon dendrites of Golgi neurons. The whole complex is surrounded by a glial envelope. It is estimated that a glomerulus contains about 100 to 300 dendritic terminals from some 20 granule cells.

Cerebellar Input

Fiber input to the cerebellum arrives via three peduncles; these are the inferior cerebellar peduncle (restiform body), the middle cerebellar peduncle (brachium pontis), and the superior cerebellar peduncle (brachium conjunctivum).

Inferior Cerebellar Peduncle

The fiber systems reaching the cerebellum via this peduncle are the following.

1. Dorsal spinocerebellar tract
2. Cuneocerebellar tract
3. Olivocerebellar tract
4. Reticulocerebellar tract
5. Vestibulocerebellar tract (both primary afferents from the vestibular end organ and secondary afferents from the vestibular nuclei)
6. Arcuatocerebellar tract
7. Trigeminocerebellar tract (from the spinal and main sensory nuclei of the trigeminal nerve)

Middle Cerebellar Peduncle

The fiber system reaching the cerebellum via this route is the corticopontocerebellar tract.

Superior Cerebellar Peduncle

The fiber input to the cerebellum via this route includes the ventral spinocerebellar tract and the tectocerebellar tract from both superior and inferior colliculi. An additional input from the locus ceruleus is now established; it projects upon Purkinje cell dendrites and exerts an inhibitory effect upon Purkinje cell activity. It has been postulated that this input from the locus ceruleus plays a role in the development of Purkinje cells. The terminals from the locus ceruleus develop prior to Purkinje cell maturation. Destruction of the locus ceruleus results in immature development of Purkinje cells. The input from all these sources brings to the cerebellum information from: 1) exteroceptors, 2) proprioceptors, 3) reticular formation of the brain stem, and 4) cerebral cortex.

The input to the cerebellum reaches the cerebellar cortex after traversing the deep core of white matter. It is customary to classify this input into the climbing fiber system and mossy fiber system.

Climbing Fiber System   The fiber tracts that constitute the climbing fiber system are not known with absolute certainty. It is, however, generally believed that the olivocerebellar tract is the major component of this system.

This climbing fiber input establishes synapses on dendrites of the principal neuron of the cerebellum (the Purkinje cell), as well as on dendrites of intrinsic neurons (Golgi, basket, and stellate). The climbing fiber input is known to exert a powerful excitatory effect on a single Purkinje cell and a much less powerful effect on the intrinsic neurons. The relationship of climbing fibers to principal neurons is so intimate that one climbing fiber is restricted to one Purkinje cell and follows the branches of the Purkinje cell dendrites like a grapevine. The climbing fiber effect on a Purkinje cell is thus one to one, all or none excitation. It is estimated that one climbing fiber establishes 1,000 to 2,000 synaptic contacts with its Purkinje cell. Stimulation of the climbing fiber system elicits a prolonged burst of high frequency action potentials from the Purkinje cell capable of overriding any ongoing activity in that cell.

Mossy Fiber System   The mossy fiber system includes all afferents to the cerebellum except those that contribute to the climbing fibers. Like the climbing fibers, mossy fibers enter the cerebellum via the core of deep white matter. They then diverge into the folia of the cerebellum, where they branch out into the granule cell layer. Within the granule cell layer, the branches divide into several subbranches or terminal rosettes which occupy the center of each glomerulus. It is estimated that each mossy fiber establishes contact with approximately 400 granule cell dendrites within a single folium and that each terminal mossy rosette contacts approximately 20 different granule cells. On the other hand, each granule cell receives synaptic contacts from four to five different mossy fiber terminals. The mossy fiber is believed to stimulate the largest number of cells to be activated by a single afferent fiber. Thus, in contrast to the climbing fiber input, which is highly specific and sharply focused upon the Purkinje cell, the mossy fiber input is diffuse and complex (Fig. 10–10). In addition to

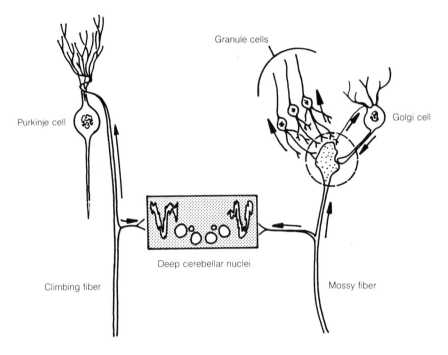

10–10 Schematic diagram comparing the climbing and mossy fiber systems within the cerebellum.

their contribution to the cerebellar cortex, both climbing and mossy fibers send collaterals to the deep cerebellar nuclei. These collaterals are excitatory in nature and help maintain a constant background discharge of these deep nuclei.

Internal Cerebellar Circuitry

A mossy fiber input excites dendrites of a group of granule cells. The discharge from these granule cells will be transmitted through their axons (parallel fibers), which bifurcate in a T configuration in the molecular layer, coming in contact with the perpendicular orientation of dendrites of Purkinje, stellate, basket, and Golgi neurons. If the excited parallel fiber bundle is wide enough to cover the Purkinje cell dendritic field, activation will result in a single row of Purkinje cells parallel to the long axis of the folium and in the related basket and stellate cells. Golgi cells will not fire, however, because their dendritic fields are wider than those of the Purkinje cells. The activation of the basket and stellate cells, the axons of which are oriented perpendicular to those of the parallel fibers and Purkinje cells in the folium, will inhibit a wide zone of Purkinje cells on each side of the row of activated Purkinje cells. Thus, this mossy fiber input will produce a row of activated Purkinje cells flanked on each side by a strip of inhibited Purkinje cells. The inhibited rows of Purkinje cells, by silencing surround activity, help the process of neural sharpening of the activated row of Purkinje cells.

If the activated bundle of parallel fibers becomes wide enough to span the dendritic field of a Golgi neuron, the Golgi cell is then excited and, through its axon in the glomerulus, will inhibit the granule cell. Thus, a mossy fiber input is completely transferred into inhibition via one of two mechanisms.

1. Mossy fiber to Golgi dendrite within the glomerulus to Golgi axon to granule cell dendrite
2. Mossy fiber to granule cell dendrite in the glomerulus to granule axon (parallel fiber) to basket, stellate, and Golgi dendrites to basket, stellate, and Golgi axons to Purkinje cell or granule cell dendrite

The mossy fiber input has both high divergence and convergence ratios. A single mossy fiber has 40 rosettes, each rosette connects with the dendritic terminals of 20 granule cells and a single granule cell connects through the parallel fibers with 100 to 300 Purkinje cells. This gives a divergence ratio of about 1:100,000 to 1:300,000 from one mossy fiber to the Purkinje cell. On the other hand, each Purkinje cell has about 100,000 dendritic spines in synaptic contact with parallel fibers (granule cells), hence a large ratio of convergence.

Similarly, a climbing fiber input will excite Purkinje cells as well as stellate, basket, and Golgi neurons. The effect on these different cells is similar to that described for the mossy fiber input and helps to focus on the activation of the Purkinje cell amidst a zone of inhibition induced by basket, stellate, and Golgi neurons. In contrast to the mossy fiber system, the convergence and divergence factors for the climbing fiber input are small (1:1).

The mossy fiber pathways conduct faster than the climbing fiber pathways. However, the ultimate inhibitory potentials produced by the mossy fiber system develop slowly so that by the time the climbing fiber input arrives in the cerebellum, the full effect of the mossy fiber inhibitory potentials has not yet developed. This allows the climbing fiber system to act on the background activity of excitation and inhibition initiated by the mossy fiber input.

Thus, of all the cells of the cerebellar cortex, only the granule cell is excitatory; all others including the Purkinje cells are inhibitory. Recent studies on the cerebellum have given the Golgi neuron a central role in cerebellar organization. Through its contact with both the mossy fibers in the glomerulus and the climbing fiber collaterals, the Golgi neuron is able to select what input will reach the Purkinje cell at any one time.

Cerebellar Output

Efferents from the cerebellum leave via the inferior and superior cerebellar peduncles.

Inferior Cerebellar Peduncle

Cerebellar efferents that travel via the inferior cerebellar peduncle are the following.

1. Cerebello-olivary fibers, of uncertain origin in the cerebellum
2. Cerebellovestibular fibers, arising from the flocculonodular lobe and the nucleus fastigi and projecting via the juxtarestiform body to all four vestibular nuclei
3. Cerebelloreticular fibers

Superior Cerebellar Peduncle

The major component of cerebellar efferents in the superior cerebellar peduncle is the cerebellorubrothalamic fiber system. This is a fiber system which originates in the deep cerebellar nuclei (dentate, globose, and emboliform), crosses in the tegmentum of the midbrain at the inferior colliculus level and projects upon the red nucleus and the ventrolateral and ventroanterior nuclei of the thalamus. A small fascicle from this crossed system descends to the inferior olive.

An uncrossed as well as a crossed component of cerebellar efferents in the superior cerebellar peduncle project upon reticular neurons in the midbrain, pons, and medulla oblongata.

The afferent input reaches the cerebellum via two systems, the mossy and climbing fiber systems. There is only one type of efferent fiber system, the axons of Purkinje cells. The majority of these axons project upon deep cerebellar nuclei; some, however, bypass the deep cerebellar nuclei to reach the lateral vestibular nucleus. The cerebellar efferents in the different peduncles mentioned above are, for the most part, axons of neurons in the deep cerebellar nuclei. The projection of Purkinje cell axons upon deep cerebellar nuclei is somatotopically organized. Those originating in the vermis of the cerebellum project upon the nucleus fastigi, the paravermal (intermediate) Purkinje axons project upon emboliform and globose nuclei, and those of the lateral hemispheres project upon the dentate nucleus (Fig. 10–11). The projections of Purkinje axons upon deep cerebellar nuclei are inhibitory.

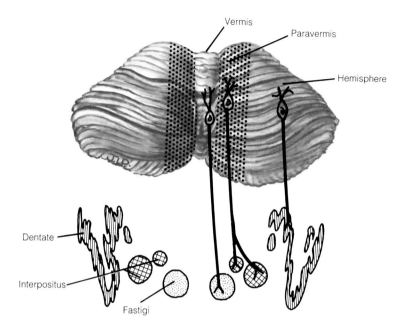

Vermis

Paravermis

Hemisphere

Dentate

Interpositus

Fastigi

10–11   Schematic diagram showing the projection of the different cerebellar zones into the deep cerebellar nuclei.

Deep Cerebellar Nuclei

The deep cerebellar nuclei are embedded in the white matter core of the cerebellum. There are four pairs of nuclei arranged from lateral to medial as follows: dentate, emboliform, globose, and fastigi.

Dentate Nucleus

The dentate nucleus (Fig. 10–12) is composed of multipolar neurons and resembles the inferior olive in configuration. It receives the axons of Purkinje cells in the lateral part of the cerebellar hemispheres and collaterals of climbing and mossy fibers. The former input is inhibitory, whereas the latter is excitatory to the dentate nucleus.

Axons of the dentate nucleus project via the superior cerebellar peduncle to the contralateral 1) ventrolateral and ventroanterior thalamic nuclei with some projection to the centromedian nucleus, 2) reticular formation of the brain stem, 3) pulvinar nucleus, 4) dorsomedial nucleus, and 5) oculomotor nucleus.

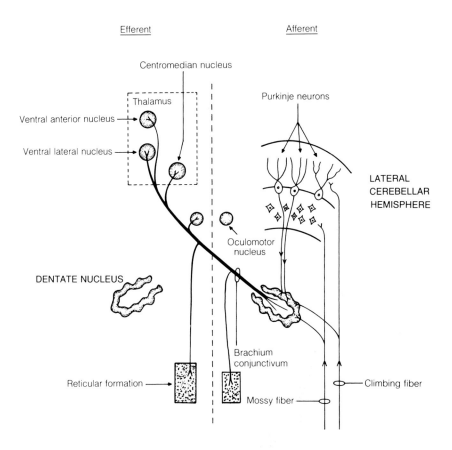

Efferent   Afferent

Centromedian nucleus

Thalamus   Purkinje neurons

Ventral anterior nucleus

Ventral lateral nucleus

LATERAL
CEREBELLAR
HEMISPHERE

Oculomotor
nucleus

DENTATE NUCLEUS

Brachium
conjunctivum

Reticular formation   Climbing fiber

Mossy fiber

10–12 Schematic diagram showing the afferent and efferent connections of the dentate nucleus.

Interposed Nuclei

These nuclei (Fig. 10–13) include the emboliform nucleus, located medial to the hilum of the dentate nucleus, and the globose nucleus, located medial to the emboliform nucleus.

The interposed nuclei receive afferent fibers from the following sources.

1. Axons of Purkinje cells in the paravermal (intermediate) zone of the cerebellum that are inhibitory in function
2. Collaterals from climbing and mossy fiber systems that are excitatory in function

Axons of interposed nuclei leave the cerebellum via the superior cerebellar peduncle to reach the contralateral 1) thalamus (ventrolateral, ventroanterior, and centromedian nuclei), 2) red nucleus, and 3) reticular formation of the brain stem.

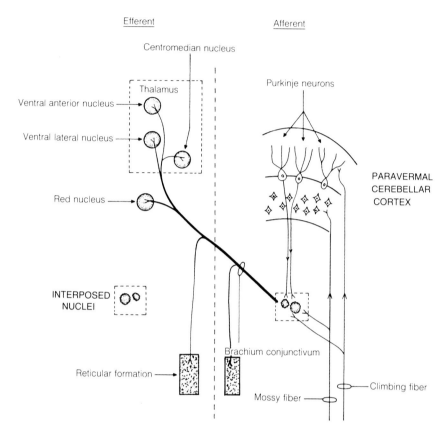

10–13 Schematic diagram showing the afferent and efferent connections of the interposed nuclei.

Fastigial Nucleus

This nucleus (Fig. 10–14) is located in the roof of the fourth ventricle medial to the globose nucleus; hence it is called the roof nucleus. It receives afferent fibers from the following sources.

1. Axons of Purkinje cells in the vermis of the cerebellum that are inhibitory in function
2. Collaterals of mossy and climbing fiber systems that are excitatory.

Axons of the fastigial nucleus project to vestibular and reticular nuclei of the brain stem via the juxtarestiform body and the uncinate fasciculus. The lateral vestibular nucleus also receives fibers directly from the vermis of the cerebellum, bypassing the fastigial nucleus.

In addition to the efferent projections of the deep cerebellar nuclei described above, all deep cerebellar nuclei have been shown to send axon collaterals to the areas of the cerebellar cortex from which they receive

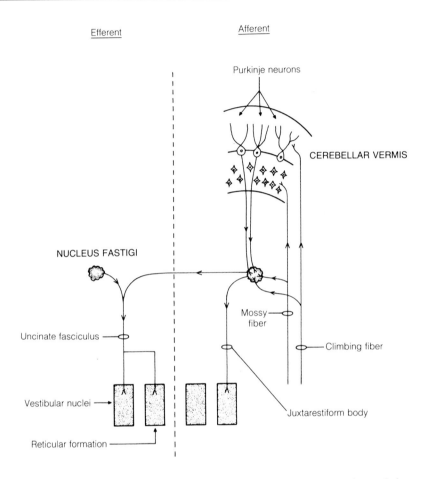

Efferent   Afferent

Purkinje neurons

CEREBELLAR VERMIS

NUCLEUS FASTIGI

Uncinate fasciculus

Mossy fiber

Climbing fiber

Vestibular nuclei

Juxtarestiform body

Reticular formation

10–14 Schematic diagram showing the afferent and efferent connections of the nucleus fastigi.

fibers; thus, the nucleus fastigi sends axon collaterals to the cerebellar vermis, the interposed nuclei to the paravermal region, and the dentate nucleus to lateral parts of the cerebellar hemispheres. Although deep cerebellar nuclei receive axons of Purkinje cells, their axon collaterals do not project directly upon Purkinje cells but upon neuronal elements in the granule cell layer via the mossy fiber system. The exact cell type in the granule cell layer that receives these axon collaterals has not been identified with certainty.

Thus, all the deep cerebellar nuclei receive a dual input; these are an excitatory input from extracerebellar sources (mossy and climbing fibers) and an inhibitory input from the cerebellum (axons of Purkinje cells). In contrast, the output of the deep cerebellar nuclei is excitatory.

Cerebrocerebellar and Cerebellocerebral Pathways

The cerebral cortex communicates with the cerebellum via a multitude of pathways, of which the following are well recognized.

1. Cortico-olivocerebellar via the inferior olivary nucleus
2. Corticopontocerebellar via the pontine nuclei
3. Corticoreticulocerebellar via the reticular nuclei of the brain stem

The first two pathways convey to the cerebellum precisely localized and somatotopically organized information. Of these two, the pathway via the pontine nuclei is quantitatively more impressive and influences the entire cerebellum. The pathway via the reticular nuclei is part of a system with diffuse input and output (reticular formation), in which information of cortical origin is integrated with information from other sources before transmission to the cerebellum.

The cerebellum influences the cerebrum mainly via the dentatorubrothalamic system, which terminates upon cortical neurons. The cerebellocerebral pathways are modest in number when compared with the cerebrocerebellar pathways (approximately 1:5). This is a reflection of the efficiency of the cerebellar machinery which makes it possible for the cerebellum to regulate cortically originating signals for movement.

Neurotransmitters

The following neurotransmitters have been identified in the cerebellum: gamma-aminobutyric acid (GABA), taurine, glutamate, aspartate, and noradrenalin.

The GABA is liberated from axons of Purkinje and basket neurons and exerts an inhibitory effect upon target neurons. Taurine is believed to be the inhibitory neurotransmitter of the superficial stellate cells; taurine levels are high in the molecular layer and drop substantially when stellate cell development is blocked by X-irradiation. Glutamate is believed to be the excitatory neurotransmitter of granule cells; glutamate levels in the granule cell layer drop substantially in the agranular cerebellum of virus-infected and mutant mice. Aspartate is probably the neurotransmitter of the climbing fiber system; aspartate levels drop in cases of olivocerebellar atrophy, in which the inferior olive (major source of climbing fibers) is atrophied. Noradrenalin is the inhibitory neurotransmitter of the locus ceruleus projection upon Purkinje cell dendrites. In addition to its presumed role in maturation of Purkinje neurons, noradrenalin seems to modulate Purkinje cell response to other cerebellar neurotransmitters. Stimulation of the locus ceruleus enhances sensitivity of Purkinje neurons to both glutamate and GABA.

Cerebellar Physiology

Cerebellar Cortex

Cerebellar neurons are characterized by high rates of resting impulse discharge. Purkinje cells discharge at the rate of approximately 20 to 40 cps, granule cells at 50 to 70 cps, and inhibitory interneurons (basket, stellate, and Golgi) at 7 to 30 cps. In the conscious monkey, the Purkinje cell has been found to discharge at rates varying between 3 and 125 cps, with a mean discharge of 70 cps. This high discharge of cerebellar neurons is derived from the nature of their synaptic drive. The activity of Purkinje cells correlates closely with the activity of mossy fibers, which also have high rates of resting discharge.

Stimulation of the mossy fiber system or the parallel fibers elicits in the Purkinje cell a brief excitatory postsynaptic potential (EPSP) (simple spike) lasting 5 to 10 msec, followed by a prolonged inhibitory postsynaptic potential (IPSP). The short EPSP is attributed to the activation of Purkinje cell dendrites by the parallel fibers. The IPSP, on the other hand, is attributed to the feed-forward inhibition of Purkinje cells by stellate and basket cells that are simultaneously activated by the beam of parallel fibers. The prolonged time course of the IPSP implies a prolonged excitatory action on these cells by the parallel fiber input.

Stimulation of the climbing fiber system elicits in the Purkinje cell an intense and prolonged reaction characterized by an initial large spike followed by several small ones. This pattern is referred to as a complex spike. This complex EPSP is followed by a prolonged IPSP. The complex spike is explained on the basis of more than one mechanism. One mechanism for this complex spike in the Purkinje cell is the repetitive discharge emanating from inferior olive neurons because of axonal collaterals within the inferior olive. Another mechanism for the complex response of Purkinje cells lies in the intrinsic property of their membranes. The IPSP that follows the complex EPSP is attributed to simultaneous activation of stellate and basket cells by the climbing fibers, which in turn inhibit the Purkinje cell by a feed-forward pathway. Both mossy and climbing fibers facilitate the Golgi cell, which in turn inhibits the granule cell and can thus contribute to Purkinje cell inhibition. After their initial activation by the mossy and climbing fiber input, intrinsic neurons (basket, stellate, and Golgi) are ultimately inhibited by Purkinje axon collaterals. The action of the recurrent Purkinje axon collaterals is thus to disinhibit the Purkinje cell.

It becomes evident from the above that the mossy and climbing input fibers are excitatory to the granule and Purkinje cells, whereas the action of cells within the cerebellum (except the granule cell) is inhibitory. It is thus not possible for cerebellar activity in response to an afferent input to be sustained. The only mechanism for sustained or reverberating activity, namely the disinhibitory pathway of the Purkinje axon collaterals, is apparently not capable of sustaining activity for a long period of time.

Several investigators have studied the effects of cerebellar stimulation in humans. The results of such stimulation are similar to those described above.

Deep Cerebellar Nuclei

Like the Purkinje cells, deep nuclei of the cerebellum have high rates of impulse discharge at rest. Also like the Purkinje cells, the deep cerebellar nuclei receive both excitatory and inhibitory inputs, the former arriving via the climbing and mossy fibers and the latter by axons of Purkinje cells. Thus, a mossy fiber input, for example, will cause first a high frequency burst followed by a lowering of the deep cerebellar nuclei frequency as a result of the inhibition arriving through the slower Purkinje cell loop. Although the pharmacology of Purkinje cell inhibition is not yet fully elucidated, it is believed to be mediated by γ-aminobutyric acid (GABA), which is present in the Purkinje cell layer.

Cerebellum and Pain

Recent studies have demonstrated that the cerebellum plays a role in pain mechanisms. Cerebellar stimulation has been shown 1) to inhibit responses in the ipsilateral sensorimotor cortex evoked by stimulation of the contralateral sciatic nerve and 2) to raise the nociceptive threshold in response to a painful shock.

Cerebellum and Epilepsy

Cerebellar stimulation has been shown to have beneficial effects on both experimentally induced epilepsy and human epilepsy. Cerebellar stimulators are now being used to treat intractable epilepsy in humans. The results of such investigations are variable and more study is needed before the role of the cerebellum in the control of epilepsy can be clearly defined.

Clinical Considerations

Cerebellar lesions in man produce manifestations which are different from those in animals. The classically described archi- , paleo- , and neocerebellar syndromes after ablation of the respective lobes of the cerebellum in experimental animals are not observed in man. Instead, one can differentiate in man manifestations of lesions in midline structures (archi- and paleocerebellum) and the cerebellar hemispheres (neocerebellum).

Experimental Animals

Archicerebellar Syndrome   The archicerebellum is related to the vestibular system. It receives fibers from the vestibular nuclei and nerve and projects to the vestibular and reticular nuclei, which in turn project to the spinal cord (vestibulospinal tracts) and the oculomotor nucleus. The function of this system is thus the regulation of postural mechanisms controlled by the vestibular and reticular systems.

Ablation of the flocculonodular lobe in experimental animals thus produces nystagmus and distubances in equilibrium.

Paleocerebellar Syndrome   The paleocerebellum is linked to muscle afferents as well as pain and pressure receptors via the spinocerebellar tracts. These tracts project to the vermis of the cerebellar cortex. The output of this system is through the fastigial nucleus to the reticular formation and spinal cord via the reticulospinal pathways.

Ablation of the paleocerebellum produces decerebrate rigidity and an increase in myotatic and postural reflexes.

Neocerebellar Syndrome   The neocerebellum receives the corticopontocerebellar pathways and projects via the interposed and dentate nuclei to the spinal cord and cerebral cortex. The paravermal part of the neocerebellum projects via the interposed nuclei to the contralateral red nucleus and the ventrolateral nucleus of the thalamus. The red nucleus projects via the rubrospinal tract to the spinal cord, while the ventrolateral nucleus projects to the cerebral cortex. The lateral part of each hemisphere, on the other hand, projects to the dentate nucleus. The dentate nucleus projects to the contralateral ventrolateral nucleus of the thalamus, which in turn projects to the cerebral cortex. The paravermal part is concerned with skilled movements of proximal limb musculature, whereas the lateral part of the hemisphere is concerned with skilled movements of distal parts of the limbs.

Ablation of the neocerebellum produces muscular hypotonia and incoordination of movement (ataxia).

Man

Midline Syndrome A picture corresponding to the archicerebellar (flocculonodular lobe) syndrome is often seen in children with a special type of tumor, the medulloblastoma. These tumors almost always arise in the most posterior part of the vermis, the nodulus, and are manifested by unsteadiness of gait and, in some cases, nystagmus.

The paleocerebellar syndrome as described in experimental animals is usually not encountered in man. However, some patients with atrophy of the cerebellum demonstrate unsteadiness of gait and increased myotatic reflexes in the lower extremities. It is believed that in such patients the anterior lobe is primarily affected by the atrophy.

Cerebellar Hemisphere Syndrome Lesions of the cerebellar hemispheres (neocerebellum) produce the following manifestations and are the most commonly encountered.

Ataxia The patient exhibits a drunken, unsteady gait.

Dysmetria The patient is unable to estimate the range of voluntary movement. In attempting to touch the tip of the finger to the tip of the nose, such a patient will shoot the finger past the nose to the cheek or ear.

Decomposition of Movement (Dyssynergia) Voluntary movements are jerky and tremulous. In attempting to touch the nose with the finger or to move the heel over the shin, the patient's movements are uneven and jerky throughout the range of motion.

Adiadochokinesia (Dysdiadochokinesia) The patient is unable to perform rapid movements such as tapping one hand with the other in alternating supination and pronation.

Intention Tremor In attempting movement of a limb, a terminal tremor is evident as the limb approaches the target.

Muscular Hypotonia The patient exhibits loss of muscular tone or resistance to passive stretching of muscles.

Dysarthria The patient exhibits a slurred, hesitating type of speech.

The cerebellum is well known for its ability to compensate for its deficits. The compensation is especially marked in children. The mechanisms underlying this ability to compensate are not known; the assumption of lost cerebellar functions by other noncerebellar structures or by remaining parts of the cerebellum are two explanations for this compensation.

Pathophysiology of Cerebellar Dysfunction

Cerebellar Signs

The incoordination of movement noted in diseases of the neocerebellum is the result of disturbances in speed, range, force, or timing of movement.

The smooth execution of voluntary acts requires a steady increase and decrease in force during movement. The lack of uniform velocity is responsible for the irregular and jerky movements (dyssynergia) of cerebellar disease.

Proper timing in intiation and termination of movement is essential in the execution of smooth movement. A delay in the initiation of each successive movement will lead to the adiadochokinesis of cerebellar disease. A delay in the termination of movement produced by a delay in intervention of antagonistic muscles to check the movement results in dysmetria and overshooting. Thus, adiadochokinesis and dysmetria are the result of an error in timing.

Intention tremor is due to defective feedback control from the cerebellum on cortically initiated movement. Normally, cerebellar feedback mechanisms control the force and timing of cortically initiated movement. Failure of these mechanisms in cerebellar disease results in tremor.

The cerebellum is able to exert its corrective influence on cortically originating movement by virtue of the input it receives from the cerebral cortex and periphery. The cerebral cortex informs the cerebellum of intended movement via the cerebrocerebellar pathways described previously. During movement, the cerebellum receives a constant flow of information, both proprioceptive and exteroceptive, from peripheral receptors (muscle spindle, Golgi tendon organ, etc.) concerning movement in progress. The cerebellum correlates peripheral information on movement in progress with central information on intended movement and corrects errors of movement accordingly.

In addition to its role as "error detector" of cortically initiated movement, the cerebellum may be involved in the initiation of movement. Recent experimental evidence suggests that deep cerebellar nuclei fire simultaneously with pyramidal cortical neurons prior to movement.

The cerebellum also influences movement via its effects on the gamma system. The cerebellum normally increases the sensitivity of muscle spindles to stretch. Cerebellar lesions are associated with a depression of gamma motor neuron activity which leads to erroneous information in the gamma system about the degree of muscle stretch. The erroneous information conveyed by the muscle spindle to the alpha motor neuron results in disturbances in discharge of the alpha motor neuron and is manifested by a disturbance in force and timing of movement.

The depression of tonic activity of gamma motor neurons in cerebellar disease is the basis of the hypotonia associated with neocerebellar syndromes.

Archi- and Paleocerebellar Signs

The archicerebellum and paleocerebellum influence spinal activity via the vestibulospinal and reticulospinal tracts. The increase in myotatic and postural reflexes associated with the anterior lobe syndrome is due to an increase in motor signals to the alpha motor neurons, with a simultaneous decrease in signals to the gamma system. Thus, the rigidity of cerebellar disease is an alpha type of rigidity.

Disturbances in Equilibrium and Gait

Disturbances in gait may be seen following involvement of all divisions of the cerebellum. When accompanied by disturbances in equilibrium, such as inability to assume upright posture, it is indicative of lesions in the posterior part of the vermis and flocculonodular lobe. Abnormalities of gait secondary to lesions in the anterior lobe are usually not associated with equilibrium disturbances. In man, ataxia of gait may be the only cerebellar manifestation of the anterior lobe syndrome.

Cerebellum and Nystagmus

Nystagmus has been reported in affections of the cerebellum without concomitant brain stem involvement. Two types of cerebellar nystagmus have been described, the spontaneous and the positional.

Spontaneous horizontal nystagmus with a quick component toward the side of the lesion occurs with asymmetric (unilateral) lesions in the posterior vermis, flocculonodular lobe, and nucleus fastigi. It is believed to represent the release of the vestibular nuclei from the posterior vermis.

Positional nystagmus has also been reported following lesions in the same sites that produce spontaneous nystagmus. It is best seen in the supine position with a quick component in the direction of gaze.

Cerebellum and Eye Movements

Complete cerebellectomy in man is associated with inability to maintain eccentric gaze, defective smooth pursuit movements, failure to suppress optokinetic nystagmus by visual fixation and moderate increase in vestibulo-ocular reflex. In unilateral cerebellar lesions, the above signs appear ipsilateral to the lesion.

Sensory Systems and Cerebellum

Although the cerebellum is generally regarded as a motor center, recent studies suggest that it has a role in sensory mechanisms. The cerebellum has been shown to receive tactile, visual, and auditory impulses. Furthermore, reciprocal connections have been demonstrated between the cerebral and cerebellar tactile, visual, and auditory areas.

Autonomic Functions

Experimental studies suggest that the cerebellum plays a role in the regulation of cardiovascular and respiratory functions, pupillary diameter, and bladder function. It has also been shown that autonomic descending fibers from the hypothalamus via the dorsal longitudinal fasciculus send collaterals to the cerebellum.

References

Brown-Gould, B.: The Organization of Afferents to the Cerebellar Cortex in the Cat: Projections from the Deep Cerebellar Nuclei. J Comp Neurol 184 (1979) 27–42.

Cody, F.W.J.; Richardson, H.C.: Mossy and Climbing Fiber Projections of Trigeminal Inputs to the Cerebellar Cortex in the Cat. Brain Res 153 (1978) 352–356.

Courville, J.; Faraco-Cantin, F.: On the Origin of the Climbing Fibers of the Cerebellum. An Experimental Study in the Cat with an Autoradiographic Tracing Method. Neuroscience 3 (1978) 797–809.

Estanol, B.; Romero, R.; Corvera, J.: Effect of Cerebellectomy on Eye Movements in Man. Arch Neurol 36 (1979) 281–284.

Ito, M.: Recent Advances in Cerebellar Physiology and Pathology. In: Advances in Neurology, Vol. 21, pp. 59–84. Ed. by R.A.P. Kark, R.N. Rosenberg, and L.J. Schut. Raven Press, New York, 1978.

Itoh, K.; Mizuno, N.: A Cerebello-Pulvinar Projection in the Cat as Visualized by the Use of Anterograde Transport of Horseradish Perodixase. Brain Res 171 (1979) 131–134.

Sasaki, K.; Jinnai, K.; Gemba, H.; Hashimoto, S.; Mizuno, N.: Projections of the Cerebellar Dentate Nucleus onto the Frontal Association Cortex in Monkeys. Exp Brain Res 37 (1979) 193–198.

11

Cerebral Cortex

The cerebral cortex is the layer of gray matter capping the white matter core of the cerebral hemispheres. Its thickness varies from 1.5 to 4.5 mm, with an average thickness of 2.5 mm. The cerebral cortex is thickest in the primary motor area and thinnest in the primary visual cortex. The cortex is irregularly convoluted, forming gyri separated by sulci or fissures. The number of neurons in the cerebral cortex is estimated at 50 billion. It is also estimated that about 5% of the area of the cerebral cortex is specialized for receiving sensory input from the eyes, ears, and skin and for projecting motor output down the pyramidal tract to bring about movement. Over 90% of the cortex serves an association function specially related to integrative and cognitive activities.

Types of Cortex

On the basis of phylogenetic development and microscopic structure, the following three types of cortices are recognized.

Isocortex (Neocortex or Homogenetic Cortex)

This cortex is six-layered and of recent phylogenetic development. It is characteristic of mammalian species, increases in size in higher mammals and comprises 90% of the cerebral cortex in man.

Isocortex in which the six layers are clearly evident (such as the primary sensory cortex) is termed homotypic cortex. Isocortex in which some of the six layers are obscured (such as the motor cortex and visual cortex) is termed heterotypic cortex. The visual cortex is also known as granular cortex or koniocortex (from the Greek *konis*, or dust). The motor cortex, in contrast, is known as agranular cortex because of the predominance of large pyramidal neurons.

Allocortex (Paleocortex, Archicortex or Heterogenetic Cortex)

This cortex is three-layered and phylogenetically older. It is found in the hippocampal formation and olfactory cortex of humans.

Mesocortex

This type of cortex is found in the cingulate gyrus and is intermediate in histology between the isocortex and allocortex.

Microscopic Structure

Cell Types

The neurons of the cerebral cortex fall into one of five types: pyramidal, stellate or granular, fusiform, horizontal cells of Cajal, and cells of Martinotti. The first and second types are the most numerous.

Pyramidal Neurons (Fig. 11–1, *A*)   These neurons derive their name from their shape. The apex of the pyramid is directed toward the cortical surface. Each pyramidal neuron has an apical dendrite directed toward the surface of the cortex and several basal dendrites which arise from the base of the pyramid. Branches of all dendrites contain numerous spines which increase the size of the synaptic area. A slender axon leaves the base of the pyramidal neuron and projects upon other neurons in the same or contralateral hemisphere or else leaves the cortex to project upon subcortical regions. The axon gives rise within the cortex to two types of axon collaterals. These are the recurrent axon collaterals (RAC), which project back upon neurons in more superficial layers, and horizontal axon collaterals (HAC), which extend horizontally to synapse upon neurons in the vicinity.

Pyramidal neurons are found in all cortical layers except layer I. They vary in size; most are between 10 and 50 μm. The largest are the giant pyramidal cells of Betz, which measure about 100 μm in height and are found in layer V of the motor cortex.

Stellate, Granule, Golgi Type II Neurons (Fig. 11–1, *B*)   These are small (4 to 8 μm) star-shaped neurons with short, extensively branched spiny dendrites and short or long axons that project upon neurons in the vicinity or in more distant laminae. Like pyramidal neurons, stellate neurons are found in all cortical laminae except lamina I. They are especially numerous in lamina IV.

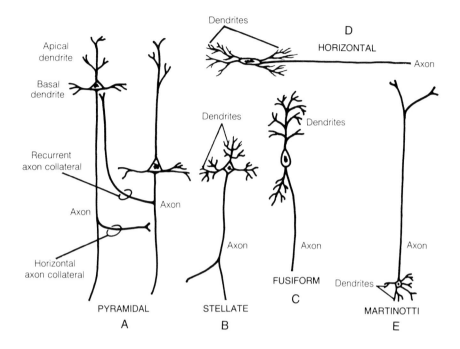

11-1   Schematic diagram of the various types of cortical neurons.

Fusiform, Spindle Neurons (Fig. 11–1, C)   These are small neurons with elongated perikarya in which the long axis is oriented perpendicular to the cortical surface. A short dendrite arises from the lower pole of the perikaryon and arborizes in the vicinity. A longer dendrite arises from the upper pole of the perikaryon and extends to more superficial layers. The axon enters the deep white matter. Fusiform neurons are found in the deeper cortical laminae.

Horizontal Cells of Cajal (Fig. 11–1, D)   These are small fusiform neurons with their long axes directed parallel to the cortical surface. A branching dendrite arises from each pole of the perikaryon and an axon arises from one pole. The dendrites and axon are oriented parallel to the cortical surface. The horizontal cells of Cajal are found only in lamina I and disappear after the neonatal period.

Cells of Martinotti (Fig. 11–1, E)   Martinotti neurons are multipolar with short branching dendrites and an axon which projects to more superficial layers, giving out horizontal axon collaterals en route. The Martinotti neurons are found in all cortical laminae except lamina I.

Table 11–1 Cortical Layers

Layer number	Cytoarchitectonic name	Myeloarchitectonic name
I	Molecular	Tangential
II	External granular	Dysfibrous
III	Pyramidal	Suprastriatal
IV	Internal granular	External of Baillarger
V	Ganglionic	Internal of Baillarger and interstriatal
VI	Multiform	Infrastriatal

Layers

The division of the neocortex into layers has been the outcome of extensive cytoarchitectonic (organization based on studies of stained cells) and myeloarchitectonic (organization based on studies of myelinated fiber preparations) studies. Although several such studies are available, the most widely used are the cytoarchitectonic classification of Brodmann and the myeloarchitectonic classification of the Vogts. According to these two classifications, the neocortex is divided into six layers (Table 11–1).

Layer I   Layer I consists primarily of a dense network of nerve cell processes among which are scattered sparse neurons (horizontal cells of Cajal) and neuroglia. The nerve cell processes in this layer comprise projection axons from extracortical sites as well as axons and dendrites of neurons in other cortical areas. This layer of the cortex is primarily a synaptic area.

Layer II   Layer II consists of a dense packing of small pyramidal and stellate neurons intermingled with axons from other cortical layers of the same and opposite hemispheres (association and commissural fibers), as well as axons and dendrites passing through this layer from deeper layers. The dendrites of pyramidal and stellate neurons in this layer project to layer I, while their axons project to deeper layers. This layer of the cortex contributes to the complexity of intracortical circuitry.

Layer III   Layer III consists of pyramidal neurons which increase in size in deeper parts of the layer. The dendrites of neurons in this layer extend to layer I, while the axons project to other layers within the same and contralateral hemisphere (association and commissural fibers) or leave the hemisphere as projection fibers to more distant extracortical sites. This layer receives primarily axons of neurons in other cortical areas (association and commissural fibers), as well as axons of neurons in extracortical regions such as the thalamus.

Layer IV Layer IV consists of densely packed small stellate cells with processes which terminate within the same layer, either upon axons of other stellate cells or upon axons of cortical or subcortical origin passing through this layer. Few of the larger stellate cells in this layer project their axons to deeper cortical layers. This layer is traversed by a dense band of horizontally oriented nerve fibers known as the external band of Baillarger. This band is particularly well developed in the visual cortex (area 17) and is known as the stripe of Gennari.

Layer V Layer V consists of large and medium-sized pyramidal cells, stellate cells, and cells of Martinotti. The largest pyramidal cells in the cerebral cortex are found in this layer (hence the name ganglionic layer). Dendrites of neurons in this layer project to the more superficial layers, while axons project upon neurons in other cortical areas or mainly in extracortical regions (projection fibers). This layer receives axons and dendrites arising in other cortical sites or in subcortical sites. It is also traversed by a dense band of horizontally oriented fibers; this is the internal band of Baillarger.

Layer VI Layer VI consists of cells of varying shapes and sizes, including the cells of Martinotti, which are prominent in this layer. Dendrites of smaller cells arborize locally or in adjacent layers, while those of large neurons reach the molecular layer. Axons of neurons in this layer project to other cortical laminae or to subcortical regions.

Layers I, V and VI are present in all types of cortex (neo-, paleo-, archicortex). Layers II, III and IV, however, are present only in neocortex and thus are considered of more recent phylogenetic development. In general, layers I to IV are considered receptive, whereas layers V and VI are efferent.

In contrast to the horizontal anatomic lamination, the vertical lamination described by Mountcastle seems to be the more functionally appropriate. The studies of Lorente de Nó, Mountcastle, Szentágothai, and others have shown that the functional unit of cortical activity is a column of neurons oriented vertically to the surface of the cortex. Each such column or module is 300 μm across and contains 4,000 neurons, 2,000 of which are pyramidal neurons. There are approximately three million such modules in the human neocortex. Each module sends pyramidal cell axons to other modules within the same hemisphere or to modules in the other hemisphere. Of interest is the fact that activation of a module tends to inhibit neuronal activity in adjacent modules.

Input to Cerebral Cortex

The input to the cerebral cortex originates in three sites (Fig. 11–2).

1. Thalamus
2. Cortex of the same hemisphere (association fibers)
3. Cortex of the contralateral hemisphere (commissural fibers)

The input from the thalamus travels via two systems. 1) The specific thalamocortical system originates in specific thalamic nuclei (ventralis anterior, ventralis lateralis, ventralis posterior, etc.) and projects upon specific cortical areas (primary motor and somesthetic cortex). This fiber system reaches the cortex as an ascending component of the internal capsule. The majority of fibers in this system project upon neurons in lamina IV, with some projecting upon neurons in lamina III (Fig. 11–3). 2) The nonspecific thalamocortical system is related to the reticular system and originates in nonspecific thalamic nuclei (intralaminar, midline, and reticular nuclei). In the cortex, fibers of this system project diffusely upon all laminae (Fig. 11–3) and establish mostly axodendritic types of synapses. This fiber system is intimately involved in the arousal response and wakefulness. An input from the locus ceruleus to the cortex has recently been confirmed. It consists of noradrenergic axons that terminate diffusely throughout all cortical areas.

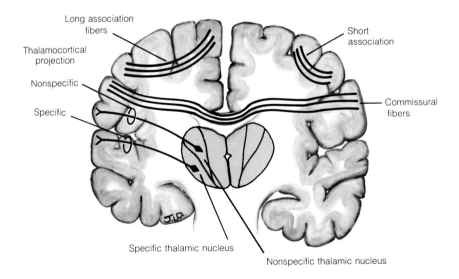

11–2 Schematic diagram showing sources of fiber input to the cerebral cortex.

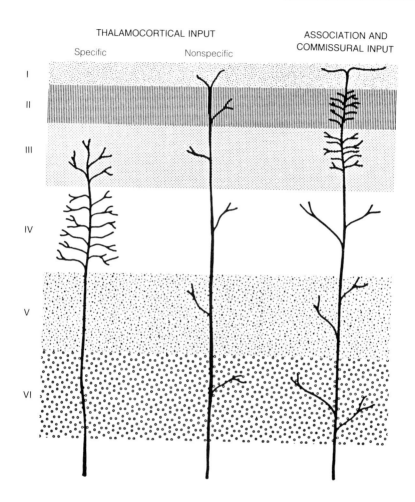

11-3 Schematic diagram of the termination pattern of the various inputs to cortical laminae.

The association fibers arise from nearby (short association fibers) and distant (long association fibers) regions of the same hemisphere. They too project diffusely in all laminae (Fig. 11–3), but mostly in laminae I to III. The long association fiber system includes such bundles as the uncinate fasciculus, the cingulum, the superior and inferior longitudinal fasciculi, and the occipitofrontal fasciculus (Fig. 11–4). The commissural fibers arise from corresponding and noncorresponding regions in the contralateral hemisphere, travel via the corpus callosum, and project upon neurons in all laminae, but mostly laminae I to III (Fig. 11–3).

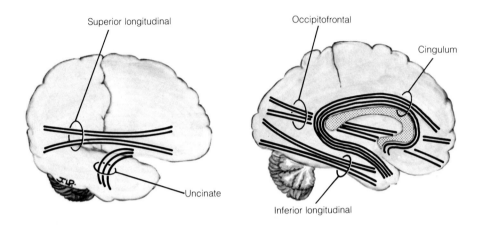

11–4 Schematic diagram showing the major long association bundles.

Studies on the topographic distribution of interhemispheric projections in the corpus callosum have shown that the genu interconnects the prefrontal and premotor cortices, the rostral half of the body of the corpus callosum interconnects the precentral gyri (primary motor areas) and the supplementary motor areas, and the caudal half of the corpus callosum interconnects the postcentral gyri (primary somesthetic areas), the parietal lobules, and the temporal and insular areas.

Output of Cerebral Cortex

Efferent outflow from the cerebral cortex is grouped into three categories (Fig. 11–5). These are the association fiber system, commissural fiber system, and corticofugal fiber system. The association and commissural fiber systems have been described in the section on input to the cortex. Essentially they represent intrahemispheric and interhemispheric connections.

The corticofugal fiber system includes all fiber tracts that leave the cerebral cortex to project upon various subcortical structures. They include the following pathways.

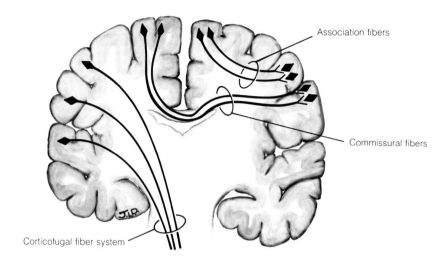

Association fibers

Commissural fibers

Corticofugal fiber system

11–5   Schematic diagram of the major groups of cortical output.

Corticospinal Pathway (Fig. 11–6)

This corticofugal fiber tract connects the cerebral cortex directly with motor neurons in the spinal cord and is concerned with highly skilled volitional movement. It arises from wide areas of the cerebral cortex but principally from the sensory motor cortex. It contains roughly a million fibers of various sizes (9 to 22 μm), about 3% of which are large in size and arise from the giant cells of Betz in lamina V of the motor cortex. The fibers of this system descend in the internal capsule, the middle part of the cerebral peduncle, the basis pontis, and the pyramids before gathering in the spinal cord as the lateral and anterior corticospinal tracts. The former constitutes the majority of the descending corticospinal fibers and decussates in the pyramids (motor decussation); the latter is smaller and crosses at segmental levels in the spinal cord. The classic notion that the corticospinal tract is of particular importance for skilled and delicate voluntary movement is in essence correct, but it is obvious that a number of other indirect tracts passing through the brain stem nuclei, reticular formation, and the cerebellum are also involved. The direct corticospinal tract most likely superimposes speed and agility on the motor mechanisms subserved by other descending indirect pathways.

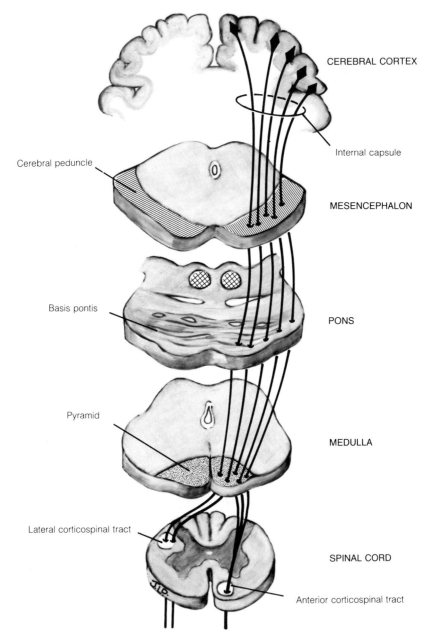

CEREBRAL CORTEX

Internal capsule

Cerebral peduncle

MESENCEPHALON

Basis pontis

PONS

Pyramid

MEDULLA

Lateral corticospinal tract

SPINAL CORD

Anterior corticospinal tract

11-6 Schematic diagram of the corticospinal pathway.

Corticoreticular Pathway (Fig. 11–7)

This fiber tract arises from most if not all parts of the cerebral cortex and accompanies the corticospinal fiber system, leaving it at different levels of the neuraxis to project upon reticular neurons in the brain stem. The corticoreticular fibers arising from one cerebral hemisphere project roughly equally to both sides of the brain stem reticular formation. Many of these fibers ultimately project upon cranial nerve nuclei in the brain stem, thus forming the corticoreticulobulbar pathway.

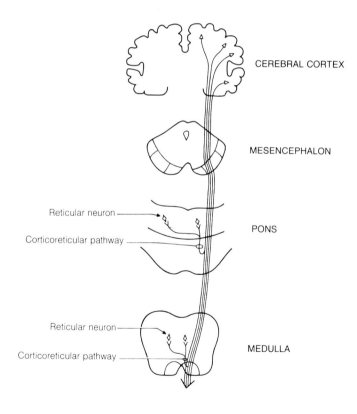

11–7 Schematic diagram of the corticoreticular pathway.

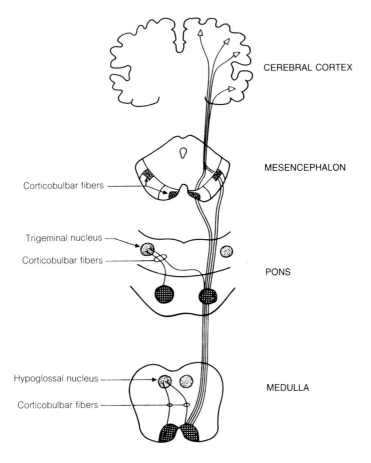

11-8 Schematic diagram of the corticobulbar pathway.

Corticobulbar Pathway (Fig. 11-8)

Direct corticobulbar fibers (without intermediate synapse on reticular neurons) are known to project from the cerebral cortex to nuclei of trigeminal (CN V), facial (CN VII), and hypoglossal (CN XII) cranial nerves. These fibers descend in the genu of the internal capsule and occupy a dorsolateral corner of the corticospinal segment of the cerebral peduncle, as well as a small area in the medial part of the base of the cerebral peduncle. In the pons, corticobulbar fibers are intermixed with the corticospinal fibers within the basis pontis. The corticobulbar input to nuclei of trigeminal and hypoglossal cranial nerves is bilateral. The input to that part of the facial nucleus which supplies upper facial muscles is also bilateral. The input to that part of the facial nucleus which supplies lower facial muscles is from

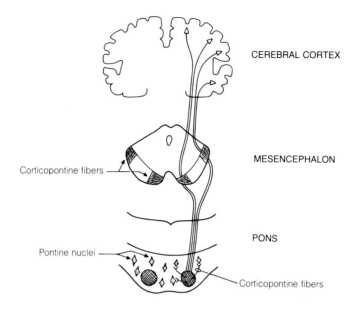

11-9   Schematic diagram of the corticopontine pathway.

the contralateral hemisphere only. Bilateral interruption of the cortico-bulbar or corticoreticulobulbar fiber system results in paresis (weakness), but not paralysis, of the muscles supplied by the corresponding cranial nerve nucleus. This condition is known as pseudobulbar palsy to distinguish it from bulbar palsy, which is a condition characterized by complete paralysis of muscles supplied by a cranial nerve nucleus as a result of a lesion of the nucleus.

Corticopontine Pathway (Fig. 11-9)

Fibers comprising this pathway arise from all parts of the cerebral cortex, but primarily from the frontal, parietal, and occipital lobes; most fibers, however, arise from the primary motor area (precentral gyrus), with relatively few from the temporal and prefrontal cortices. These fibers descend in the internal capsule and occupy the most medial and lateral parts of the cerebral peduncle before reaching the basis pontis, where they project upon pontine nuclei. The corticopontine fibers constitute by far the largest component of the corticofugal fiber system. It is estimated that each corticopontine pathway contains approximately 19 million fibers. With approximately the same number of pontine neurons on each side of the basis pontis, the ratio of corticopontine fibers to pontine neurons becomes 1:1. Corticopontine fibers terminate in sharply delineated lamellae extending rostrocaudally. Various cortical regions project to separate parts of the pontine nuclei, although considerable overlap takes place between some projection areas. Pontine neurons which receive corticopontine fibers give rise to the pontocerebellar pathway discussed in the chapter on the pons. The corticopontine pathway is thus one of several pathways that link the cerebral cortex with the cerebellum for the coordination and regulation of movement. Lesions of the corticopontine pathway at its sites of origin in the cortex or along its course will result in incoordinated movement (ataxia) contralateral to the lesion. The ataxia observed in some patients with frontal or temporal lobe pathology is thus explained as an interruption of the corticopontine pathway.

Corticothalamic Pathway

The corticothalamic pathway arises from cortical areas that receive thalamic projections and thus constitutes a feedback mechanism by which the cerebral cortex influences thalamic activity.

The thalamocortical relationship is such that a thalamic nucleus which projects to a cortical area receives in turn a projection from that area. Examples of such reciprocal connections include the dorsomedial thalamic nucleus and prefrontal cortex, anterior thalamic nucleus and cingulate cortex, ventrolateral thalamic nucleus and motor cortex, posteroventral thalamic nucleus and postcentral gyrus, medial geniculate nucleus and auditory cortex, and lateral geniculate nucleus and visual cortex.

Corticothalamic fibers descend in various parts of the internal capsule and enter the thalamus in one bundle known as the thalamic radiation, which also includes the reciprocal thalamocortical fibers.

Corticohypothalamic Pathway

The corticohypothalamic fibers arise primarily from the frontal cortex.

Corticostriate Pathway

Fibers in this pathway arise from wide areas of the cortex and project mainly upon the ipsilateral caudate and putamen. They travel via the internal or external capsule. A crossed corticostriate projection has recently been described arising from the prefrontal cortex. Bilateral cortical projections to the striatum have also been described arising from the supplementary motor cortex and from area 5 of the parietal cortex. There is so much overlap in striatal terminations from the cortex that no one part of the striatum is under the sole control of one cortical area. Corticostriate projections may reach the striatum directly or indirectly via thalamic nuclei or as collaterals from such corticofugal pathways as the cortico-olivary and corticopontine tracts.

Other Corticofugal Pathways

These include cortical projections to several sensory brain stem nuclei, such as the nuclei gracilis and cuneatus, trigeminal nuclei, and others. Most of these fibers serve a feedback purpose. The questionable corticosubthalamic projection has recently been confirmed arising from the primary sensory cortical areas. A corticotectal projection has also been described recently arising from the frontal eyefields (area 8 of the frontal cortex) in addition to an already established origin in the occipital cortex.

Intracortical Circuitry

Cortical neurons may have descending, ascending, horizontal, or short axons. The descending axons contribute to the association and the corticofugal fiber systems outlined above. The ascending, horizontal, and short axons play important roles in intracortical circuitry. Neurons with ascending axons are the cells of Martinotti. The horizontal cells of Cajal have horizontal axons. Short axons arborizing in the vicinity of the cell body are seen in stellate neurons. Pyramidal neurons have horizontal and recurrent axon collaterals which terminate at all levels of the cortex and contribute significantly to intracortical connections. The axon collaterals of pyramidal neurons may project upon a stellate cell or a Martinotti cell that in turn may influence other cortical neurons and thus provide for rapid dispersion of activity throughout a population of neurons. This fact was recognized by Cajal, who referred to it as *avalanche conduction*. Recurrent collaterals of pyramidal neurons may contribute to excitatory as well as inhibitory circuits. The inhibitory circuit is mediated through a recurrent collateral-interneuron pathway analogous to the Renshaw pathway in the spinal cord.

Possible reverberating circuits within the cortex are illustrated in the following pathways.

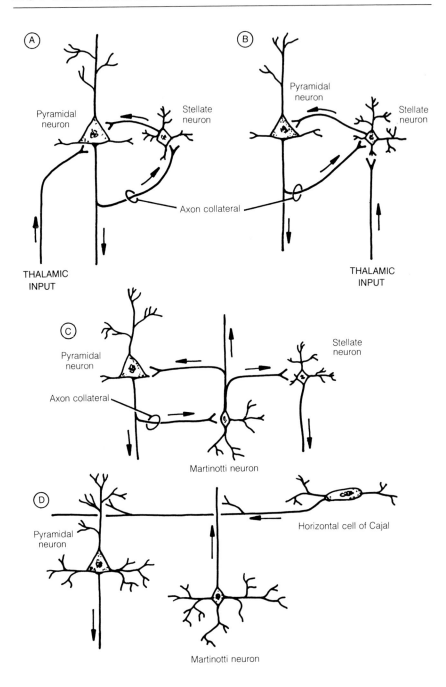

11-10 Schematic diagram of various internal neuronal loops within the cerebral cortex.

1. A thalamic input projects upon the basal dendrites of a pyramidal neuron with axon collaterals to a stellate (granule) neuron and through short axons back to the pyramidal neuron (Fig. 11–10, *A*).
2. A thalamic input projects upon a stellate (granule) neuron. The short axon of the stellate neuron projects upon a pyramidal neuron. The axon collateral of the pyramidal neuron projects back upon the same or another stellate neuron (Fig 11–10, *B*).
3. Axon collaterals of a pyramidal neuron project upon Martinotti neurons with ascending axons to either a stellate (granule) neuron or a pyramidal neuron (Fig. 11–10, *C*).
4. Axons of horizontal cells of Cajal project upon dendrites of pyramidal neurons and axons of Martinotti neurons (Fig. 11–10, *D*). This pathway plays a minimal role in intracortical circuits in the adult, since the horizontal cells of Cajal disappear after neonatal life.

From the above, it can be seen that an input to the cortex is spread both horizontally and vertically via the various intracortical connections. The complexity of these interconnections is far from clear definition and is the basis of the complexity of human brain function.

Cortical Cytoarchitectonic Areas

Different parts of the cortex vary in relation to the following parameters.
1. Thickness of the cortex
2. Thickness of the different laminae of the cortex
3. Neuronal morphology
4. Nerve fiber lamination

Based on the above variations, different investigators have parceled the cortex into from 20 to 200 areas, depending on the criteria used. The classification of Brodmann, published in 1909, remains the most widely used. It contains 52 cytoarchitectonic areas. More important than the cytoarchitectonic classification is the functional classification of the cortex into several motor and sensory areas. The account that follows will focus on functional areas of the cortex. Brodmann's terminology will be used since it is the most frequently cited. The commonly used classification of cortical areas into purely sensory and motor is somewhat misleading and inaccurate. There is ample evidence to suggest that motor responses can be elicited from so-called sensory areas. This has prompted the use of the term sensory motor cortex to refer to previously designated sensory and motor areas.

However, for didactic purposes, the motor and sensory areas of the cortex will be discussed separately.

Cortical Sensory Areas

Sensory function in the cortex is localized mainly in three lobes: parietal, occipital, and temporal. There are six primary sensory areas in the cortex.

1. Primary somesthetic (general sensory) area in the postcentral gyrus of the parietal lobe
2. Primary visual area in the occipital lobe
3. Primary auditory area in the temporal lobe
4. Primary gustatory (taste) area in the parietal lobe
5. Primary olfactory (smell) area in the temporal lobe
6. Primary vestibular area in the temporal lobe

Each of these areas receives a specific sensory modality (smell, taste, vision, etc.). Sensory modalities reaching each of these areas (except olfaction) pass through the thalamus (specific thalamic nucleus) prior to reaching the cortex. Each of the above sensory areas is designated as a primary sensory area. Adjacent to the primary somesthetic, visual, and auditory areas are secondary sensory areas. The secondary sensory areas are found by recording evoked potentials in the respective areas following an appropriate peripheral stimulus (sound, light, etc). In general, the secondary sensory areas are smaller in size than the primary areas and their ablation is without effect on the specific sensory modality.

Primary Somesthetic (General Sensory) Area (SI)

This area (Fig. 11–11) corresponds to the postcentral gyrus of the parietal lobe (areas 1, 2, and 3 of Brodmann). In 1916 Dusser de Barenne applied strychnine, a central stimulant drug, to the postcentral gyrus of monkeys and noted that the animals scratched their skin. Subsequent work by Head on World War I soldiers with head injuries and by the neurosurgeons Cushing and Penfield has added tremendously to knowledge about the function of this area.

Although the primary somesthetic area is concerned basically with sensory modalities, it is possible to elicit motor responses following its stimulation.

The primary somesthetic area receives nerve fibers from the posteroventral lateral and posteroventral medial nuclei of the thalamus. These fibers convey general sensory (touch, pain, and temperature) as well as proprioceptive sensory modalities (position, vibration, and two-point discrimination). The bulk of thalamic input terminates upon neurons in area 3 of Brodmann. The contralateral half of the body is represented in a precise but disproportionate manner (sensory homunculus) in the somesthetic area (Fig. 11–12). The pharynx, tongue, and jaw are represented

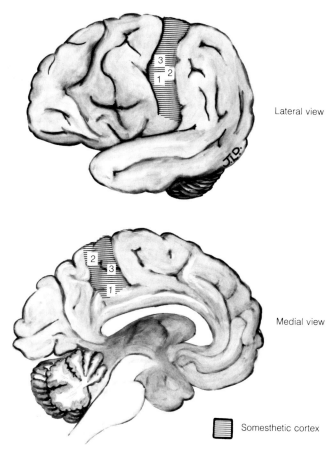

11–11 Schematic diagram of the primary somesthetic cortex.

in the most ventral portion of the lateral surface of the somesthetic area, followed in ascending order by the face, hand, arm, trunk, and thigh. The leg and foot are represented on the medial surface of this area. The anal and genital regions are represented in the most ventral portion of the medial surface just above the cingulate gyrus. The representation of the face, lips, hand, thumb, and index fingers is disproportionately large in comparison with their relative size in the body. This is a reflection of the functional importance of these parts in sensory function.

Stimulation of the primary somesthetic cortex in conscious patients elicits sensations of numbness and tingling, a feeling of electricity, and a feeling of movement without actual movement.

Ablation of the postcentral gyrus will result, in the immediate postoperative period, in loss of all modalities of sensation (touch, pressure, pain,

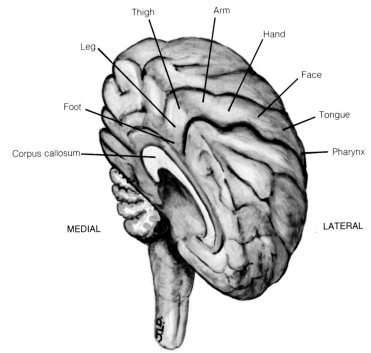

Thigh
Arm
Hand
Leg
Face
Foot
Tongue
Corpus callosum
Pharynx
MEDIAL
LATERAL

11–12 Schematic diagram of the sensory homunculus.

and temperature). Soon, however, pain and temperature sensations will return. It is believed that pain and temperature sensations are determined at the thalamic level, whereas the source, severity, and quality of such sensations are perceived in the postcentral gyrus. Thus, the effects of postcentral gyrus lesions would be 1) complete loss of discriminative touch and proprioception and 2) crude awareness of pain, temperature and touch.

Neurophysiologic studies of the somesthetic cortex have revealed the following information. 1) The functional cortical unit appears to be associated with a vertical column of cells which is modality-specific. Neurons within a cortical unit are activated by the same peripheral stimulus and are related to the same peripheral receptive field. 2) Area 3 is activated by cutaneous stimuli, whereas area 2 receives proprioceptive impulses. 3) Somatosensory neurons responding to joint movement show a marked degree of specificity in that they respond to displacement in one direction. 4) Fast and slow adapting neuronal pools have been identified in response to hair displacement or cutaneous deformation. 5) Fibers mediating cutaneous sensations terminate rostrally, while those mediating proprioceptive sensations terminate more caudally in the somesthetic area.

A secondary somesthetic (S II) area has been described in subprimate species and probably exists in man, although its function is not yet clear.

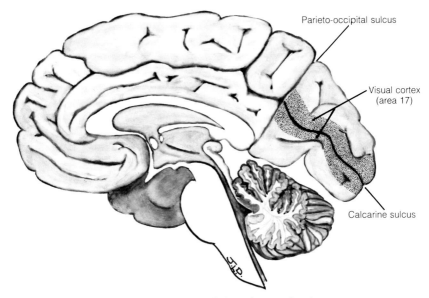

11–13 Schematic diagram of the primary visual cortex.

It is located on the superior bank of the lateral sulcus within the postcentral gyrus and extending on the insula. Body representation in this area is the reverse of that in the primary area, so that the two face areas are adjacent to each other.

Primary Visual Cortex

This area (Fig. 11–13) corresponds to the calcarine gyrus on the medial surface of the occipital lobe on each side of the calcarine sulcus (area 17 of Brodmann). In sections of fresh cortex, this area is characterized by the appearance of a prominent band of white matter which can be identified by the naked eye and is named the band of Gennari, after the Italian medical student who described it. The band of Gennari represents a thickened external band of Baillarger in layer IV of the cortex. In myelin preparations, the band of Gennari appears as a prominent dark band in the visual cortex, also known as the striate cortex. The term striate refers to the presence in unstained preparations of the thick white band of Gennari.

The primary visual area receives fibers from the lateral geniculate nucleus. These fibers originate in the retina, synapse in the lateral geniculate

LEFT   RIGHT

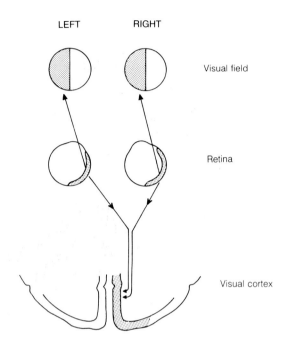

Visual field

Retina

Visual cortex

11–14   Schematic diagram of retinal representation in the visual cortex.

nucleus, and reach the visual cortex via the optic (geniculocalcarine) radiation. Each visual cortex receives fibers from the ipsilateral half of each retina (Fig. 11–14) which convey information about the contralateral half of the visual field. Thus, lesions of one visual cortex are manifested by loss of vision in the contralateral half of the visual field (homonymous hemianopia). The projections from the retina into the visual cortex are spatially organized in such a way that macular fibers occupy the posterior part of the visual cortex, while peripheral retinal fibers occupy the anterior part (Fig. 11–15). Fibers originating from the superior half of the retina terminate in the superior part of the visual cortex; those from the inferior half of the retina terminate in the inferior part (Fig. 11–16). The representation of the macula in the visual cortex is disproportionately large in comparison with its relative size in the retina. This is a reflection of its important function as the retinal area of keenest vision.

    Stimulation of the visual cortex elicits a crude sensation of bright flashes of light; patients with irritative lesions (such as tumors) of the visual cortex experience visual hallucinations which consist of bright light. Conversely, lesions that destroy the visual cortex of one hemisphere result in loss of

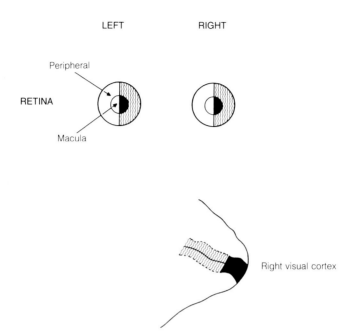

11–15 Schematic diagram of retinal representation in the visual cortex.

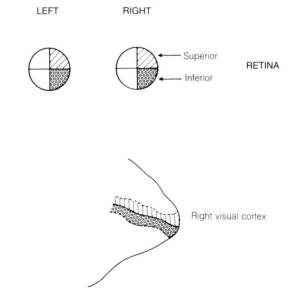

11–16 Schematic diagram of retinal representation in the visual cortex.

vision in the contralateral half of the visual field. If the destructive lesion is of vascular origin, such as occurs in occlusions of the posterior cerebral artery, central (macular) vision in the affected visual field is spared. This phenomenon is known clinically as macular sparing and is attributed to the collateral arterial supply of the posterior visual cortex (macular area) from the patent, contralateral posterior cerebral artery.

In the last decade, elegant neurophysiologic studies of single neurons in the visual cortex have revealed the following information.

1. The visual cortex is organized into units that correspond to specific areas in the retina.
2. These units respond to linear stripe (straight line) configurations.
3. For each unit, a particular orientation of the stimulus is most effective. Some units respond only to vertically oriented stripes, while others respond only to horizontally oriented stripes. Some units respond at onset of illumination, while others respond at cessation of illumination.
4. Units are of two varieties, simple and complex. Simple units react only to stimuli in corresponding fixed retinal receptive fields. Complex units are connected to several simple cortical units. It is presumed that the complex units represent an advanced stage in cortical integration.
5. Units that respond to the same stimulus pattern and orientation are grouped together in vertical columns similar to those described for the somesthetic cortex.
6. Visual columns respond poorly if at all to diffuse retinal illumination.
7. Visual units respond optimally to moving stimuli.
8. Most cortical units receive fibers from corresponding receptive fields in both retinae, thus allowing for single image vision of corresponding points in the two retinae.

Adjacent to the primary visual area is the secondary visual (association, prestriate) area. This corresponds to areas 18 and 19 of Brodmann (Fig. 11–17). The primary visual cortex projects bilaterally and reciprocally to the secondary visual areas. Units in the secondary visual area are all of the complex type. The secondary visual area is connected with the frontal eye fields (area 8 of Brodmann), as well as with the superior colliculus and motor nuclei of extraocular muscles. Thus, it plays a key role in conjugate eye movement induced by visual stimuli. The secondary visual area is also connected via association and commissural fibers with the angular gyrus and with many parts of the ipsi- and contralateral hemispheres. Connections to the contralateral hemisphere play an important role in transfer of monocular learned behavior into the opposite hemisphere. The secondary visual area is also concerned with the recognition of what is seen. Stimulation of this area (as occurs in irritative lesions in humans) elicits hallucinations of formed images, in contrast to that of the bright, crude flash or spark experienced after stimulation of the primary visual cortex. Con-

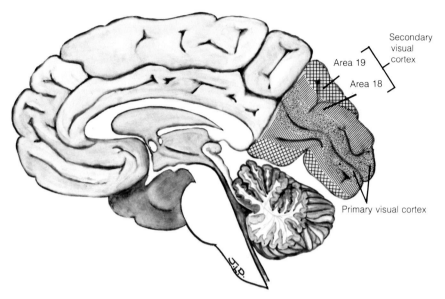

11–17 Schematic diagram of the primary and secondary visual cortices.

versely, ablation of this area results in the phenomenon of visual agnosia, in which the patient is able to see objects but is unable to recognize them.

Color vision is localized inferiorly in the secondary (association) visual cortex. No color representation is found in the superior association visual cortex. Thus in unilateral inferior association visual cortex lesions, the patient loses color vision in the contralateral half field of vision (central hemiachromatopsia). Bilateral lesions of the inferior association visual cortex result, in addition to achromatopsia, in loss of facial recognition (prosopagnosia). Depth perception is localized to the upper visual association cortex. Lesions in the upper visual association cortex result in disturbances in depth of vision contralaterally. The evidence for depth perception localization is not as firm as that for color vision.

Primary Auditory Cortex

The primary auditory cortex (Fig 11–18) corresponds to the transverse temporal gyri of Heschl (areas 41 and 42 of Brodmann) located in the temporal lobe within the lateral fissure.

The primary auditory cortex receives fibers from the medial geniculate nucleus. These fibers originate in the peripheral organ of Corti and establish several synapses in the neuraxis, both homolateral and contralateral to their side of origin, before reaching the medial geniculate nucleus of the

Lateral fissure (widely opened)

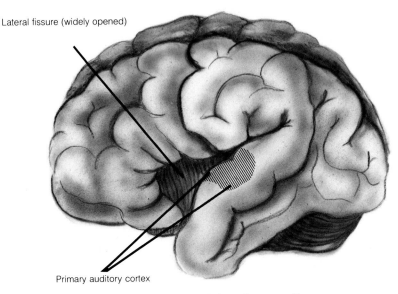

Primary auditory cortex

11–18   Schematic diagram of the primary auditory cortex.

thalamus. The primary auditory cortex, therefore, receives fibers from both organs of Corti, predominantly from the contralateral side. Stimulation of the primary auditory cortex produces crude auditory sensations such as buzzing, humming, or knocking. Such sensations are referred to clinically as tinnitus. Lesions of the auditory cortex result in 1) impairment in sound localization in space and 2) diminution of hearing bilaterally, but mostly contralaterally.

Adjacent to the primary auditory cortex is the association auditory cortex (areas 22 and 24 of Brodmann). This area is believed to be concerned with the comprehension of spoken sound. Area 22 in the dominant hemisphere is also known as Wernicke's area. Lesions of this area are associated with a receptive type of aphasia, a disorder of communication characterized by the inability of the patient to comprehend spoken words. The primary auditory cortex is connected with the association auditory cortex. Other important connections include the auditory cortex of the contralateral hemisphere, the primary somesthetic cortex, frontal eye fields, Broca's area of speech in the frontal lobe, and the medial geniculate nucleus. The association auditory cortex is connected via the anterior commissure with the prefrontal cortex and via the corpus callosum with the prefrontal, premotor, parietal, and cingulate cortices.

Physiologic studies of the auditory cortex have revealed that it does not play a major role in sound frequency discrimination, but rather in the temporal patterns of acoustic stimuli. Frequency discrimination of sound is a function of subcortical structures of the acoustic system. The optimal stimulus that fires auditory cortical units seems to be a changing frequency of sound stimuli rather than a steady frequency stimulus.

Primary Gustatory Cortex

The cortical receptive area for taste is located in the parietal operculum, ventral to the primary somesthetic area and in close proximity to the cortical areas receiving sensory afferents from the tongue and pharynx. It corresponds to area 43 of Brodmann. Irritative lesions in this area in man have been shown to give rise to hallucinations of taste, usually preceding the onset of an epileptic attack. Such a prodromal symptom preceding an epileptic fit focuses attention on the site of the irritative lesion. Conversely, ablation of this area produces impairment of taste contralateral to the site of the lesion. The gustatory cortex receives fibers from the posteroventral medial nucleus of the thalamus, upon which converge sensory fibers from the face and mouth, including taste fibers. Although crude taste sensations can be perceived at the thalamic level, discrimination among different taste sensations is a cortical function.

Primary Olfactory Cortex

The primary olfactory cortex is located in the tip of the temporal lobe and consists of the prepyriform cortex and the periamygdaloid area. The primary olfactory cortex receives fibers from the lateral olfactory stria and has an intimate relationship with adjacent cortical regions comprising part of the limbic system. Such relationships, as well as the role of olfaction in emotion and behavior, are discussed in the chapter on the limbic system. Adjacent to the primary olfactory cortex is the entorhinal cortex, which is considered the association or secondary olfactory cortical area.

Irritative lesions in the region of the olfactory cortex give rise to olfactory hallucinations which are usually disagreeable. As in the case of taste, such hallucinations frequently precede an epileptic fit. Since olfactory hallucinations frequently occur in association with lesions in the uncus of the temporal lobe (including the olfactory cortex), they are referred to clinically as uncinate fits.

The olfactory system is the only sensory system in which fibers reach the cortex without passing through the thalamus.

Basic olfactory functions needed for reflex action reside in subcortical structures. The discrimination of different odors, however, is a function of the olfactory cortex.

Primary Vestibular Cortex

Data are scant about the anatomic location as well as the physiologic properties of the primary vestibular cortex. It is, however, generally agreed that the vestibular cortex is located in two adjacent areas. The first is near or in the face area of the primary somesthetic cortex (parietal lobe) and the second is in close proximity (anterior) to the primary auditory area (temporal lobe). Although the primary vestibular cortex is believed to receive contralateral vestibular fibers, this has not been demonstrated with certainty. It is assumed that the vestibular cortex functions in the conscious appreciation of orientation in space. Stimulation of the vestibular cortex in man produces a hallucination of body movement (vertigo). This hallucination is more marked following stimulation of the vestibular cortex of the temporal lobe.

Cortical Motor Areas

Motor function in the cortex is located primarily in the frontal lobe. The following motor areas are generally recognized.

1. Primary motor area
2. Supplementary motor area
3. Premotor area
4. Frontal eye fields
5. Motor speech area

Primary Motor Area (MI)

The primary motor area (Fig. 11–19) corresponds to the precentral gyrus (area 4 of Brodmann). The contralateral half of the body is represented in the primary motor area in a precise but disproportionate manner, giving rise to the motor homunculus in the same way as that described for the primary somesthetic cortex. Stimulation of the motor cortex in conscious man gives rise to discrete and isolated contralateral movement limited to a single joint or a single muscle. Bilateral responses are seen in the head muscles. The primary motor cortex thus functions in the initiation of highly skilled fine movements, such as buttoning one's shirt or sewing.

The representation of bodily regions in the contralateral motor cortex does not seem to be rigidly fixed. Thus, repetitive stimulation of the thumb area will produce movement of the thumb, followed after a while by immobility of the thumb and movement at the index finger or even the wrist. This has been interpreted to mean that in the thumb area of the cortex the motor units controlling the index finger and wrist have a higher threshold for stimulation than those controlling the thumb.

Precentral gyrus
(primary motor cortex)

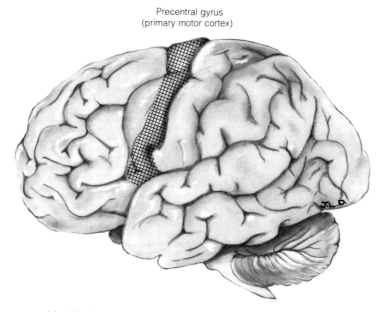

11–19   Schematic diagram of the primary motor cortex.

The motor area receives fibers from the ventrolateral and ventral anterior nuclei of the thalamus. The former is the main projection area of the cerebellum, the latter of the basal ganglia. The motor area is also connected to the somesthetic cortex, the premotor cortex, and the contralateral motor cortex. Its output contributes to the association, commissural, and corticofugal fiber systems discussed earlier. The primary motor cortex is the site of origin of about 40% of the fibers in the pyramidal tract. Furthermore, all of the large-diameter axons (approximately 3% of the pyramidal fibers) originate from the giant motor neurons (of Betz) in the primary motor cortex. Ablation of the primary motor cortex results in flaccid (hypotonic) paralysis in the contralateral half of the body, associated with loss of all reflexes. With time, there is recovery of stereotyped movement at proximal joints, but the function of distal muscles concerned with skilled movement remains impaired.

Although the primary motor cortex is not the sole area from which movement can be elicited, it is nevertheless characterized by initiating highly skilled movement at a lower threshold of stimulation than the other motor areas.

Epileptic patients with a lesion in the primary motor cortex frequently manifest a seizure (epileptic) pattern which consists of progression of the epileptic movement from one part of the body to another in a characteristic sequence corresponding to body representation in the motor cortex. Such a phenomenon is known clinically as a "Jacksonian march," after the English neurologist Hughlings Jackson.

Neurophysiologic studies of motor cortex neurons reveal that action potentials can be recorded from motor neurons in the cortex about 60 to 80 msec preceding muscle movement. Furthermore, two types of neurons in the motor cortex have been identified. These are a larger neuron with a phasic pattern of firing and a smaller neuron that fires in a tonic pattern. From experiments on conscious animals performing specific tasks, it has been shown that the frequency of firing is highly correlated with the force exerted to perform a specific movement. Motor neurons supplying a given muscle are usually grouped together in a columnar fashion. Although some motor neurons can be stimulated from a wide area, each has a so-called "best point" from which it can be most easily stimulated. Such best points usually are confined to a cylindric area of cortex about 1 mm in diameter.

Supplementary Motor Area

The supplementary motor area is located on the medial surface of the frontal lobe, anterior to the medial extension of the primary motor cortex (area 4). It corresponds roughly to the medial extensions of area 6 and part of area 8 of Brodmann. A homunculus has been defined for the supplementary motor area in which hand and arm are represented rostral to the leg and trunk. Stimulation in man gives rise to complex movement in preparation for the assumption of characteristic postures. Recently, cells were identified in the supplementary motor area in response to movements of both proximal and distal extremity muscles, ipsi- and contralateral. Supplementary motor area neurons differ from primary motor area neurons in that only a small percentage (5%) of supplementary motor area neurons contribute axons to the pyramidal tract and these neurons have insignificant input from the periphery and are activated bilaterally. Studies on fiber connections of the supplementary motor area have shown extensive connections with cortical and subcortical structures. Projections to the supplementary motor area have been described from the primary and association cortices of the frontal and parietal lobes as well as from the thalamus. The supplementary motor area has been shown to project to the contralateral supplementary motor area as well as to the striatum, thalamus, red nuclei, pontine nuclei, dorsal column nuclei, and the spinal cord. Available anatomic and physiologic data suggest that the supplementary motor area could be the site where external inputs and commands are matched with internal needs and drives to facilitate formulation (programming) of a strategy of voluntary movement. The threshold of stimulation of the supplementary motor area is higher than that of the primary motor cortex and the responses elicited are ipsi- or bilateral.

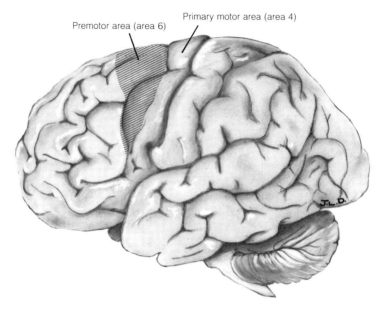

Premotor area (area 6) Primary motor area (area 4)

11–20 Schematic diagram of the premotor cortex.

Ablation of the supplementary motor area gives rise to a transient grasp reflex, hypertonia, increase in myotatic reflexes, clonus, and the Babinski sign. Thus, involvement of the supplementary motor cortex may be responsible for the above signs, known to accompany lesions of the motor cortex in man.

Premotor Area

The premotor area (Fig. 11–20) is located in the frontal lobe just anterior to and encroaching upon the primary motor area. It corresponds to area 6 of Brodmann. Stimulation of the premotor area elicits a stereotyped gross movement that requires coordination among many muscles, such as turning the head, twisting the trunk, and limb movement at proximal joints. The threshold of stimuli which elicit responses from this area is higher than that required for the primary motor cortex. The premotor area exerts influence on movement via the primary motor area or directly through its projections to the pyramidal and extrapyramidal systems. The projection of the visual and auditory cortices to the premotor area suggests that the premotor area provides a route, at cortical level, whereby visual and auditory information may influence the activity of the primary motor area. The premotor area is activated when a new motor program is established or when the motor program is changed on the basis of sensory information received, for example, when the subject is exploring the environment or objects. Ablation of the premotor cortex in man may produce a deficit in the execution of skilled, sequential, and complex movement such as walking. Such a deficit is known clinically as apraxia. In such a syndrome, the patient has difficulty in walking, although there is no voluntary motor paralysis. The grasp reflex attributed to lesions of the premotor area in the older literature is now believed to be due to involvement of the supplementary motor cortex.

Some neuroscientists consider the separation of the motor cortex into primary motor and premotor areas somewhat artificial. However, closer consideration of this issue justifies this separation on the basis of the threshold of stimuli that elicit motor responses (much lower in the primary motor area) as well as the type of movement elicited from stimulation (discrete from the primary motor area *versus* coordinated, complex movement from the premotor area).

In clinical situations, however, both areas are more often than not involved together in disease processes, be it vascular occlusion, or hemorrhage leading to stroke or a tumor invading this region of the cortex. In such situations, the clinical manifestations can be classified into those seen immediately after the onset of the pathology and those that follow after a few days or weeks. The former consist of loss of all reflexes and hypotonia of affected muscles. Within hours or days, however, stereotyped movement, particularly in proximal muscles, returns, hypotonia changes to hypertonia and areflexia to hyperactive myotatic reflexes, and a Babinski sign appears. The discrete movements in distal muscles, however, remain impaired. Such a clinical picture is often seen following a stroke involving this region of the cortex.

Frontal Eye Fields

The frontal eye fields (Fig. 11–21) are located in the middle frontal gyrus anterior to the primary motor and premotor areas. They correspond to area 8 of Brodmann and the immediately adjacent cortex. Stimulation of this area elicits conjugate (binocular) division of both eyes to the contralateral side (Fig. 11–22). In clinical situations, this phenomenon is observed as part of an epileptic seizure when the irritating focus is in or near area 8 of Brodmann. Conversely, ablation of area 8 on one side will result in conjugate deviation of the eyes to the homolateral side (Fig. 11–22) as a result of the unopposed action of the intact area 8. In clinical situations, such a phenomenon is seen in patients with occlusion of a major cerebral artery and infarction (death) of cortical tissue in the frontal cortex. Such patients manifest paralysis of face and extremities contralateral to the cortical lesion and a conjugate deviation of the eyes toward the cortical lesion.

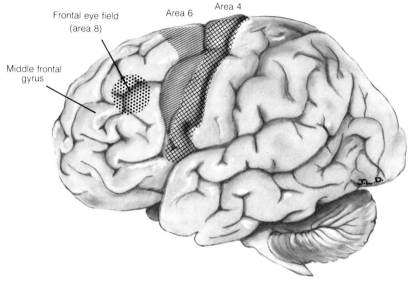

11–21 Schematic diagram of the frontal eye fields.

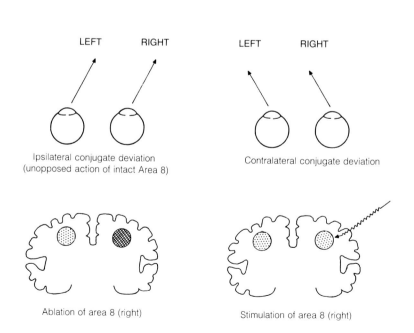

11–22 Schematic diagram of the effect of stimulation and lesions in the frontal eye fields on conjugate eye movements.

The frontal eye fields elicit conjugate deviation of the eyes through their action on nuclei of extraocular muscles in the brain stem. The exact pathway has not been fully defined; it is believed, however, that the frontal eye fields influence nuclei of extraocular muscles through an indirect path via the intermediary of reticular neurons in the brain stem.

The frontal eye fields receive fibers from the occipital lobe (primary and association visual cortices). Stimulation of the occipital cortex elicits conjugate eye movements similar to those elicited from the frontal eye fields. Under normal conditions, visual stimuli seem to trigger the frontal eye fields via the occipital cortex.

Motor Speech Area

The motor area for speech (Broca's area) (Fig. 11–23) is located in the inferior frontal gyrus rostral to the face, tongue, lip, and pharynx areas of the primary motor area. It corresponds to areas 44 and 45 of Brodmann in the dominant hemisphere. Lesions affecting the motor speech area result in the inability of the patients to express themselves in oral or written language. Such patients can comprehend language but cannot express themselves using language (motor or expressive aphasia). If you ask such a patient to name an object such as a pencil, the patient will not be able to name it. On the other hand, if you display this pencil along with another

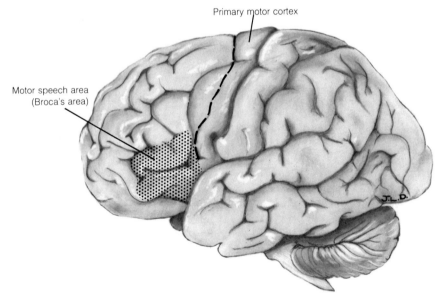

11–23 Schematic diagram of Broca's area of speech.

object such as a coin or eraser and ask the patient to point to the pencil, it will be correctly done.

Electrophysiologic studies and cerebral blood flow studies have confirmed the role of Broca's area in speech expression. Records made from scalp electrodes placed over Broca's area have revealed a slow negative potential of several seconds in duration appearing over Broca's area 1 to 2 sec prior to uttering of words. Stimulation of Broca's area in conscious patients may inhibit speech or may result in utterance of vowel sounds. Studies on cerebral blood flow have shown a marked increase in flow in Broca's area during speech.

Other Cortical Areas

In addition to the previously discussed motor and sensory areas, the cerebral cortex contains other functionally important areas. These include the prefrontal cortex and the major association cortex.

Prefrontal Cortex

The prefrontal cortex (Fig. 11–24) refers to the area of the cortex comprising the pole of the frontal lobe. It corresponds to areas 9, 10, and 11

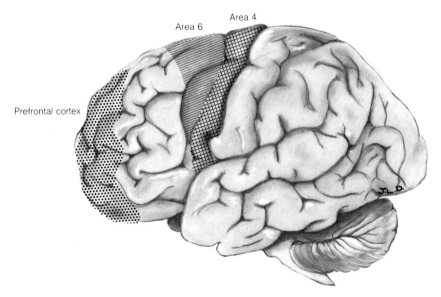

11–24 Schematic diagram of the prefrontal cortex.

of Brodmann. Motor responses are as a rule not elicited by stimulation of this area of the frontal lobe. The prefrontal cortex is well developed only in primates and especially so in man. It is believed to play a role in affective behavior and judgment. Bilateral lesions in the prefrontal cortex result in inappropriate judgmental behavior and emotional lability. Such patients usually neglect their appearance, laugh or cry inappropriately, and have no appreciation of norms of social behavior and conduct. They are uninhibited and highly distractable. Surgical ablation of the prefrontal cortex (prefrontal lobotomy) was resorted to in the past to treat patients with mental disorders such as schizophrenia, and intractable pain. In the latter group, the effect of the operation was not to relieve the sensation of pain but rather to alter the affective reaction (suffering) of the patient to pain. Such patients continue to feel pain but become indifferent to it. The ablation of the prefrontal area in patients with mental illness has largely been replaced by administration of psychopharmacologic drugs.

Major Association Cortex

The major association cortex (Fig. 11–25) refers to the supramarginal and angular gyri in the inferior parietal gyrus. It corresponds to areas 39 and 40 of Brodmann. The major association cortex is connected with all the

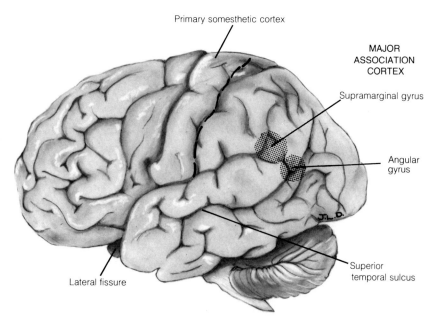

11–25 Schematic diagram of the major association cortex.

sensory cortical areas and thus functions in higher order and complex multisensory perception. Its relation to the speech areas in the temporal and frontal lobes gives it an important role in communication skills. Patients with lesions in the major association cortex of the dominant hemisphere present a conglomerate of manifestations that include receptive and expressive aphasia; inability to write (agraphia); inability to synthesize, correlate, and recognize multisensory perceptions (agnosia); left-right confusion; difficulty in recognizing the different fingers (finger agnosia); and inability to calculate (acalculia). These symptoms and signs are grouped together under the term "Gerstmann's syndrome."

Involvement of the major association cortex in the nondominant hemisphere is usually manifested by disturbances in drawing (constructional apraxia) and in the awareness of body image. Such patients have difficulty in drawing a square or circle or copying a complex figure. They often are unaware of a body part and thus neglect to shave one half of the face or dress one half of the body.

Cortical Electrophysiology

Electrical Responses of Cortical Neurons

Two basic types of responses have been recorded from cortical neurons; these are the all or none response and the graded response.

The all or none response of cortical neurons to a threshold stimulus is primarily triggered by a critical membrane depolarization initiating an increase in sodium conductance (further depolarization) and "regenerative action" which augments the inward flow of sodium. This process is arrested by the subsequent sodium inactivation process and a state of increased potassium conductance, during which the membrane recovers its resting potential. The all or none response is followed by after-potentials which are lower in amplitude and longer in duration. The amplitude and duration of the after-potentials vary with different types of neurons.

The graded responses include the depolarizing excitatory and hyperpolarizing inhibitory postsynaptic potentials (EPSPs and IPSPs) which precede the all or none response.

Evoked Potentials

The evoked potentials represent the electrical responses recorded from a population of neurons in a particular cortical area following stimulation of the input to that area.

The most studied of the evoked potentials is the primary response recorded from the cortical surface and elicited by a single shock to a major thalamocortical pathway. This response is characterized by a diphasic, positive-negative wave and is generated primarily by synaptic currents in cortical neurons.

Evoked potentials elicited by a volley of impulses in thalamocortical pathways are of two varieties, recruiting responses and augmenting responses.

Recruiting responses are recorded following 6 to 12 cps stimulation of a nonspecific thalamocortical pathway (*e.g.*, from intralaminar nuclei). They are characterized by a long latency (multisynaptic pathway), a predominantly surface negative response which increases in amplitude to a maximum by the fourth to the sixth stimulus of a repetitive train. This is followed by a decrease in amplitude (waxing and waning). Such a response has a diffuse cortical distribution. This pattern of response is generally attributed to an oscillator network at cortical as well as thalamic levels in which cortical and thalamic elements provide both positive and negative feedback.

Augmenting responses are recorded following low frequency (6 to 12 cps) stimulation of a specific thalamocortical pathway (*e.g.*, from ventrolateral thalamic nucleus). They are characterized by a short latency (monosynaptic pathway), a diphasic, positive-negative configuration which increases in amplitude and latency during the initial four to six stimuli of the train. The response to subsequent stimuli remains augmented, but waxes and wanes in amplitude. This type of response is localized in the primary cortical area to which the stimulated specific thalamocortical pathway projects.

Electroencephalography (EEG) (Fig. 11–26)

Electroencephalography is the recording of spontaneous cortical activity from the surface of the scalp. This procedure is very commonly used in the investigation of diseases of the brain. Its usefulness is mainly in the diagnoses of epilepsy and localized (focal) brain pathology (*e.g.*, brain tumors). In recent years and with the advent of the concept of brain death, the electroencephalogram has been used to confirm a state of electrical brain silence. In such a condition, repeated electroencephalographic tracings will show no evidence of cortical potentials (flat EEG).

The spontaneous rhythmic activity of the cortex is classified into four types.

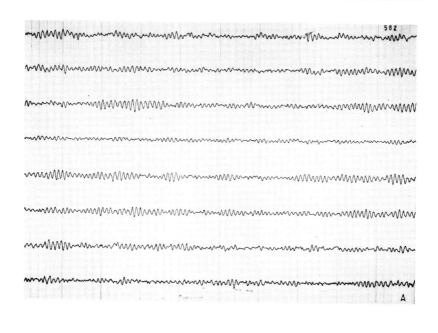

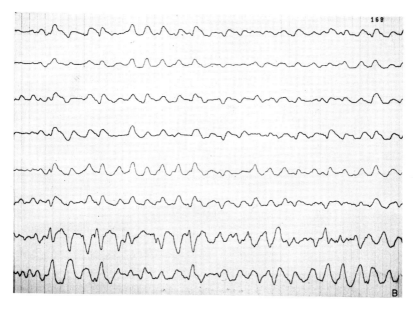

11-26 Electroencephalograms showing the normal alpha pattern (*A*), slow delta pattern (*B*), and spike potentials (*C*).

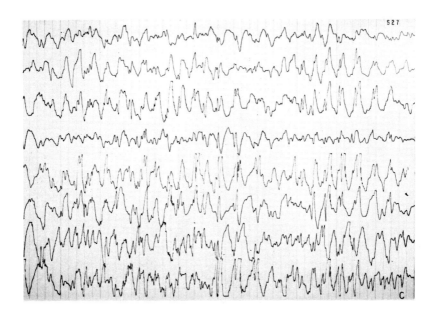

(**Fig. 11–26** continued)

1. Alpha rhythm with a range of frequency from 8 to 13 cps. This type is most developed over the posterior part of the hemisphere.
2. Beta rhythm with a range of frequency faster than 13 cps (17 to 30 cps). This activity can be seen over wide regions of the cortex and is especially apparent in records from patients receiving sedative drugs.
3. Theta rhythm with a range of frequency from 3 to 7 cps.
4. Delta rhythm with a range of frequency from 0.5 to 3 cps.

The EEG pattern varies in different age groups. The EEG is dominated by slow activity (theta and delta) in childhood. The alpha rhythm increases in amount with the advent of puberty. In the adult, delta activity and excessive theta activity usually denote cerebral abnormality.

The EEG of unconscious patients is dominated by generalized slow frequencies. The EEG in epileptic patients is characterized by the presence of spike potentials. Two EEG patterns have been associated with sleep. The first is a slow pattern (delta and theta) associated with the early phase of sleep. The second is a fast pattern (beta) associated with a later and deeper stage of sleep. This second pattern is associated with rapid eye movements (REM) and dreaming, hence this stage of sleep has been called REM sleep or D-sleep (dreaming).

References

Brinkman, C.; Porter, R.: Supplementary Motor Area in the Monkey: Activity of Neurons during Performance of a Learned Motor Task. J Neurophysiol 42 (1979) 681–709.

Brodal, P.: The Corticopontine Projection in the Rhesus Monkey. Origin and Principles of Organization. Brain 101 (1978) 251–283.

Cherubini, E.; Novak, G.; Hull, C.D.; Buchwald, N.A.; Levine, M.S.: Caudate Neuronal Responses Evoked by Cortical Stimulation: Contribution of an Indirect Corticothalamic Pathway. Brain Res 173 (1979) 331–336.

Damasio, A.; Yamada, T.; Damasio, H.; Corbett, J.; McKee, J.: Central Achromatopsia: Behavioral, Anatomic and Physiologic Aspects. Neurology 30 (1980) 1064–1071.

Eccles, J.C.: The Modular Operation of the Cerebral Neocortex Considered as the Material Basis of Mental Events. Neuroscience 6 (1981) 1839–1856.

Fallon, J.H.; Zeigler, B.T.S.: The Crossed Cortico-Caudate Projection in the Rhesus Monkey. Neurosci Lett 15 (1979) 29–32.

Jinnai, K.; Matsuda, Y.: Neurons of the Motor Cortex Projecting Commonly on the Caudate Nucleus and the Lower Brain Stem in the Cat. Neurosci Lett 13 (1979) 121–126.

Leichnetz, G.R.; Spencer, R.F.; Hardy, S.G.P.; Astruc, J.: The Prefrontal Corticotectal Projection in the Monkey; An Anterograde and Retrograde Horseradish Peroxidase Study. Neuroscience 6 (1981) 1023–1041.

Markowitsch, H.J.; Pritzel, M.; Divac, I.: Cortical Afferents to the Prefrontal Cortex of the Cat: A Study with the Horseradish Peroxidase Technique. Neurosci Lett 11 (1979) 115–120.

Orgogozo, J.M.; Larsen, B.: Activation of Supplementary Motor Area during Voluntary Movements in Man Suggests It Works as a Supramotor Area. Science 206 (1979) 847–850.

Roland, P.E.; Skinhøj, E.; Lassen, N.A.; Larsen, B.: Different Cortical Areas in Man in Organization of Voluntary Movement in Extrapersonal Space. J Neurophysiol 43 (1980) 137–150.

Romansky, K.V.; Usunoff, K.G.; Ivanov, D.P.; Galabov, G.P.: Corticosubthalamic Projection in the Cat: An Electron Microscopic Study. Brain Res 163 (1979) 319–322.

Van Hoesen, G.W.; Yeterian, E.H.; Lavizzo-Mourey, R.: Widespread Corticostriate Projections from Temporal Cortex of the Rhesus Monkey. J Comp Neurol 199 (1981) 205–219.

Yeterian, E.H.; Van Hoesen, G.W.: Cortico-Striate Projections in the Rhesus Monkey: The Organization of Certain Cortico-Caudate Connections. Brain Res 139 (1978) 43–63.

12

Limbic System and Rhinencephalon

The concept of the limbic system is derived from the limbic lobe. The latter term, coined by Broca in 1878, refers to a number of structures on the medial and basal surfaces of the hemisphere forming a limbus (border) around the brain stem. The limbic lobe and all of the structures connected to it comprise the limbic system, which plays a major role in visceral function, emotional behavior, and memory.

The rhinencephalon or smell brain is the anterior part of the limbic cortex. It is primarily concerned with olfaction, but has some reciprocal relationships with parts of other limbic system regions.

Rhinencephalon (Smell Brain)

The rhinencephalon (Fig. 12–1) constitutes a relatively small part of the limbic system in man. It consists of the following structures.

1. Olfactory nerve rootlets
2. Olfactory bulb
3. Olfactory tract
4. Olfactory striae
5. Primary olfactory cortex

Olfactory Nerve Rootlets

The olfactory nerve is composed of unmyelinated thin processes (rootlets) of the olfactory hair cells in the nasal mucosa. Fascicles of the olfactory nerve pierce the cribriform plate of the ethmoid bone, enter the cranial cavity and terminate upon neurons in the olfactory bulb.

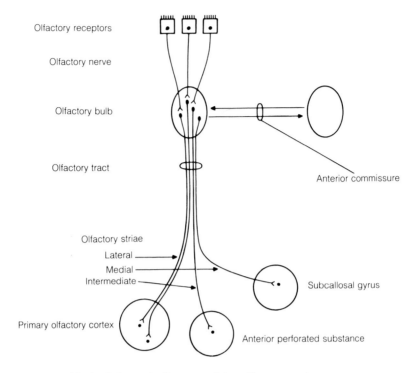

12–1   Schematic diagram of the olfactory pathways.

Olfactory Bulb

The olfactory bulb is the main relay station in the olfactory pathways.

Lamination and Cell Types (Fig. 12–2)   In histologic sections, the olfactory bulb appears laminated into the following layers.

Olfactory Nerve Layer   This layer is composed of incoming olfactory nerve fibers.

Glomerular Layer   In this layer, synaptic formations occur between the olfactory nerve axons and dendrites of the olfactory bulb neurons (mitral and tufted neurons).

External Plexiform Layer.   This layer consists of tufted neurons, some granule cells, and a few mitral cells with their processes.

Mitral Cell Layer   This layer is composed of large neurons (mitral neurons).

Granule Layer   Composed of small granule neurons and processes of granule and mitral cells, this layer also contains incoming fibers from other cortical regions.

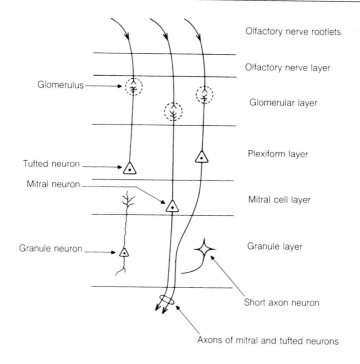

Glomerulus

Tufted neuron

Mitral neuron

Granule neuron

Olfactory nerve rootlets

Olfactory nerve layer

Glomerular layer

Plexiform layer

Mitral cell layer

Granule layer

Short axon neuron

Axons of mitral and tufted neurons

12-2 Schematic diagram of the olfactory bulb showing laminae and types of cells.

The mitral and tufted cells are considered the principal neurons of the olfactory bulb. Their dendrites establish a synaptic relationship with the olfactory nerve fibers within the glomeruli.

The granule cells are considered to be the intrinsic neurons of the olfactory bulb. These cells have vertically oriented dendrites but no axon and exert their action on other cells solely by dendrites. The olfactory bulb contains two other varieties of intrinsic neurons. These are the periglomerular short axon cells in close proximity to the glomeruli in the glomerular layer and the deep short axon cells located in the granule layer.

The olfactory bulb receives fibers (input) from the following sources.

1. Olfactory hair cells in the nasal mucosa
2. Contralateral olfactory bulb
3. Primary olfactory cortex
4. Diagonal band of Broca
5. Anterior olfactory nucleus

The output from the olfactory bulb is composed of axons of the mitral and tufted cells (principal neurons) which project to the following areas.

1. Contralateral olfactory bulb
2. Subcallosal gyrus
3. Anterior perforated substance
4. Primary olfactory cortex

Neuronal Population   Quantitative studies in the rabbit have revealed that there are 50 million olfactory hair cells in the nasal mucosa. Since there is a 1:1 ratio between olfactory receptor cells and olfactory nerve fibers, it follows that there are 50 million olfactory nerve fibers entering the olfactory bulb. The number of principal neurons in the olfactory bulb is estimated to be 50,000 (48,000 tufted and 2,000 mitral cells), suggesting a convergence ratio of 1,000 olfactory nerve fibers upon a single principal neuron. There are more intrinsic neurons than principal neurons in the olfactory bulb. The ratio varies from 25 periglomerular cells per 1 principal neuron to 200 granule cells per 1 principal neuron.

Olfactory Tract

The olfactory tract is the outflow pathway of the olfactory bulb. It is composed of the axons of principal neurons (mitral and tufted cells) of the olfactory bulb and centrifugal axons originating from the contralateral olfactory bulb, as well as from central brain regions. The olfactory tract also contains the scattered neurons of the anterior olfactory nucleus, the axons of which contribute to the olfactory tract. At its caudal extremity, just anterior to the anterior perforated substance, the olfactory tract divides into the olfactory striae.

Olfactory Striae

At its caudal extremity, just rostral to the anterior perforated substance, the olfactory tract divides into three striae.

1. Lateral olfactory stria
2. Medial olfactory stria
3. Intermediate olfactory stria.

Each of the striae is covered by a thin layer of gray matter, the olfactory gyri.

The lateral olfactory stria projects to the primary olfactory cortex in the temporal lobe. The medial olfactory stria projects upon the medial olfactory area, also known as the septal area, located on the medial surface of the frontal lobe, ventral to the genu and rostrum of the corpus callosum and anterior to the lamina terminalis. The medial olfactory area is closely related to the limbic system and hence is concerned with emotional responses elicited by olfactory stimuli. It does not play a role in the perception of olfactory stimuli. The medial and intermediate striae are poorly developed in man. The intermediate stria blends with the anterior perforated substance. The thin cortex at this site is designated the intermediate olfactory area. The three areas of olfactory cortex are interconnected by the diagonal band of Broca, a bundle of subcortical fibers in front of the optic tract.

Primary Olfactory Cortex

The primary olfactory cortex is located within the uncus of the temporal lobe and is composed of the prepyriform cortex, periamygdaloid area, and part of the entorhinal area. The prepyriform cortex is the region on each side of and beneath the lateral olfactory stria; hence, it is also called the lateral olfactory gyrus. It is considered the major part of the primary olfactory cortex. The primary olfactory cortex is relatively large in some animals, like the rabbit, but in man it occupies a small area. The primary olfactory cortex in man is concerned with the conscious perception of olfactory stimuli. In contrast to all other primary sensory cortices (vision, audition, taste, and somatic sensibility), the primary olfactory cortex is unique in that afferent fibers from the receptors reach it directly without passing through a relay in the thalamus.

The primary olfactory cortex contains two types of neurons. These are 1) principal neurons (pyramidal cells) with axons which leave the olfactory cortex and project to nearby or distant regions and 2) intrinsic neurons (stellate cells) with axons which remain within the olfactory cortex.

The major input to the primary olfactory cortex is from 1) the olfactory bulb via the lateral olfactory stria and 2) other central brain regions.

The output from the olfactory cortex is via axons of principal neurons which project to nearby areas surrounding the primary olfactory cortex, as well as to more distant areas, such as the thalamus and hypothalamus, which play an important role in behavior and emotion.

Quantitative studies of the primary olfactory cortex have revealed that 1) there is a predominance of principal type neurons (compared with the intrinsic variety) and 2) the number of principal neurons far exceeds the number of fibers in the lateral olfactory stria. Thus, in contrast to the olfactory bulb, in which there is a high convergence ratio, the input to output ratio in the primary olfactory cortex is low. This is similar to the pattern in the neocortex and in the climbing fiber system of the cerebellar cortex.

Studies on the intrinsic organization of the primary olfactory cortex have revealed the following observations. 1) The lateral olfactory stria establishes synapses with dendrites of the principal pyramidal neurons, whereas

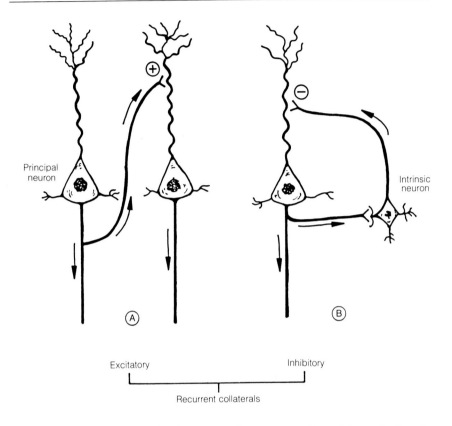

12–3 Schematic diagram showing types of recurrent collateral fibers in the olfactory cortex.

the input from other brain regions projects upon both principal and intrinsic neurons. 2) Principal neurons have both excitatory and inhibitory recurrent collateral influence upon other principal neurons in the primary olfactory cortex. The inhibitory recurrent collaterals exert their influence through an intermediary inhibitory intrinsic neuron. The excitatory recurrent collaterals exert their effect directly upon dendrites of other principal neurons (Fig. 12–3). Although the concept of inhibitory recurrent collaterals is well established in the central nervous system (Renshaw cell circuit in the spinal cord and Purkinje collaterals in the cerebellum), the excitatory recurrent collateral concept is unique to the primary olfactory cortex and, as will be seen later, to the hippocampus. There is some evidence to suggest that such a recurrent collateral pathway may also be found in the neocortex. 3) Principal neurons are continuously active, providing a constant background activity which is modulated by incoming olfactory stimuli.

Rhinencephalon and Other Brain Regions

The primary terminal stations of the three olfactory striae have connections with each other and with a number of cortical and subcortical areas concerned with visceral function (hippocampus, thalamus, hypothalamus, epithalamus, and brain stem reticular formation). Through these connections, the rhinencephalon exerts an influence on visceral function (salivation, nausea, etc.), as well as behavioral reactions.

Abnormalities in Olfaction

Rhinencephalic structures can be affected in several sites with resultant derangement in the sense of smell.

Olfactory receptors are involved in common colds, resulting in bilateral diminution or loss of smell (anosmia). Olfactory nerve fibers may be affected in their course through the cribriform plate of the ethmoid bone in fractures of the plate.

The olfactory bulb and tracts may be involved in inflammatory processes of the meninges (meningitis) or tumors in the frontal lobe or the anterior cranial fossa. Unilateral loss of smell may be the earliest clinical manifestation in such processes and should be evaluated by the physician.

Pathologic processes in the region of the primary olfactory cortex (the uncus of the temporal lobe) usually give rise to hallucinations of smell (uncinate fits). The odor experienced in such cases is often described as unpleasant. Such hallucinations may herald an epileptic seizure or be part of it. They may also be a manifestation of a tumor in that region.

Limbic Lobe

As described by Broca in 1878, the limbic lobe refers to the gray matter in the medial and basal parts of the hemisphere that forms a limbus (border) around the brain stem. Thus, the limbic lobe is a synthetic lobe with component parts which are derived from different lobes of the brain. There is no general agreement on all the parts that enter into the formation of the limbic lobe. The following, however, are generally accepted as limbic lobe components (Fig. 12–4).

1. Subcallosal gyrus (anterior and inferior continuation of the cingulate gyrus)
2. Cingulate gyrus
3. Parahippocampal gyrus
4. Uncus

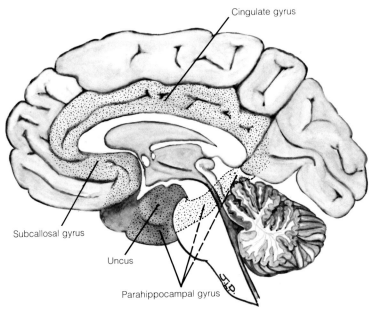

Cingulate gyrus

Subcallosal gyrus

Uncus

Parahippocampal gyrus

12–4   Schematic diagram showing the components of the limbic lobe.

Originally, the limbic lobe was assigned a purely olfactory function. Recently, it has been established that only a minor part of the limbic lobe has olfactory function. The rest of the limbic lobe, which forms part of the limbic system, plays a role in emotional behavior and memory.

Limbic System

The limbic system is defined as the limbic lobe and all cortical and subcortical structures related to it. These include the following.

1. Septal nuclei
2. Amygdala
3. Hypothalamus (particularly mamillary body)
4. Thalamus (particularly anterior thalamic nucleus)
5. Brain stem reticular formation
6. Epithalamus
7. Hippocampal formation

This conglomerate of neural structures, which constitute the old part of the brain and are highly interconnected, seems to play a role in the following.

1. Emotional behavior

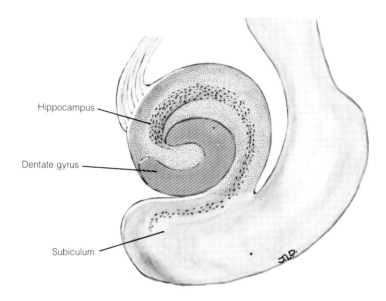

12–5   Schematic diagram showing the components of the hippocampal formation.

2. Memory
3. Integration of homeostatic responses, such as those related to preservation of the species, securing food, *fight or flight* response, etc.
4. Sexual behavior
5. Motivation

The underlying mechanisms for these different functions are very complex and are inadequately understood.

The presentation of the limbic system in this chapter will focus on the following components: hippocampal formation, amygdala, and septal area. Major pathways that connect these key structures with other components of the limbic system will be described.

Hippocampal Formation

The hippocampal formation (Fig. 12–5) is an infolding of the parahippocampal gyrus into the inferior (temporal) horn of the lateral ventricle and consists of three regions: the hippocampus, dentate gyrus, and subiculum. The dentate gyrus occupies the interval between the hippocampus and the parahippocampal gyrus. Its name is derived from its toothed or beaded surface. The subiculum is the part of the parahippocampal gyrus in direct continuity with the hippocampus.

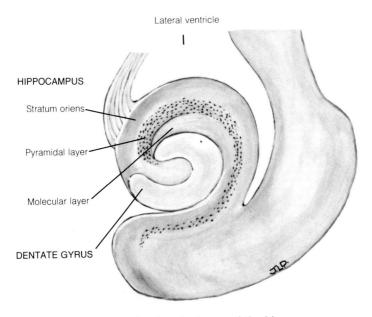

Lateral ventricle

HIPPOCAMPUS

Stratum oriens

Pyramidal layer

Molecular layer

DENTATE GYRUS

12–6 Schematic diagram showing the layers of the hippocampus.

Of the three components of the hippocampal formation, the hippocampus is the largest in man, and the best studied. Therefore, it will be presented as the prototype of this segment of the limbic system.

The hippocampus is a C-shaped structure in coronal sections, bulging into the inferior horn of the lateral ventricle. It resembles in shape a ram's horn; hence it is known as Ammon's horn (cornu Ammonis) after the Egyptian deity who had a ram's head. The hippocampus is closely associated with the adjacent dentate gyrus (Fig. 12–5) and together they form an S-shaped structure.

Lamination and Divisions   Although Ramon y Cajal described seven laminae in the hippocampus, it is customary to combine the different laminae into three major layers (Fig. 12–6). These are the molecular layer, pyramidal cell layer, and stratum oriens (polymorphic layer).

The pyramidal cell layer is divided into two zones. These are a zone in which the pyramidal cells are compact and a zone (rostral to the compact zone) in which the pyramidal cells are less compact. The boundary between the compact and less compact zones of the pyramidal layer separates the two divisions of the hippocampus (Fig. 12–7) into the superior division (compact zone) and the inferior division (less compact zone).

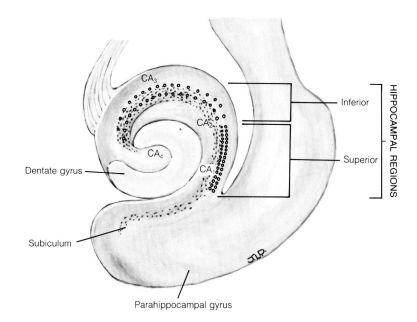

12-7 Schematic diagram showing the division of the hippocampus into superior and inferior regions and four fields (CA_1-CA_4).

The hippocampus has been subdivided further into fields designated as cornu Ammonis 1, 2, 3, and 4 (CA_1-CA_4). CA_1 corresponds to the superior division and CA_3 to the inferior division. CA_2 and CA_4 comprise the transition zones between the hippocampus and the dentate gyrus. Field CA_1 (also known as Sommer's sector) is of interest to the neuropathologist because its pyramidal neurons are highly sensitive to anoxia and ischemia.

Neuronal Population (Fig. 12-8) There are basically two types of neurons in the hippocampus, the principal neurons (pyramidal cell) and intrinsic neurons (polymorphic cell, basket cell).

Principal Neurons The pyramidal neurons in the pyramidal cell layer are the principal neurons of the hippocampus. They are the only neurons with axons which contribute to the outflow tract from the hippocampus. Pyramidal neurons vary in size and density in different regions of the hippocampus. They are smaller and more densely packed in the superior region than those in the inferior region. The largest neurons in the inferior region are referred to as the giant pyramidal cells of the hippocampus.

Basal dendrites of pyramidal neurons are oriented toward the ventricular surface; apical dendrites are oriented toward the molecular layer. Both types arborize extensively and are rich in dendritic spines.

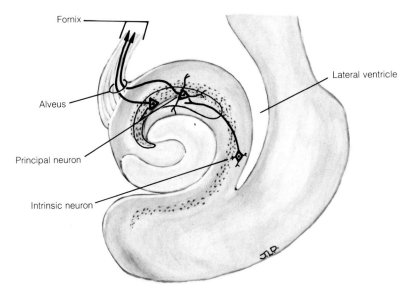

Fornix

Lateral ventricle

Alveus

Principal neuron

Intrinsic neuron

12–8 Schematic diagram showing the major types of neurons in the hippocampus and their interrelationships.

Axons of pyramidal cells are directed toward the ventricular surface where they gather together to form the alveus and fimbria and finally join the fornix as the outflow tract from the hippocampus. Recurrent axon collaterals terminate within the stratum oriens or reach the molecular layer. They exert a facilitatory influence.

It is estimated that the hippocampus of man contains 1,200,000 principal neurons on each side, a figure close to the number of pyramidal tract fibers.

Intrinsic Neurons   These neurons have axons which remain within the hippocampus. Because of the irregularity of their perikarya and dendrites, they are referred to as polymorphic neurons. They are located in the stratum oriens (Fig. 12–6). Their irregularly oriented dendrites arborize locally, while their axons ramify between pyramidal neurons and arborize around perikarya of pyramidal neurons in a basket formation (hence the term basket cells). They are inhibitory to pyramidal cell activity. There are no estimates available of the exact number of intrinsic neurons in the hippocampus. It is estimated, however, that one basket cell is related to about 200 to 500 pyramidal cells. Thus, it is believed that the intrinsic neurons are much fewer in number than the principal neurons.

Afferent Pathways (Fig. 12–9)   The hippocampus receives fibers from the following sites.

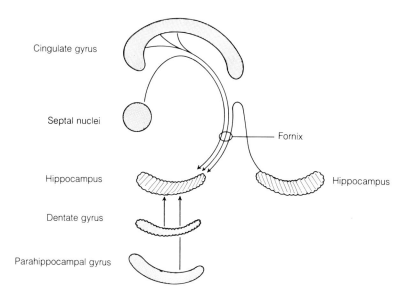

Cingulate gyrus

Septal nuclei

Fornix

Hippocampus

Hippocampus

Dentate gyrus

Parahippocampal gyrus

12-9   Schematic diagram showing the major afferent connections of the hippo-campus.

Parahippocampal Gyrus   Fibers from the parahippocampal gyrus arise mainly from the entorhinal area. They reach the hippocampus via two routes. One goes through (perforates) the adjacent subicular area en route to the hippocampus and dentate gyrus and is therefore called the perforant path. Another arrives in the hippocampus at the ventricular surface where the alveus (axons of pyramidal neurons) is formed and is therefore called the alvear path.

Dentate Gyrus   Axons of small pyramidal neurons (granule cells) in the dentate gyrus reach the hippocampus via the mossy fiber pathway.

Contralateral Hippocampus   The two hippocampi are in communication via the hippocampal commissure (commissure of the fornix).

Cingulate Gyrus   Fibers from the cingulate gyrus reach the hippocampus via the cingulum (association fiber bundle).

Septal Area   Fibers from the septal nuclei reach the hippocampus via the fornix. Compared to the input from the entorhinal area, the septal input is modest.

Recently confirmed afferent connections include the following.

Hypothalamus   Fibers from the hypothalamus originate from cell groups in the vicinity of the mamillary body and exert a strong inhibitory influence on the hippocampus.

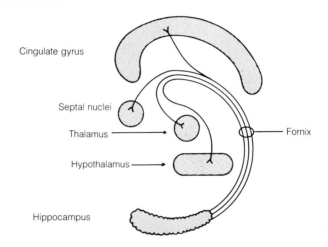

12-10 Schematic diagram showing the major efferent connections of the hippocampus.

Thalamus   Thalamic input to the hippocampus has been shown to originate in the anterior thalamic nucleus.

Locus Ceruleus   Noradrenergic fibers from the locus ceruleus have been traced to the hippocampus and dentate gyrus.

Raphe Nuclei   Serotonergic fibers from the raphe nuclei have also been traced to the hippocampus.

Efferent Pathways (Fig. 12-10)   The efferent fibers from the hippocampus travel via the fornix. They are axons of pyramidal (principal) neurons of the hippocampus. Axons which gather together at the ventricular surface of the hippocampus to enter the alveus converge further on to form a flattened band of white matter, the fimbria. Traced posteriorly on the floor of the inferior horn of the lateral ventricle, the fimbria continues as the crus of the fornix, which begins at the posterior limit of the hippocampus beneath the splenium of the corpus callosum. The crus joins its counterpart from the other side to form the body of the fornix. At the conversion of the two crura, a small hippocampal commissure joins the hippocampi of the two sides. The body of the fornix separates into two columns, each of which curves ventrally in front of the interventricular foramen and continues through the hypothalamus, dividing it into medial and lateral areas. Most of the fibers terminate in the mamillary bodies. A bundle of fibers leaves the column of the fornix below the interventricular foramen and projects into the anterior nucleus of the thalamus. The above components constitute the postcommissural portion of the fornix. Some of these fibers have been traced to the periaqueductal gray matter of the mesencephalon. Other fibers separate from the columns of the fornix above the anterior commissure (precommissural portion of the fornix) and project into the septal area and the anterior part of the hypothalamus. Each fornix contains 1,200,000 axons of pyramidal hippocampal neurons in man.

The fornix distributes fibers to the following brain regions.

1. Cingulate gyrus
2. Septal nuclei
3. Preoptic region of the hypothalamus
4. Lateral region of the hypothalamus
5. Mamillary body of the hypothalamus
6. Anterior nucleus of the thalamus
7. Periaqueductal gray matter of the mesencephalon

There is also some evidence to suggest that the hippocampus pyramidal neurons project fibers to the adjacent subiculum.

The application of new methods for pathway tracing has permitted a more reliable study of the origin of fornix fibers. These studies have shown that most of the fibers of the fornix are derived from the subiculum and not the hippocampus. The subiculum has been shown to be the source of fibers to the hypothalamus, anterior thalamic nucleus, and most of the fibers to the septal area. The fibers originating in the hippocampus have been traced to the septal area, cingulate gyrus, and subiculum. The significance of hippocampal projections becomes more evident when one examines the system of relays that exists between some of these projection sites. Figures 12–11 and 12–12 are simplified schemas of only two such relay systems.

Synaptic Connections (Fig. 12–13) Using Golgi preparations, electron microscopy, and electrophysiology, the following synaptic connections have been established within the hippocampus.

Parahippocampal Gyrus The input from the parahippocampal gyrus (perforant path) establishes axodendritic synapses on the distant portion of the apical dendrites of pyramidal cells in the molecular layer, exerting an excitatory influence on pyramidal neurons. The input through the alvear path from the parahippocampal gyrus establishes axodendritic excitatory synapses on the basal dendrites of pyramidal neurons.

Dentate Gyrus The input from the dentate gyrus (mossy fiber pathway) establishes axodendritic synapses on apical dendrites of pyramidal neurons close to the site of origin of the dendrites from the perikaryon. The boutons of mossy axons contain two types of vesicles. These are the ordinary acetylcholine (clear) vesicles and large dense core vesicles. They too are excitatory to the apical dendrites. Each mossy terminal has synaptic connections with numerous dendrites.

Basket Cell The local input from intrinsic (basket) neurons in the stratum oriens establishes axosomatic synapses upon perikarya of pyramidal neurons. They are believed to exert an inhibitory effect on pyramidal

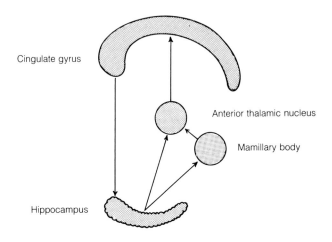

12-11 Simplified schematic diagram of one of the hippocampal relay systems.

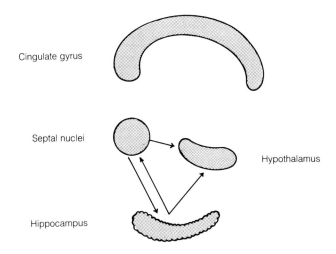

12-12 Simplified schematic diagram of one of the hippocampal relay systems.

neurons. The basket cells receive excitatory recurrent collaterals from axons of pyramidal neurons.

Recurrent Collaterals   The recurrent axon collaterals from the axons of pyramidal neurons establish axodendritic synapses on apical dendrites of pyramidal neurons. They are excitatory to pyramidal neurons.

The inputs to the hippocampus from the parahippocampal gyrus, dentate gyrus, commissural connections, and the recurrent axon collaterals of pyramidal neurons are all excitatory. On the other hand, the basket cell is inhibitory.

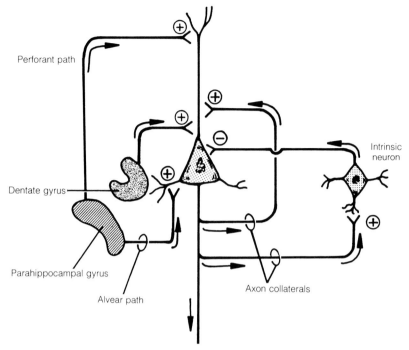

Perforant path

Dentate gyrus

Parahippocampal gyrus

Alvear path

Intrinsic neuron

Axon collaterals

12–13 Schematic diagram of the sources and types of synaptic formation within the hippocampus.

Functional Considerations   When considering the functions of the hippocampus, it is important to emphasize the complex relationships of the hippocampus with other brain regions as outlined previously. The effects of stimulation or ablation of the hippocampus cannot be evaluated in isolation from the elaborate systems of hippocampal communication.

Contrary to older concepts, the hippocampus is no longer believed to play a role in olfaction. The hippocampus is very well developed in man, who is microsmatic; it is also present in the whale, which is anosmatic. No direct pathways from the primary olfactory cortex can be traced to the hippocampus, although a multisynaptic pathway through the primary olfactory cortex and the parahippocampal gyrus (entorhinal area) exists. Olfactory bulb stimulation results in excitatory postsynaptic potential (EPSP) activity, but no action potential firing in the hippocampus. This is consistent with a polysynaptic pathway from the olfactory bulb to the hippocampus. The suggestion has been made that this subthreshold EPSP activity may be comparable to a conditional stimulus that plays a role in memory and learning.

Action potentials, on the other hand, have been recorded in the hippocampus following stimulation of various areas both centrally and peripherally. Hippocampal responses have been elicited after visual, acoustic, gustatory, and somatosensory stimulation, as well as following stimulation of various cortical and subcortical areas. Such responses are characteristically labile and are easily modified by a variety of factors.

Stimulation and ablation of the hippocampus gives rise to changes in behavioral, endocrine, and visceral functions. The same effects may follow either ablation or stimulation.

The hippocampus has been implicated in the processes of attention and alertness. Stimulation of the hippocampus in animals produces glancing and searching movements associated with bewilderment and anxiety.

Bilateral ablation of the hippocampus in man (usually involving adjacent regions as well) results in loss of recent memory and inability to store newly learned facts. Unilateral ablation of the hippocampus in man does not affect memory to any significant degree. The relationship of the hippocampus to memory deficits has been re-examined in view of recent anatomic data on hippocampal connections. In spite of the voluminous literature on the subject, no final conclusion has been reached about which structure(s) in the temporal lobe are involved in post-traumatic memory deficits.

The hippocampus has a low threshold for seizure (epileptic) activity; however, the spread of such epileptic activity to the nonspecific thalamic system, and hence all over the cortex, is not usual. This may explain why temporal lobe epilepsy (psychomotor epilepsy) in man does not become generalized and is usually not associated with the loss of consciousness encountered in generalized epilepsy.

Amygdala

The amygdalar (from the Greek *amygdala,* for almonds) nuclei resemble almonds in shape and are located in the tip of the temporal lobe beneath the cortex of the uncus. There are two main groups of nuclei, the corticomedial and the basolateral. The basolateral group is large and well developed in the human. Several neurotransmitters have been demonstrated in the amygdala. These include acetylcholine, GABA, noradrenalin, serotonin, dopamine, substance P, and enkephalin. Fiber connections of the amygdala are complex and poorly understood.

Afferent Pathways (Fig. 12–14)   The amygdala receive direct fibers from the olfactory bulb. These reach the corticomedial group of amygdaloid nuclei by way of the lateral olfactory stria. The basolateral group receives indirect olfactory fibers from the pyriform cortex. Other sources of afferent fibers include the cingulate gyrus, thalamus (from both the specific and nonspecific thalamic nuclei), hypothalamus, prefrontal cortex, and brain stem reticular formation, as well as from the somatosensory, visual, and auditory systems.

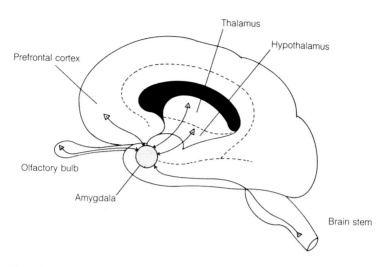

12–14   Schematic diagram of the major afferent connections of the amygdala.

Efferent Pathways   There are two main efferent pathways from the amygdala, the stria terminalis (dorsal amygdalofugal pathway) and the ventrofugal bundle (ventral amygdalofugal pathway).

Stria Terminalis (Fig. 12–15)   The stria terminalis is the main outflow tract of the amygdala. It arises predominantly from the corticomedial group of amygdalar nuclei. From its sites of origin, it follows a C-shaped course caudally, dorsally, anteriorly, and ventrally along the medial surface of the caudate nucleus to reach the region of the anterior commissure, where it branches out to supply the following areas.

1. Septal nuclei
2. Anterior olfactory nucleus
3. Anterior nuclei of the hypothalamus
4. Ventromedial nucleus of the hypothalamus
5. Bed nucleus of the stria terminalis (a scattered group of nuclei at the rostral extremity of the stria terminalis)
6. Habenular nuclei via the stria medullaris thalami

Ventral Amygdalofugal Pathway   This ventral outflow tract takes its origin from both nuclear groups of the amygdala, as well as from the periamygdaloid cortex. It proceeds along the base of the brain and distributes fibers to the following areas.

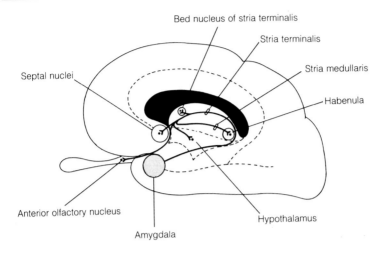

12–15 Schematic diagram of the major efferent connections of the amygdala.

1. Pyriform cortex
2. Dorsomedial nucleus of the thalamus
3. Midbrain reticular formation and substantia nigra
4. Claustrum
5. Anterior olfactory nucleus
6. Caudate
7. Putamen
8. Hypothalamus
9. Prefrontal cortex
10. Reticular formation of the pons and medulla

The two amygdaloid nuclei communicate with each other through the stria terminalis and anterior commissure. Fibers leave one amygdaloid nucleus and travel via the stria terminalis to the level of the anterior commissure, where they cross and join the other stria terminalis and return to the contralateral amygdaloid nucleus. Nuclear groups within each amygdaloid nuclear complex communicate with each other via short fiber systems.

Functional Considerations The functions of the amygdala are somewhat elusive. Stimulation and ablation experiments usually involve adjacent neural structures. The intricate neural connectivity of the amygdala makes it difficult to ascribe an observed behavior purely to the amygdala. The following manifestations, however, have been noted to occur after stimulation or ablation of the amygdala.

Autonomic Effects Changes in heart rate, respiration, blood pressure, and gastric motility have been observed following amygdalar stimulation.

Both an increase and decrease in these functions have been observed, depending on the area stimulated.

Orienting Response Animals with amygdalar lesions manifest reduced responsiveness to novel events in their visual environment. Their responsiveness, however, is improved if they are rewarded for the response. Stimulation of the amygdala, on the other hand, enhances the orienting response to novel events. Such animals will arrest ongoing activity and will orient their bodies to the novel situation.

Emotional Behavior and Food Intake There seem to be two regions in the amygdala that are antagonistic to each other with regard to emotional behavior and eating. Lesions in the dorsomedial region of the amygdala result in aphagia, decreased emotional tone, fear, sadness, and aggression. Lesions of the lateral region of the amygdala, on the other hand, produce hyperphagia, happiness, and pleasure reactions. Stimulation of rostral and lateral regions of the amygdala is associated with fear and flight. Stimulation of the caudal and medial regions produces a defense and aggression reaction. The attack behavior elicited by amygdalar stimulation differs from that elicited by hypothalamic stimulation in its gradual build-up and gradual subsidence upon onset and cessation of stimulation. Attack behavior elicited from the hypothalamus, in contrast, begins and subsides almost immediately after onset and cessation of the stimulus. Of interest also is the fact that prior septal stimulation will prevent the occurrence of aggressive behavior elicited from both the amygdala and hypothalamus.

Arousal Response Stimulation of dorsal regions of the amygdala produces an arousal response similar to, but independent of, the arousal response that follows stimulation of the reticular activating system of the brain stem. The amygdalar response is independent from the reticular activating system response, since it can be elicited following lesions in the reticular formation of the brain stem. Stimulation of ventral regions of the amygdala, on the other hand, produces the reverse effect (decrease in arousal and sleep). The net total effect of the amygdala, however, is facilitatory, since ablation of the amygdala results in a sluggish, hypoactive animal which is placid and tame. Such animals avoid social interaction and may become social isolates.

Sexual Activity Stimulation of the amygdala has been associated with a variety of sexual behavior including erection, ejaculation, copulatory movements, and ovulation. Bilateral lesions of the amygdala produce hypersexuality and perverted sexual behavior.

Motor Activity Stimulation of the amygdala also produces complex rhythmic movements related to eating, such as chewing, smacking of lips, licking, and swallowing.

It should be pointed out that many, if not all, of the above functions can be observed after stimulation or ablation of other brain regions, notably the hypothalamus and septal regions. It is proposed that the amygdala play an integrative role in all of the above functions.

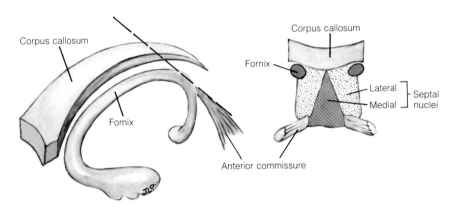

12–16 Schematic diagram of the location and divisions of the septal nuclei.

Septal Area

The septal area refers to a group of nuclei located below the rostral part of the corpus callosum and in front of the anterior commissure in the medial wall of the anterior horn of the lateral ventricle. It is made up of medium-sized neurons which are grouped into medial and lateral nuclei (Fig. 12–16). The lateral septal nucleus receives most of the septal afferents and the medial nucleus gives rise to most of the septal efferents.

Afferent Pathways (Fig. 12–17) The septal area receives fibers from the hippocampus, amygdala, hypothalamus, and midbrain.

Hippocampus Fibers from the hippocampus reach the septal area via the fornix. The hippocampal-septal relationship seems to be organized topographically in such a way that specific areas of the hippocampus project upon specific regions of the septum (CA_1 of the hippocampus to medial septal region; CA_3 and CA_4 of the hippocampus to lateral septal region). The hippocampal-septal relationship assumes more importance when one considers that septal projection to the hippocampus is from the medial septal region to CA_3 and CA_4 of the hippocampus. When one adds to this the intrinsic connection between the medial and lateral septal regions and between CA_1 and CA_3-CA_4 of the hippocampus, it becomes evident that a neural circuit is established connecting these two limbic regions, as illustrated in Figure 12–18.

Amygdala Fibers from the amygdala reach the septal area via the stria terminalis.

Hypothalamus Fibers from the hypothalamus reach the lateral septal area via the medial forebrain bundle (MFB).

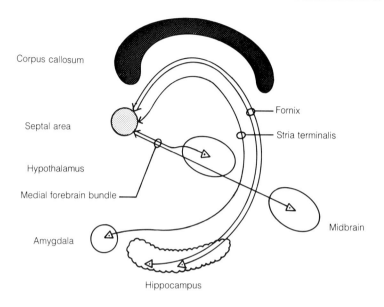

12–17   Schematic diagram of the major afferent connections of the septal nuclei.

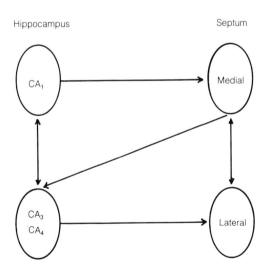

12–18   Schematic diagram showing the reciprocal relationship between the hippocampus and septal nuclei.

Midbrain   Fibers from the midbrain reach the septal area via the medial forebrain bundle. They arise primarily from the periaqueductal gray region and the ventral tegmental area.

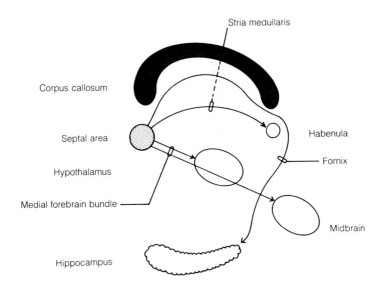

12–19 Schematic diagram of the major efferent connections of the septal nuclei.

The pattern of termination of septal input varies with the different sources of input. The majority of hippocampal fibers terminate as axodendritic synapses and very few as axosomatic synapses. In contrast, the majority of axosomatic synapses are of hypothalamic origin. Although very few hippocampal fibers terminate on somas of septal neurons, they are capable of forming such synapses and do so if the hypothalamic input which normally forms such synapses is interrupted. This is an illustration of central nervous system plasticity, of which the septal area is the outstanding example.

Afferent fibers recently confirmed include those from the subiculum, nucleus fastigi of the cerebellum, and cingulate gyrus.

Efferent Pathways (Fig. 12–19) The septal area projects to the following neural structures: hippocampus, hypothalamus, habenular nucleus, and midbrain.

Hippocampus Fibers from the medial septal region reach CA_3 and CA_4 of the hippocampus via the fornix. The neural circuit between the septal area and the hippocampus has been described.

Hypothalamus Septal efferents reach the hypothalamus via the medial forebrain bundle and project primarily upon the lateral nuclear group of the hypothalamus.

In addition, the medial septal area is connected with the supraoptic and paraventricular nuclei of the hypothalamus. This connection is believed to be important in the regulation of oxytocin release.

Habenular Nucleus Fibers reach the habenular nucleus via the stria medullaris thalami. The septal-habenular relationship is topographically organized.

Midbrain Projections to the midbrain also course through the medial forebrain bundle.

Efferent connections recently confirmed include those to the thalamus (anterior and dorsomedial nuclei), cingulate gyrus, and amygdala.

Functional Considerations The functional importance of the septal area lies in providing a site of interaction between limbic and diencephalic structures. The connection of the hippocampus with the hypothalamus via the septal region is one such illustration.

Stimulation and ablation experiments have provided the following information about the role of the septal region.

Emotional Behavior Lesions of the septal area in some animal species such as rats and mice produce rage reactions and hyperemotionality. These behavioral alterations are usually transitory and disappear 2 to 4 weeks following the lesion.

Water Consumption Animals with lesions in the septal area tend to consume increased amounts of water. There is evidence to suggest that this is a primary effect of the lesion due to disruption of a neural system concerned with water balance in response to change in total fluid volume. Chronic stimulation of the septal area tends to decrease spontaneous drinking even in animals deprived of water for a long time.

Activity Animals with septal lesions demonstrate a high initial state of activity in response to a novel situation. This heightened activity, however, rapidly declines almost to immobility.

Learning Animals with septal lesions tend to learn tasks quickly and to perform them effectively once learned.

Reward Stimulation of several regions of the septal area gives rise to pleasure or rewarding effects.

Autonomic Effects Stimulation of the septal region has an inhibitory effect on autonomic function. Cardiac deceleration ensues after septal stimulation and is reversed by the drug atropine, suggesting that septal effects are mediated via the cholinergic fibers of the vagus nerve.

Septal Syndrome Destruction of the septal nuclei gives rise to behavioral overreaction to most environmental stimuli. Behavioral changes occur in sexual and reproductive behavior, feeding, drinking, and the rage reaction.

Kluver-Bucy Syndrome

This is a clinical syndrome observed in man and other animals following bilateral lesions in the temporal lobe that involve the amygdala, hippocampal formation, and adjacent neural structures. The syndrome is man-ifested by the following.

1. Visual agnosia
2. Oral tendencies (tendency to examine all objects by mouth)
3. Hypersexuality (normal as well as perverted sexual activity). Such pa-tients and animals manifest heightened sexual drives toward either sex of their own or of other species and even inanimate objects.
4. Docility
5. Lack of emotional response
6. Increased appetite
7. Memory deficit

Temporal Lobe Epilepsy

Another manifestation of temporal lobe lesions in man which involve the amygdala and hippocampus is temporal lobe epilepsy, also known as psy-chomotor seizures. During the seizure, the patient may manifest one or more of the following.

1. Olfactory hallucinations, consisting of transient and recurrent episodes of unpleasant olfactory experiences such as smelling burning rubber
2. Auditory hallucinations
3. Visual hallucinations
4. Rhythmic movements related to feeding (chewing, licking, swallowing)
5. Complex motor acts such as walking, undressing, or twisting movements of trunk and extremities
6. Amnesia which may last several hours or days
7. Aggressive behavior. During attacks of temporal lobe epilepsy, such patients may commit violent, even criminal, acts.

Overview of Limbic System

It is evident that the limbic system is a highly complex system intercon-nected by a multiplicity of pathways and reciprocal circuitries among its component parts and among those parts and other brain regions, notably the hypothalamus. In spite of the apparent complexity of these connections, there seems to be some order in their hierarchy. All components of the limbic lobe and of the amygdala receive fibers from and send fibers to the association cortex. The limbic lobe is in turn reciprocally interconnected with all subcortical parts of the limbic system. Finally, the subcortical parts of the limbic system are reciprocally interconnected with the hypothalamus. Thus, a hierarchy of connections is established by which the hypothalamus is reciprocally connected with the subcortical limbic system, which is reciprocally connected with the limbic lobe, which is reciprocally connected with the association cortex. It is also evident that there is a lot of overlap in the functions of different components of the limbic system with those of the hypothalamus. At best, one can define the functions of the limbic system in the most general terms as subserving the following functions.

1. Homeostatic mechanisms both for preservation of the individual (flight or defensive response, eating, drinking) and preservation of the species (sexual and social behavior)
2. Emotional behavior (including fear, rage, pleasure, sadness, etc.)
3. Memory for recent events
4. Matching up sensory input with hypothalamic drive and putting it into the context of the situation. In this respect, the Kluver-Bucy syndrome is an example of mismatch manifested by placing inedible objects in the mouth, docility in the presence of threatening situations, and sexual advances toward inanimate objects.

References

Baleydier, C.; Mauguiere, F.: The Duality of the Cingulate Gyrus in Monkey. Neuroanatomical Study and Functional Hypothesis. Brain 103 (1980) 525–554.

Ben-Ari, Y.; Zigmond, R.E.; Shute, C.C.D.; Lewis, P.R.: Regional Distribution of Choline Acetyltransferase and Acetylcholinesterase within the Amygdaloid Complex and Stria Terminalis System. Brain Res 120 (1977) 435–445.

Emson, P.C.; Björklund A.; Lindvall, O.; Paxinos, G.: Contributions of Different Afferent Pathways to the Catecholamine and 5-Hydroxytryptamine-Innervation of the Amygdala: A Neurochemical and Histochemical Study. Neuroscience 4 (1979) 1347–1357.

Girgis, M.: Kindling as a Model for Limbic Epilepsy. Neuroscience 6 (1981) 1695–1706.

Hopkins, D.A.; Holstege, G.: Amygdaloid Projections to the Mesencephalon, Pons and Medulla Oblongata in the Cat. Exp Brain Res 32 (1978) 529–547.

Horel, J.A.: The Neuroanatomy of Amnesia. A Critique of the Hippocampal Memory Hypothesis. Brain 101 (1978) 403–445.

Kosel, K.C.; Van Hoesen, G.W.; West, J.R.: Olfactory Bulb Projections to the Parahippocampal Area of the Rat. J Comp Neurol 198 (1981) 467–482.

Lopes da Silva, F.H.; Arnolds, D.E.A.T.: Physiology of the Hippocampus and Related Structures. Ann Rev Physiol 40 (1978) 185–216.

Meibach, R.C.; Siegel, A.: Efferent Connections of the Septal Area in the Rat: An Analysis Utilizing Retrograde and Anterograde Transport Methods. Brain Res 119 (1977) 1–20.

Ottersen, O.P.; Ben-Ari, Y.: Afferent Connections to the Amygdaloid Complex of the Rat and Cat. I. Projections from the Thalamus. J Comp Neurol 187 (1979) 401–424.

Swanson, L.W.; Cowan, W.M.: An Autoradiographic Study of the Organization of the Efferent Connections of the Hippocampal Formation in the Rat. J Comp Neurol 172 (1977) 49–84.

13

Autonomic
Nervous System

The autonomic nervous system, one of the three main subdivisions of the nervous system, functions involuntarily and is concerned with the regulation of visceral activity. It controls the activity of smooth and cardiac muscles, as well as glands. It regulates and coordinates such visceral functions as respiration, circulation, digestion, glandular secretion, reproduction, and the maintenance of body temperature.

Components of the autonomic nervous system are located within the central and peripheral nervous systems. Because of its nature and the functions it serves, the autonomic nervous system is also known as the involuntary nervous system, vegetative nervous system, and visceral nervous system.

The older concept of the autonomic nervous system as a purely efferent system has been altered. The newer concept of this system includes both afferent and efferent components. The receptors of this system are located in visceral organs and walls of blood vessels. Afferent fibers have their cell bodies in spinal or cranial ganglia and enter the spinal cord or brain stem via the dorsal root or the appropriate cranial nerve. The efferent component leaves the neuraxis via ventral roots or the appropriate cranial nerves. There are generally two neuronal chains in the efferent outflow, a preganglionic neuron and a postganglionic neuron. The preganglionic neuron has its cell body within the central nervous system. The postganglionic neuron is located outside the central nervous system; its axons terminate upon an effector organ (smooth muscle, cardiac muscle, or gland). The postganglionic neurons are aggregated in autonomic ganglia and outnumber preganglionic neurons. Preganglionic axons are myelinated and of small diameter (less than 4 μm). Postganglionic axons are unmyelinated.

Somatic and Autonomic Nervous Systems

Although the somatic and autonomic nervous systems often act together, there are certain anatomic and physiologic differences between them.

1. In the somatic nervous system, the axon of a motor neuron goes directly to the effector organ (skeletal muscle). In the autonomic nervous system, the preganglionic neuron terminates upon the postganglionic neuron, which in turn terminates upon the effector organ (Fig. 13–1).

2. In the somatic motor system, the synaptic region between the axon and the effector organ is well defined and localized (motor endplate of skeletal muscle). In the autonomic nervous system, the synaptic region between the postganglionic neuron and the effector organ (smooth muscle, cardiac muscle, or gland) is more diffuse.

3. Conduction of impulses is faster in the somatic nervous system than in the autonomic nervous system. The slow conduction in the autonomic nervous system is due to the small nerve fibers comprising the system and to synaptic delay.

4. The neurotransmitter substance in the somatic nervous system is acetylcholine. The transmitters in the autonomic nervous system are acetylcholine and norepinephrine (noradrenalin). Acetylcholine is liberated 1) at the junction of preganglionic and postganglionic neurons and 2) at the junction of the postganglionic neuron and effector organ in the parasympathetic division of the autonomic nervous system. Norepinephrine is liberated at the junction of the postganglionic neuron and effector organ in the sympathetic division of the autonomic nervous system. In addition to these classically recognized neurotransmitters of the autonomic nervous system, there is mounting evidence to suggest the presence of nonadrenergic and noncholinergic autonomic neurotransmission mechanisms. Such mechanisms have been found in the gastrointestinal tract, lung, bladder, and some blood vessels. They have been shown to use adenosine triphosphate (ATP), polypeptides, 5-hydroxytryptamine (5-HT), dopamine, and GABA as neurotransmitters.

5. The effector organ in the somatic nervous system (skeletal muscle) will atrophy when it is denervated. Denervation in the autonomic nervous system does not lead to atrophy of the effector (smooth muscle, cardiac muscle, or gland).

6. The somatic nervous system exerts an excitatory action on its effectors. The autonomic nervous system may either excite or inhibit an effector.

The two systems are not independent. They do act together in a complementary fashion. For example, when body temperature drops, the somatic nervous system reacts by contracting skeletal muscles (shivering), thus generating heat; the autonomic nervous system reacts by constricting cutaneous blood vessels, thus reducing heat loss.

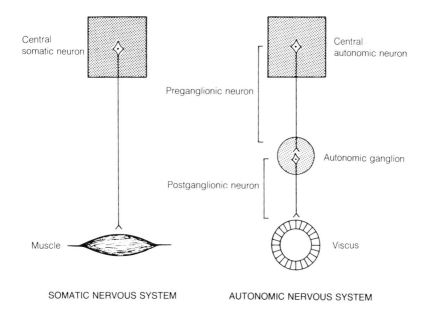

13-1 Schematic diagram comparing the anatomic organization of the somatic and autonomic nervous systems.

Divisions of Autonomic Nervous System

The autonomic nervous system has two divisions, the sympathetic and the parasympathetic. The two divisions differ in several ways.

1. They originate from different parts of the central nervous system.
2. The peripheral ganglia associated with each division have different distributions in relation to the effector organ.
3. The transmitter released at the effector organ is different for each division.
4. The action exerted by one division on an effector organ is usually opposed to the action of the other division.

Sympathetic Division

Since the neurons of origin of the sympathetic division of the autonomic nervous system are located in the intermediolateral cell column of the thoracic and upper lumbar spinal cord (T_1-L_2), this division is also known as the thoracolumbar division.

Axons of sympathetic neurons are small in diameter and myelinated. They leave the spinal cord with the ventral root, join the spinal nerve

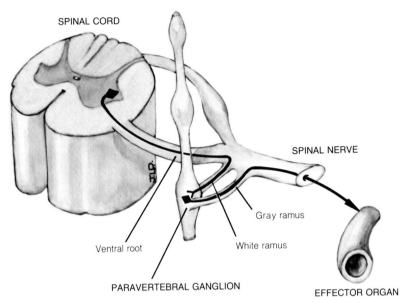

SPINAL CORD

SPINAL NERVE

Gray ramus

Ventral root

White ramus

PARAVERTEBRAL GANGLION

EFFECTOR ORGAN

13–2 Schematic diagram showing the anatomic organization of the sympathetic nervous system.

trunk, and subsequently enter the white ramus communicantes (connecting the nerve trunk with the chain of sympathetic ganglia) to reach the chain of sympathetic ganglia located in the paravertebral region. This preganglionic fiber may follow one of two pathways.

1. It may synapse upon neurons in the sympathetic ganglia. In this case, a postganglionic fiber will leave the ganglion and return to the spinal nerve (via a gray ramus communicantes) to reach the effector organ (Fig. 13–2).

2. It may pass through the ganglia (without synapsing) and join the splanchnic nerve to reach a peripherally located sympathetic ganglion (prevertebral), such as the celiac or mesenteric ganglion, where the synapse takes place. Prevertebral ganglia are scattered in the thorax, abdomen, and pelvis. The postganglionic fibers arising from prevertebral ganglia reach their effector organs via the blood vessels supplying these effector organs (Fig. 13–3). The adrenal gland is supplied directly by preganglionic neurons. The cells of the medulla of the adrenal gland are in effect the postganglionic neurons.

The chains of paravertebral ganglia are situated on each side of the vertebral column and are connected together by nerves (sympathetic trunk). Many fibers ascend or descend in the trunk to reach several ganglia. A single preganglionic neuron in the intermediolateral cell column of the spinal cord may project upon several postganglionic neurons (Fig. 13–4)

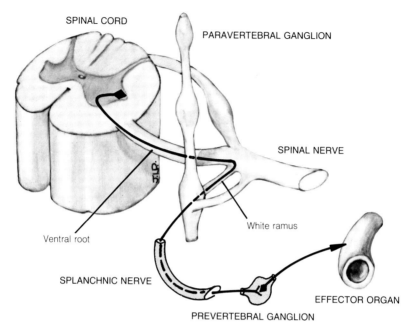

SPINAL CORD

PARAVERTEBRAL GANGLION

SPINAL NERVE

White ramus

Ventral root

SPLANCHNIC NERVE

EFFECTOR ORGAN

PREVERTEBRAL GANGLION

13–3 Schematic diagram showing the anatomic organization of the sympathetic nervous system.

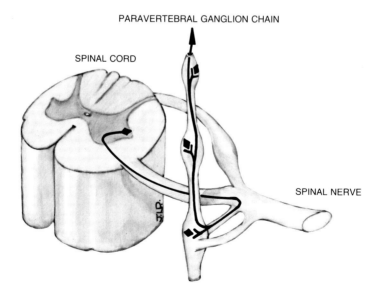

PARAVERTEBRAL GANGLION CHAIN

SPINAL CORD

SPINAL NERVE

13–4 Schematic diagram showing how an axon from an intermediolateral column neuron establishes synapses in several paravertebral ganglia.

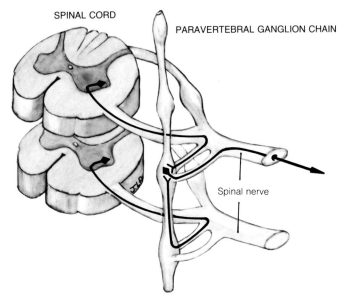

SPINAL CORD

PARAVERTEBRAL GANGLION CHAIN

Spinal nerve

13–5 Schematic diagram showing how a single postganglionic neuron in a para-vertebral ganglion receives axons from several neurons in the intermediolateral cell column.

in the paravertebral chain (diversion). A single preganglionic neuron may synapse with as many as 30 postganglionic neurons. On the other hand, a single postganglionic neuron in the paravertebral chain of ganglia may receive preganglionic fibers from several sympathetic neurons (Fig. 13–5) in the spinal cord (conversion).

The peripherally located (prevertebral) ganglia are unpaired and receive preganglionic fibers from both sides of the spinal cord. The principles of conversion and diversion of input described above also apply to this group of ganglia.

The sympathetic outflow from the thoracic region innervates structures in the head, thorax, upper extremities, and abdomen. The outflow from the lumbar spinal cord innervates the lower extremities and pelvic structures.

As stated previously, the neurotransmitter substance at the postganglionic-effector junction in the sympathetic division of the autonomic nervous system is norepinephrine (adrenalin in the adrenal medulla). This division is therefore called adrenergic. An exception exists in the sympathetic innervation of sweat glands and skeletal muscle blood vessels, where the neurotransmitter is acetylcholine.

The effector organs supplied by the sympathetic division are the smooth muscles of all organs, cardiac muscle, and glands. Smooth muscles of the intestine and of excretory organs, as well as the digestive glands, are inhibited by the sympathetic system. All other effectors are facilitated.

The sympathetic division is not essential for life, but is needed for the proper response of the organism to stressful situations. Activation of the sympathetic division will result in acceleration of the heart, elevation of blood sugar, increased blood flow to skeletal muscles, piloerection, pupillary dilatation, and elevation of blood pressure. The mass reaction prepares the animal for the *fight or flight* response. The structural and biochemical characteristics of the sympathetic division permit this generalized reaction to be sustained. The diversion of preganglionic input to the postganglionic neuron and the multiplicity of junctions at the postganglionic-effector site allow for the widespread effect. The slow deactivation of the transmitter norepinephrine by monoamine oxidase (MAO) and catechol-o-methyl transferase (COMT) permits the sustained action.

Parasympathetic Division

The neurons of origin of the parasympathetic division of the autonomic nervous system are located in two regions, the brain stem and the sacral spinal cord. Thus, this division is also known as the craniosacral division.

The parasympathetic outflow from the brain stem leaves the central nervous system via the following cranial nerves.

1. Oculomotor (CN III)
2. Facial (CN VII)
3. Glossopharyngeal (CN IX)
4. Vagus (CN X)

The preganglionic neurons originate in the following brain stem nuclei.

1. Edinger-Westphal nucleus of the oculomotor nerve
2. Superior salivatory nucleus of the facial nerve
3. Inferior salivatory nucleus of the glossopharyngeal nerve
4. Dorsal motor nucleus of the vagus

The parasympathetic outflow of the sacral region originates from autonomic ganglia in the intermediolateral cell column of the second to the fourth sacral segments. The preganglionic axons leave the spinal cord with the ventral roots and join pelvic nerves.

Preganglionic axons of the parasympathetic division are characteristically longer than those of the sympathetic division (Fig. 13–6).

The postganglionic neurons are located in the walls of or in very close proximity to the effector organs. They comprise the following peripheral ganglia.

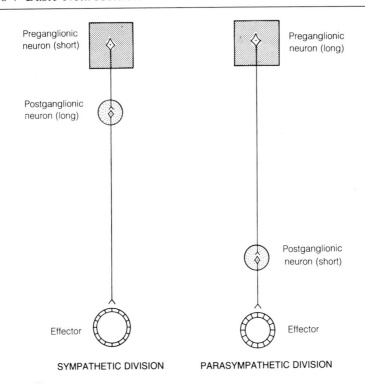

13–6 Schematic diagram comparing the anatomic organization of the sympathetic and parasympathetic divisions of the autonomic nervous system.

1. Ciliary ganglion (oculomotor outflow)
2. Pterygopalatine (sphenopalatine) and submaxillary ganglia (facial nerve outflow)
3. Otic ganglion (glossopharyngeal outflow)
4. Terminal ganglia in the thorax and abdomen (vagal outflow)
5. Terminal ganglia in the pelvic region (sacral outflow)

The cranial outflow via cranial nerves supplies the following structures.

1. Sphincter pupillae muscle of the pupil and ciliary muscle of the iris (via the oculomotor nerve)
2. Lacrimal, submaxillary and submandibular glands (via the facial nerve)
3. Parotid gland (via the glossopharyngeal nerve)
4. Thoracic and abdominal viscera (via the vagus nerve)

The sacral outflow via the pelvic nerves supplies the descending colon and pelvic organs and is involved in the mechanisms of urination and defecation.

The transmitter substance at the postganglionic junction of the parasympathetic division is acetylcholine. This division is thus also known as the cholinergic division.

In contrast to the sympathetic division, the parasympathetic division is geared to localized action for a short time. The following are the anatomic and biochemical substrates of such action.

1. Preganglionic neurons exert their action on a few postganglionic neurons.
2. Postganglionic neurons establish synaptic junctions with a limited number of effector organs.
3. The neurotransmitter acetylcholine is rapidly deactivated by the enzyme cholinesterase.

The role of the parasympathetic division is conservation and restoration of body energy. Activation of this division brings about lowering of blood pressure, decrease in heart rate and increase in activity of the gastrointestinal system.

Autonomic Centers of Central Nervous System

Autonomic centers are scattered throughout the central nervous system.

Spinal Cord

The autonomic centers in the spinal cord, as noted previously, are located in the intermediolateral cell column of T_1-L_2 for the sympathetic division and S_2-S_4 for the parasympathetic division. These centers receive both facilitatory and inhibitory influences from suprasegmental structures via the reticulospinal pathways. In turn, spinal centers influence suprasegmental centers via the spinoreticular pathways.

Brain Stem

In addition to the anatomically delineated autonomic centers outlined under the parasympathetic division, the brain stem contains the following autonomic centers.

1. Cardiovascular center in the medulla oblongata
2. Salivatory center in the medulla oblongata
3. Respiratory center in both medulla oblongata and pons

These different centers are scattered in the reticular formation of the brain stem; most of them have been delineated on physiologic grounds. They exert their influence via reticular pathways to the appropriate cranial nerves or to the spinal autonomic centers.

Cerebellum

The cerebellum exerts its effects on autonomic function via the reticular formation.

Hypothalamus

The role of the hypothalamus in autonomic function has already been outlined in the chapter on the diencephalon. Hypothalamic effects are mediated mainly via three pathways: the dorsal longitudinal fasciculus, mamillotegmental tract, and hypothalamotegmental tract.

The hypothalamic role in autonomic function is evident in its effects on the following.

1. Arterial pressure
2. Heart rate
3. Sweating
4. Temperature
5. Pupillary size
6. Blood sugar level
7. Food and water intake
8. Rage
9. Sexual behavior
10. Sleep and wakefulness

Cerebral Cortex, Basal Ganglia and Thalamus

The neocortex, limbic system, corpus striatum, and thalamus play a role in autonomic function. The autonomic function of the limbic system has been outlined in the chapter on the limbic system. The role of the other structures is not fully understood. They are known, however, to exert a regulating effect on lower centers.

Synaptic Transmission

Synaptic transmission in the autonomic nervous system occurs at two sites, 1) the junction of preganglionic and postganglionic neurons and 2) the junction of postganglionic neuron and effector organ.

The neurotransmitter between the pre- and postganglionic neuron in both divisions of the autonomic nervous system is acetylcholine, whereas the neurotransmitters between the postganglionic neuron and effector organ are acetylcholine in the parasympathetic division and norepinephrine in the sympathetic division. Exceptions to this occur in the sympathetic

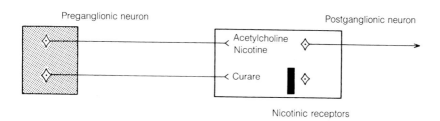

13–7 Schematic diagram illustrating the concept of nicotinic receptors.

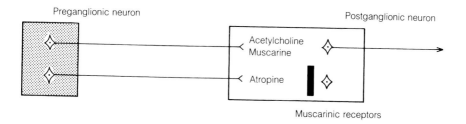

13–8 Schematic diagram illustrating the concept of muscarinic receptors.

supply of sweat glands and skeletal muscle blood vessels, where the neurotransmitter is acetylcholine. The transmitter in the adrenal medulla is adrenalin. Adrenal medullary cells pour their secretions directly into the blood stream.

Preganglionic-Postganglionic Junction

Acetylcholine liberated at the terminals of preganglionic neurons acts on two types of cholinergic receptors, the nicotinic receptors and the muscarinic receptors. Nicotinic receptors are stimulated by nicotine (hence their name), as well as by acetylcholine. They are blocked by curare (Fig. 13–7). Muscarinic receptors, on the other hand, are stimulated by acetylcholine and muscarine (hence their name). They are blocked by atropine (Fig. 13–8).

Stimulation of the preganglionic axon gives rise to one of the following responses: 1) short latency excitatory postsynaptic potential (EPSP), 2) long latency EPSP, and 3) long latency inhibitory postsynaptic potential (IPSP).

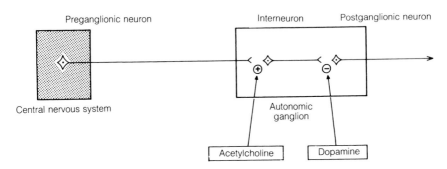

13-9   Schematic diagram showing the mechanism of the long latency IPSP (⊖) elicited by stimulation of preganglionic neurons.

The short latency EPSP is mediated by nicotinic receptors. The long latency EPSP is mediated by muscarinic receptors. The long latency IPSP, on the other hand, is believed to be mediated via an interneuron which liberates dopamine, an adrenergic substance which acts on the postganglionic neuron (Fig. 13-9).

Postganglionic-Effector Junction

The synaptic junction between the postganglionic neuron and effector organ in the autonomic nervous system is not as well defined as that of the somatic system. From available observations, it appears that the unmyelinated postganglionic nerve fibers lose their Schwann sheaths as they approach the junction and develop swellings which contain vesicles and mitochondria. In some species and certain sites, such axonal terminals appear to fit into depressions in the postsynaptic end of the junction. The neurotransmitter is released into the extracellular space and acts upon receptor sites in the effector organ.

Stimulation of the postganglionic axon gives rise to either EPSPs or IPSPs.

The neurotransmitters liberated at the postganglionic-effector junction are acetylcholine (parasympathetic division) and norepinephrine (sympathetic division). There are, therefore, two types of receptors at this site: cholinergic receptors and adrenergic receptors.

The cholinergic receptors of the muscarinic variety are blocked by atropine. An example of such receptors are those in the heart. Vagal stimulation results in inhibition of cardiac action with slowing of the heart rate. This action is blocked by the administration of atropine.

Adrenergic receptors are of two types, alpha receptors and beta receptors. Both receptors react to adrenalin. Alpha receptors are more responsive to norepinephrine than to isoproterenol and are blocked by phenoxybenzamine (alpha blocker).

Beta receptors are more responsive to isoproterenol than to norepinephrine and are blocked by dichloroisoproterenol (beta blocker). Beta receptors have been divided into beta 1 and beta 2 receptors. The heart contains the former, whereas most other effector organs contain the latter.

Stimulation of alpha receptors gives rise to vasoconstriction, sweating, piloerection, intestinal relaxation, and pupillary dilatation. Stimulation of beta receptors gives rise to cardiac acceleration, increase in strength of cardiac contraction, relaxation of bronchial and skeletal muscle blood vessels, gastrointestinal hypomotility, and relaxation of the detrusor muscle of the urinary bladder.

Clinical Correlates

The processes involved in synaptic transmission occur in the following sequence.

1. Synthesis of transmitter substance
2. Storage of transmitter in nerve endings
3. Release of transmitter
4. Binding of transmitter to receptor sites
5. Inactivation of transmitter by reuptake or metabolism

In clinical practice, drugs that will either stimulate or inhibit each of the above processes have been used to interfere with autonomic function. Examples of such drugs are isoproterenol (Isuprel), which stimulates beta receptors; propranolol (Inderal), a beta receptor blocker; reserpine, which interferes with norepinephrine storage; phentolamine (Regitine), which blocks alpha receptors; and metaraminal (Levophed), which stimulates alpha receptors.

Diffuse abnormalities in autonomic function are encountered in clinical practice. Disseminated degeneration of autonomic neurons occurs in elderly patients (Shy-Drager syndrome). Familial dysautonomia, a disorder in autonomic function in infants and children, is characterized by absence of tears, a drop in blood pressure on assumption of erect posture, marked elevation of blood pressure with emotional states, excessive sweating, excessive salivation, and marked changes in temperature.

Denervation Supersensitivity

Denervation of the effector organ by severance of the postganglionic axon or of the postganglionic neuron by severance of the preganglionic axon results in a state of supersensitivity of the postsynaptic membrane to the transmitter or related substances. This phenomenon, which appears in a week or two, is usually more marked at the postganglionic neuron-effector organ junction than at the pre- and postganglionic junction. Several theories have been proposed to explain this phenomenon; none, however, is satisfactory. The following factors may play a role in inducing this supersensitive state.

1. There may be a defect in the reuptake of the transmitter due to the pathology at the nerve terminal.

2. An increase in the number of available receptor sites in the effector organ will enhance the response to the transmitter. Such an increase in the number of receptors has actually been observed following denervation.

Autonomic Control of Visceral Function

Bladder Function

The urinary bladder receives dual autonomic innervation from the sympathetic and parasympathetic divisions. The two divisions have an antagonistic effect on bladder function. The sympathetic supply relaxes the smooth muscles of the fundus and contracts those of the internal sphincter. The parasympathetic supply has the reverse effect. It is doubtful, however, whether the sympathetic supply has an important role to play in bladder function. Thus, bladder function is mainly controlled by the parasympathetic outflow from the sacral spinal cord (S_2–S_4).

Filling of the bladder stimulates receptors in its wall which will activate visceral afferents to the sacral cord. This will activate the preganglionic neurons in the intermediolateral cell column. Impulses originating above the level of the axons of preganglionic neurons will activate the postganglionic neurons in peripheral autonomic ganglia close to the bladder, the axons of which terminate upon smooth muscles of the bladder wall (detrusor muscle) and the internal sphincter. This results in contraction of the bladder wall and relaxation of the sphincter to allow micturition. Interruption of the parasympathetic supply to the bladder causes detrusor muscle areflexia and urinary retention. On the other hand, interruption of the sympathetic supply may result in stress urinary incontinence.

Superimposed on the involuntary mechanism is a voluntary mechanism that controls the act of micturition. This voluntary mechanism is mediated by several pathways. The first pathway is from the frontal cortex to the pontine and mesencephalic reticular formation and is necessary for the voluntary control of micturition. Interruption of this pathway results in precipitous voiding due to involuntary detrusor muscle contraction and involuntary sphincter relaxation. The second pathway is from the pontine and mesencephalic reticular formation to the parasympathetic centers of the spinal cord via the reticulospinal tract. Its integrity is necessary for coordinated micturition (detrusor muscle contraction and sphincter relaxation). Interruption of this pathway results in involuntary, dyssynergic bladder and sphincter contractions. These patients are incontinent because of involuntary detrusor muscle contraction, yet urine flow is partially obstructed by contractions of the external sphincter. The third pathway is the corticospinal tract from the frontal cortex to the parasympathetic sacral nuclei. This pathway is necessary for voluntary interruption of the urinary stream.

Gastrointestinal Function

The gastrointestinal tract receives dual innervation with antagonistic effects from the sympathetic and parasympathetic divisions. These effects are exerted on the following: 1) smooth muscle fibers of the wall, 2) sphincter, and 3) glands.

Sympathetic stimulation relaxes the smooth muscles of the intestinal wall (decreased peristalsis) and contracts the sphincters. Parasympathetic stimulation has the reverse effect. In addition, parasympathetic stimulation increases the secretion of intestinal glands. Because of the effect of the parasympathetic division on glandular secretion, vagotomy (cutting of the vagus nerve) is sometimes performed for the treatment of peptic ulcer. Congenital absence of postganglionic neurons in the wall of the rectum or rectosigmoid (Hirschsprung's disease) results in the loss of peristaltic activity in the constricted part of the intestine. The normal portion of the intestine proximal to the affected region will have normal peristaltic activity and will dilate greatly. Such patients present with symptoms and signs of intestinal obstruction such as abdominal distention and vomiting.

Cardiac Function

The heart also receives dual and antagonistic innervation from both the sympathetic and parasympathetic divisions.

These effects are exerted upon the sinoatrial (SA) node, atrial and ventricular walls, and the atrioventricular (AV) node. The net effect of sympathetic stimulation is acceleration of the cardiac rate and increase in contractility. Parasympathetic stimulation has the reverse effect.

References

Blaivas, J.G.: Management of Bladder Dysfunction in Multiple Sclerosis. Neurology 30, No. 7, Pt. 2 (1980) 12–18.

Brodal, A.: Neurological Anatomy in Relation to Clinical Medicine, Ed. 3, pp. 698–787. Oxford University Press, London, 1981.

Burnstock, G.; Hökfelt, T.; Gershon, M.D.; Iversen, L. L.; Kosterlitz, H.W.; Szurszewski, J.H.; Non-Adrenergic, Non-Cholinergic Autonomic Neurotransmission Mechanisms. Neurosci Res Program Bull 17 (1979) 379–519.

Leek, B.F.: Abdominal and Pelvic Visceral Receptors. Brit Med Bull 33 (1977) 163–168.

14

Special Senses

Olfaction

Olfactory stimuli are received by the olfactory receptors in the nasal wall and are conveyed via olfactory nerve fibers through the cribriform plate of the ethmoid bone to the olfactory bulb inside the cranial cavity. After synaptic transmission in the glomeruli of the olfactory bulb, the impulses are carried by mitral and tufted cell axons (which form the olfactory tract) to the primary olfactory area in the tip of the temporal lobe. The anatomy and physiology of this pathway have been outlined in the chapter on the rhinencephalon and limbic system. Attention in this chapter will be focused on the receptor area in the nasal cavity.

Olfactory Mucosa (Fig. 14–1)

Olfactory stimuli are received in the olfactory epithelium located in the mucous membrane of the upper part of the nasal septum and the roof and upper part of the lateral wall of the nasal cavity, including the superior concha. Man is a microsmatic animal in which the surface area of the olfactory mucous membrane in both nostrils is small (approximately 5 cm^2). The olfactory epithelium contains three types of epithelial cells; these are receptor cells, supporting cells, and basal cells. Interspersed among epithelial cells are ducts of Bowman's glands.

Receptor Cells Olfactory receptor cells are bipolar sensory neurons. Their perikarya are located in the lower part of the olfactory epithelium. Each cell has a single dendrite that reaches the surface of the epithelium and forms a knob-like expansion which extends beyond the epithelial surface. From this expansion, 10 to 20 cilia project into a layer of fluid covering the epithelium. From the basal part of the perikaryon, a nonmyelinated

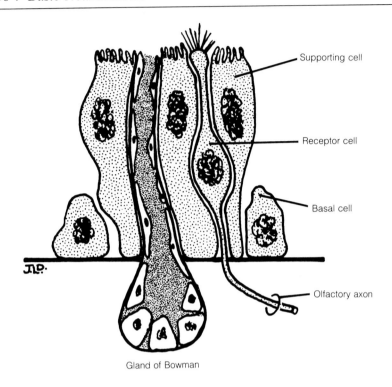

Supporting cell

Receptor cell

Basal cell

Olfactory axon

Gland of Bowman

14–1 Schematic diagram of the cellular components of the olfactory mucosa.

axon emerges and joins with axons of adjacent receptor cells to form the olfactory nerve. Olfactory nerve bundles penetrate the cribriform plate of the ethmoid bone to reach the olfactory bulb. It is estimated that there are more than 100 million receptor cells in the olfactory mucosa. Olfactory receptor cells decrease in number with age, which explains the diminution of olfactory acuity in older people.

Supporting Cells   These are columnar epithelial cells which separate the olfactory receptor cells. Their nuclei are lined up toward the surface of the epithelium, above the perikarya of receptor cells. The surface of supporting cells is specialized into microvilli projecting into the fluid layer covering the epithelium.

Basal Cells   These polygonal cells, limited to the basal part of the epithelium, are the source of new epithelial cells. Mitotic activity persists in these cells through maturity.

Bowman's Glands   These are located beneath the epithelium and send their ducts in between epithelial cells to pour their secretions on the surface of the epithelium, bathing the cilia of receptor cells and microvilli of supporting cells. The secretion of Bowman's gland plays an important role in dissolving odorous substances and diffusing them to receptor cells.

Olfactory Mechanisms

Olfaction is a chemical sense. For a substance to be detected, it should have the following physical properties.

1. Volatility, so that it can be sniffed
2. Water solubility, so that it can diffuse through the olfactory epithelium
3. Lipid solubility, so that it will interact with the lipids of the membranes of olfactory receptors

After an odorous substance is dissolved in the fluid bathing the surface of the olfactory mucosa, it interacts with receptors on the surface of the receptor cell. This interaction causes a change in membrane permeability. The ion flux that ensues gives rise to a slow surface negative wave (receptor or generator potential) which can be detected at the surface of the receptor cell. An all or none action potential, on the other hand, can be detected in the axons of receptor cells.

The olfactory receptors have a marked variability in their sensitivity to different odors. They can detect methyl mercaptan (garlic odor) in a concentration of less than one-millionth of a milligram per liter of air, whereas ethyl ether is detected in a concentration of 5.8 mg per liter of air.

Olfactory receptors adapt rather quickly to a continuous stimulus. Although the olfactory mucosa can discriminate among a large number of different odors, their ability to detect changes in concentration of an odorous substance is rather poor. It is estimated that the concentration of an odorous substance must change by 30% before it can be detected by receptor cells. The mechanism of discrimination is poorly understood, but is probably due to a spatial pattern of stimulation of the receptor cells.

The sense of olfaction is lost (anosmia) or diminished (hyposmia) in man in connection with several conditions. These include common colds, trauma to the olfactory mucosa or nerve, and tumors in the base of the frontal lobe. The olfactory hallucinations that occur in diseases of the temporal lobe have been outlined in the chapter on the rhinencephalon and limbic system.

Taste

Taste receptors are located within taste buds in the tongue (circumvallate and fungiform papillae), as well as in the soft palate, oropharynx, and

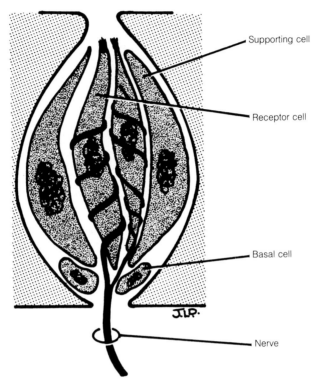

Supporting cell

Receptor cell

Basal cell

JLP.

Nerve

14-2 Schematic diagram of the cellular components of the taste bud.

epiglottis. Taste sensations are conveyed centrally via the facial (CN VII), glossopharyngeal (CN IX), and vagus (CN X) cranial nerves.

Taste Buds

Taste buds (Fig 14-2) are barrel-like structures distributed in the epithelium of the tongue, soft palate, and epiglottis. Each taste bud is composed of receptor cells, supporting cells, basal cells, and nerve fibers.

Receptor Cells Two types of receptor cells can be identified in taste buds; these are clear receptor cells and dense receptor cells. Clear receptor cells contain clear vesicles; dense receptor cells contain dense core vesicles. Both cell types presumably function as receptors. They are believed to represent two stages in the development of receptor elements, the dense cell being the more mature one. The apex of each receptor cell is modified into microvilli which increase the receptor surface and project into an opening, the taste pore. There are approximately 4 to 20 receptor cells located in the center of each taste bud. Receptor elements decrease in number with age.

Supporting Cells   These are spindle-shaped cells which surround the receptor cells and are located at the periphery of the taste bud. They have both an insulating and a secretory function. They are believed to secrete the substance that bathes the microvilli in the taste pore.

Basal Cells   These are located at the base of the taste bud and, by division, replenish the receptor cells that are continually lost.

Nerve Fibers   These are terminal nerve fibers of the facial, glossopharyngeal, and vagus nerves. They are peripheral processes of sensory neurons in the geniculate ganglion of the facial nerve and in the inferior ganglia of the glossopharyngeal and vagus nerves. They enter the taste bud at its base and wind themselves around the receptor cells in close apposition with receptor cell membranes. Synaptic vesicles cluster on the inner surfaces of receptor cell membranes at sites of apposition with nerve terminals.

Physiology of Taste

Like olfaction, the sense of taste is a chemical sense. Although man can taste a large number of substances, only four primary taste sensations are identified: sour, salty, sweet, and bitter.

Most taste receptors respond to all four primary taste modalities at varying thresholds, but respond preferentially at a very low threshold to only one or two. Thus, taste buds at the tip of the tongue respond best to sweet and salty substances, and those at the lateral margins and posterior part of the tongue respond best to sour and bitter substances, respectively. The ability of taste buds to detect changes in concentration of a substance is poor, similar to the response of olfactory receptors. A difference in taste intensity remains undetected until the concentration of a substance has changed by 30%.

The mechanism by which a substance is tasted is not well understood. It has been established, however, that contact of a substance with the surface of taste receptors will induce a change in the electrical potential of the membrane (receptor or generator potential). This receptor potential will in turn produce an action potential in the nerve terminals in apposition to the receptor cell surface. The mechanisms by which a receptor potential triggers an action potential are not well defined.

Central Transmission

As outlined previously, the nerve terminals in the taste buds are peripheral processes of sensory neurons in ganglia belonging to the facial, glossopharyngeal, and vagus cranial nerves. The nerve terminals of the facial nerve supply taste buds in the anterior two-thirds of the tongue; those of the glossopharyngeal nerve supply taste buds in the posterior one-third of the tongue, as well as those in the soft palate and oropharynx; and those of the vagus nerve supply taste buds in the epiglottis.

Central processes of sensory neurons in the ganglia of the facial, glossopharyngeal, and vagus nerves contribute to the tractus solitarius in the brain stem and terminate upon the gustatory (taste) portion of the nucleus solitarius. Axons of neurons in the nucleus solitarius project upon a number of reticular nuclei before crossing the midline to reach the ventral posteromedial (VPM) nucleus of the thalamus, giving on their way collateral branches to such nuclei as the nucleus ambiguus and salivatory nuclei for reflex activity. From VPM, axons project to the cerebral cortex to terminate upon neurons in the inferior part of the somesthetic cortex, just anterior to the face area.

Vision

Light rays falling on the eye pass through its refractive media (cornea, lens and anterior and posterior chambers) before reaching the visual receptor cells (the rods and cones) in the retina. The refractive media help focus the image on the retina.

Retinal Structure

The retina (Fig. 14–3) is an outward extension of the brain to which it is connected by the optic nerve. The human retina is made up of the following 10 layers, starting with the outermost layer.

1. Layer of pigment epithelium
2. Layer of rods and cones
3. External limiting membrane
4. Outer nuclear layer
5. Outer plexiform layer
6. Inner nuclear layer
7. Inner plexiform layer
8. Layer of ganglion cells
9. Optic nerve layer
10. Internal limiting membrane

Layer of Pigment Epithelium   This is a single layer of melanin-containing, pigmented cuboidal cells firmly bound to the choroid layer. The function of this layer is not fully understood; it probably plays a role in light absorption.

Layer of Rods and Cones   This layer contains the light-sensitive parts of the photoreceptors, the rods and cones. The human retina contains

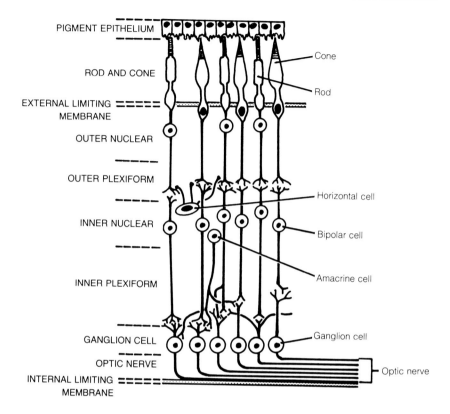

PIGMENT EPITHELIUM

ROD AND CONE

Cone

Rod

EXTERNAL LIMITING
MEMBRANE

OUTER NUCLEAR

OUTER PLEXIFORM

INNER NUCLEAR

Horizontal cell

Bipolar cell

INNER PLEXIFORM

Amacrine cell

GANGLION CELL

Ganglion cell

OPTIC NERVE

Optic nerve

INTERNAL LIMITING
MEMBRANE

14–3   Schematic diagram of the layers of the retina and their cellular components.

approximately 100 million rods and five million cones. The rods and cones differ in their distribution along the retina. In humans, a modified region called the fovea contains only cones and is adapted for high visual acuity. At all other points along the retina, rods greatly outnumber cones.

Rods   The rod photoreceptor cell is a modified neuron having as components the cell body, axonal process, and photosensitive process.

The *cell body* contains the nucleus. This part of the rod is located in the outer nuclear layer.

The *axonal process* is located in the outer plexiform layer.

The *photosensitive process* is located in the layer of rods and cones. The photosensitive process of the rod is made up of two segments, outer and inner, connected by a narrow neck containing cilia. The outer segment has been shown by electron microscopy to be filled with stacks of double membrane discs containing the visual pigment rhodopsin. Its function is to trap the light that reaches the retina. The visual pigment molecules are positioned within the disc membranes in such a way as to maximize the probability of their interacting with the path of incident light. The extensive invagination of the disc membranes increases the total surface area available for visual pigment. Rhodopsin is composed of a vitamin A aldehyde, retinal, combined with the protein scotopsin. Exposure to light breaks the bond between retinal and the protein. This chemical change triggers a change in the electrical potential and produces a generator (receptor) potential. The stacked discs in the outer segment are shed continually and are replaced by the infolding of the cell membrane. The outer segments are separated and supported by processes from the layer of pigment epithelium.

The inner segment of the rod contains mitochondria, glycogen, endoplasmic reticulum, and Golgi apparatus. It is the site of formation of the protein scotopsin, which subsequently moves to the outer segment. The inner segment is connected to the cell body of the rod fiber, which traverses the external limiting membrane.

Cones   Cones have the same structural components as the rods (cell body, axonal process, and photosensitive process).

The photosensitive processes of cones, like those of rods, contain outer and inner segments. The discs in the outer segments, unlike those of rods, remain attached to the cell membrane and are not shed. The pigment they contain is made up of retinal and the protein cone opsin.

External Limiting Membrane   This is a sieve-like sheet fenestrated to allow the passage of processes that connect the photosensitive process of rods and cones with their cell bodies. It also contains the outer processes of Muller's (supporting) cells.

Outer Nuclear Layer   This layer contains the cell bodies of rods and cones with their nuclei. Cone nuclei are ovoid and limited to a single row close to the external limiting membrane. Rod nuclei are rounded and distributed in several layers.

Outer Plexiform Layer   This layer contains axonal processes of rods and cones, as well as dendrites of bipolar cells and processes of horizontal cells.

Inner Nuclear Layer   This layer contains cell bodies and nuclei of bipolar cells and association cells (horizontal and amacrine), as well as supporting (Muller's) cells.

This layer has three zones, an outer zone containing horizontal cells, an intermediate zone containing bipolar cells, and an inner zone containing amacrine cells.

Three types of bipolar cells are recognized. They are rod bipolar cells related to several rod axons, midget bipolar cells related to one cone axon, and flat bipolar cells related to several cone axons.

The horizontal association cells are larger than the bipolar cells. Their axons and dendrites are located in the outer plexiform layer. Their axons establish synapses with rod and cone axons, whereas their dendrites establish relationships with cone axons. Thus, they connect cones of one area with cones and rods of another area.

The amacrine association cells are pear-shaped. They have a single process that terminates on bipolar and ganglion cell processes in the inner plexiform layer.

Muller's supporting cells send their processes to the outer plexiform layer.

Inner Plexiform Layer   This layer contains axons of bipolar cells, dendrites of ganglion cells, and processes of the association (amacrine) cells.

Layer of Ganglion Cells   This layer is composed of the perikarya of multipolar ganglion cells. Two types of ganglion cells are recognized on the basis of their dendritic connections. These are a monosynaptic (midget) ganglion cell related to a single bipolar (midget) cell and a diffuse (polysynaptic) ganglion cell related to several bipolar cells. The axons of ganglion cells form the optic nerve. In man, the number of ganglion cells is estimated to be one million.

Optic Nerve Layer   This layer is composed of axons of ganglion cells that form the optic nerve, as well as some Muller's fibers. Axons of ganglion cells in this layer are unmyelinated but have a glial sheath around them. They run toward the posterior pole of the eye, where they form the optic disc and penetrate the sclera to form the optic nerve.

Internal Limiting Membrane   This is formed by the expanded inner ends of the processes of Muller's cells. Muller's cells, the cell bodies of which are located in the inner nuclear layer, send processes both outward to the external limiting membrane and inward to the internal limiting membrane. They are thus homologous to glial cells of the central nervous system.

The above retinal structure is maintained throughout the retina except at two sites, the fovea centralis in the central area of the retina and ora serrata at the periphery of the retina.

In both sites, the structure of the retina is modified. Absent from both areas are the 1) ganglion cell layer, 2) inner plexiform layer, and 3) bipolar cell layer.

The fovea centralis represents the area of greatest visual acuity and its center contains only cones arranged in multiple rows. The cones of the fovea are slender and resemble rods in structure. Near the ora serrata, at the periphery of the retina, rods predominate.

Synaptic Organization

The human retina is considered to be a simple retina in which there is relatively little processing of information, as compared to complex retinae (frog) in which information processing is more extensive.

The different types of cells encountered in the retina can be divided into three categories.

1. Input elements (rods and cones)
2. Output elements (ganglion cells)
3. Intrinsic elements (bipolar, horizontal and amacrine cells)

It is estimated that the human retina contains 100 million rods, five million cones, and one million ganglion cells. This provides an input to output ratio of 100:1 for rods and 5:1 for cones. This difference correlates well with the function of cones, namely high acuity vision. The input to output ratio is lowest (approximately 1:1) in the fovea centralis, where visual acuity is highest.

Synaptic interaction in the retina takes place in two layers, the outer plexiform layer and the inner plexiform layer.

Outer Plexiform Layer   In the outer plexiform layer (Fig. 14–3), synaptic interaction takes place both vertically and horizontally. The vertical interaction is represented by the rod and cone terminals on bipolar cell dendrites. The horizontal interaction is represented by the interaction of horizontal cell processes with both rod and cone axons.

Axon terminals of rods (rod spherules) are smaller than cone terminals; the latter are flat or pyramidal in shape and large (cone pedicle).

Receptor-Bipolar Cell Interaction   As stated previously, there are three varieties of bipolar cells. 1) A rod bipolar cell forms synapses with several rod spherules, 2) a midget bipolar cell forms synapses with one cone pedicle, and 3) a flat bipolar cell forms synapses with several cone pedicles.

Horizontal Cell-Receptor Interaction   Horizontal cell processes form synapses with several cones or rods, relating cones of one area to rods and cones of another area. Processes of horizontal cells are not classified as either axons or dendrites and possibly transmit bidirectionally.

Inner Plexiform Layer   In the inner plexiform layer (Fig. 14–3), synaptic interaction takes place between bipolar and ganglion cells (vertical interaction), as well as among amacrine, bipolar, and ganglion cells (horizontal interaction).

Bipolar-Ganglion Cell Interaction   Rod bipolar cells project upon several ganglion cells. Midget bipolar cells relate to one ganglion cell (midget ganglion cell). Flat bipolar cells relate to several ganglion cells.

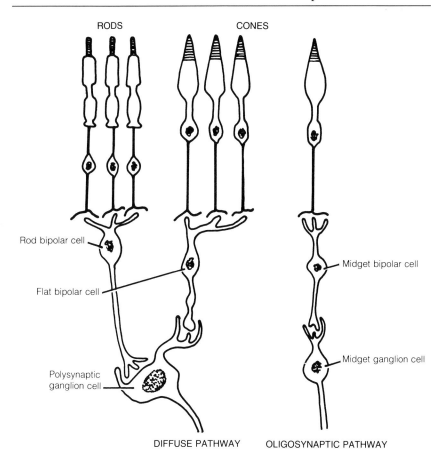

RODS   CONES

Rod bipolar cell

Flat bipolar cell

Midget bipolar cell

Polysynaptic
ganglion cell

Midget ganglion cell

DIFFUSE PATHWAY   OLIGOSYNAPTIC PATHWAY

14–4 Schematic diagram of the types of synaptic activity within the retina.

Amacrine, Bipolar and Ganglion Cell Interaction Amacrine cells relate to axons of bipolar cells, as well as to dendrites and perikarya of ganglion cells. Amacrine cell processes, like horizontal cell processes, probably conduct bidirectionally.

It is apparent from the above that synaptic activity in the retina has the following characteristics.

1. It is oriented both vertically (receptor-bipolar-ganglion cell axis) and horizontally (via horizontal and amacrine cell connnections).
2. It is carried out by both diffuse (flat bipolar- or rod bipolar-polysynaptic ganglion cell) and oligosynaptic (midget bipolar-midget ganglion cell) pathways (Fig. 14–4).

Photochemistry and Physiology

The retina contains two types of photoreceptors, the rods and cones. The rods are highly sensitive to light, have a low threshold of stimulation and are thus best suited for dim light vision. Such vision, however, is poor in detail and does not differentiate colors (achromatic).

The cones, on the other hand, have a high threshold of stimulation and function best in strong illumination (daylight). They provide the substrate for acute vision, as well as color vision.

Upon exposure to light, the visual pigments in the outer segments of the rods and cones (rhodopsin and cone opsin, respectively) break down into two components, retinal (colorless pigment) and the protein opsin.

By a mechanism which is not fully understood, the degradation of visual pigment triggers a change in the electrical potential of the photoreceptors (receptor or generator potential). The generator potential of rods and cones (unlike similar potentials in other receptors) is in the hyperpolarizing direction. This unique response of the photoreceptors has been attributed to the fact that the photoreceptor membrane is depolarized in the resting state (darkness) by a constant leak of electrical current (sodium ion permeability) in the outer segment. Exposure to light will reduce the permeability of the membrane to sodium ions, reduce the electrical current and hyperpolarize the membrane. Thus, hyperpolarizing currents in photoreceptors are produced by turning off depolarizing sodium ion conductance, whereas the orthodox hyperpolarization (IPSP) seen in other neurons is produced by turning on hyperpolarizing potassium ion conductance in the neuronal membrane.

The generator potential of photoreceptors leads to hyper- or depolarization of the bipolar and horizontal cells. Neither of these cell types, however, is capable of triggering a propagated action potential.

On the basis of their hyper- or depolarizing response, two types of bipolar cells are identified. One type responds by hyperpolarization to a light spot in the center of its receptive field and by depolarization to a light spot in the area surrounding the center (surround). The other type responds in a reverse fashion by depolarization to a light spot in the center of its receptive field and by hyperpolarization to the surround. The bipolar cell is the first of the retinal elements to show this variation of response in relation to the spatial position of the stimulus in its receptive field.

The amacrine cell responds to a light stimulus by a propagated, all or none action potential. It is the first cell of the retinal elements to generate a propagated action potential.

Ganglion cells discharge continuously at a slow rate in the absence of any stimulus. Upon superimposition of a circular beam of light, ganglion cells may behave in a variety of ways. Some cells increase their discharge in response to the superimposed stimulus ("on" cells); others inhibit their discharge in response to the superimposed stimulus, but discharge again with a burst when the stimulus is turned off ("off" cells); and still others increase their discharge when the stimulus is turned both on and off ("on-off" cells). Furthermore, the behavior of ganglion cells, like that of bipolar cells, is regulated by the spatial position of the stimulus in their receptive field. "On" cells, which increase their discharge in response to a spot of light in the center of their receptive field, will inhibit their discharge when light is shone in the area surrounding the center. The same principle applies to "off" cells, which inhibit their discharge in response to a light stimulus in the center of the receptive field, but increase their discharge when the stimulus is shown in the surround.

Furthermore, some ganglion cells respond only to a steady stimulus of light in their receptive field, whereas others respond only to a change in intensity of illumination; still others respond only to a moving stimulus and in a particular direction.

Dark and Light Adaptation

When an individual moves from an environment of bright light to dim light or darkness, the retina adapts and becomes more sensitive to light. This process is called dark adaptation and takes about 20 min to become maximally effective. The time required for maximal adaptation to darkness can be shortened by wearing red glasses. Light waves in the red end of the spectrum do not effectively stimulate the rods; they remain dark-adapted. Nor do they interfere with cone stimulation, so the individual can still see in bright light. The process of dark adaptation has two components, a fast one attributed to adaptation of cones and a slower one attributed to adaptation of rods.

Conversely, when an individual moves from a dark environment to a bright one, it takes time to adapt to the bright environment. This process is called light adaptation and takes about 5 min to be effective.

Night Blindness

Night blindness (nyctalopia) is encountered in individuals with vitamin A deficiency. As mentioned previously, photoreceptor pigment is formed of two substances, vitamin A aldehyde (retinal) and the protein opsin. In vitamin A deficiency, the total amount of visual pigment is reduced, thus decreasing the sensitivity to light of both rods and cones. Although this reduction does not interfere with bright light (daylight) vision, it does significantly affect dark light (night) vision because the amount of light is not enough to excite the depleted visual pigment. This condition is treatable by administration of vitamin A.

Color Vision

Color vision is a function of the retina, lateral geniculate nucleus, and cerebral cortex.

In the retina, the cone receptors and the horizontal cells, as well as ganglion cells, take part in the integration of color vision. According to the Young-Helmholtz theory of color vision, retinal cone receptors are of three varieties. There are those that respond maximally to wavelengths in the red end of the spectrum, those that respond maximally to wavelengths in the green end of the spectrum, and those that respond maximally to wavelengths in the blue range of the spectrum. A monochromatic color (red, green or blue) stimulates maximally one variety of cones and to a variable but lesser degree the other varieties of cones. Blue light, for example, stimulates blue cones maximally, green cones much less so, and red cones not at all. This pattern is interpreted centrally as blue color. Two monochromatic colors stimulating two types of cones equally and simultaneously will be interpreted as a different color; thus, if green and red lights stimulate green and red cones simultaneously and equally, they will be interpreted as yellow. Simultaneous and equal stimulation by red, green and blue lights will be interpreted as white.

The horizontal cells respond to a particular monochromatic color by either depolarization or hyperpolarization. A red-green horizontal cell responds by depolarization to red light and by hyperpolarization to green light. Such a cell will be turned off by equal and simultaneous stimulation by red and green. There are also yellow-blue horizontal cells, which accounts for the four hues, namely red, green, blue, and yellow. The depolarization and hyperpolarization responses of horizontal cells also explains why red and green and blue and yellow are complementary colors which, when mixed together in proper amounts, result in the cancellation of color.

Ganglion cells of the retina respond in an "on-off" manner to monochromatic light. Thus, there are green "on" and red "off" ganglion cells, red "on" and green "off" ganglion cells, blue "on" and yellow "off" ganglion cells, etc.

Furthermore, there are color-sensitive neurons in the lateral geniculate nucleus and occipital cortex which respond maximally to color in one part of the spectrum. They also play a role in color discrimination. The color-contrast cells in the striate cortex form a distinct population separate from cells concerned with brightness contrast. As with cells concerned with brightness discrimination, the color-contrast cells can be divided into simple, complex, and hypercomplex cells.

Color Blindness

Some individuals exhibit a deficiency in or lack of a particular color cone. Such individuals have color weakness or color blindness, respectively. Most

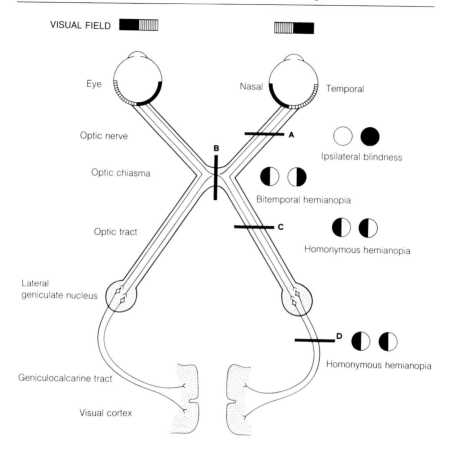

14–5 Schematic diagram of the visual pathway showing clinical manifestations of lesions in various sites.

color blind individuals are red-green blind; a minority are blue color blind. Among the red-green blind group, there is a preponderance of green color blindness.

Color blindness for red and green is inherited by an X-linked recessive gene; thus, there are more male red-green color blind individuals than female. Color blindness for blue is inherited by an autosomal gene.

Visual Pathways (Fig. 14–5).

Axons of ganglion cells in the retina gather together at the optic disc in the posterior pole of the eye, penetrate the sclera, and form the optic nerve. The point of exit of ganglion cell axons from the retina, the optic disc, is devoid of receptor elements (blind spot). There are approximately one million axons in the optic nerve. Outside the sclera, the optic nerve is covered by extensions of the meninges that ensheathe the brain. Marked increase in intracranial pressure from tumors or bleeding inside the cranial cavity or increase in cerebrospinal fluid pressure around the nerve sufficient to interfere with venous return from the retina will result in swelling of the optic disc (papillaedema). This swelling can be seen using a special instrument, an ophthalmoscope, which views the retina through the pupil.

The optic nerve enters the cranial cavity through the optic foramen. Thus, tumors of the optic nerve (optic glioma) may be diagnosed by taking X-ray views of the optic foramen, which appears enlarged in such conditions.

Lesions of the optic nerve produce unilateral blindness on the side of the lesion (Fig. 14–5, *A*).

The two optic nerves come together at the optic chiasma, where partial crossing of optic nerve fibers takes place. Optic nerve fibers from the nasal half of each retina cross at the optic chiasma. Fibers from the temporal halves remain uncrossed. The optic chiasma is related to the hypothalamus above and pituitary gland below. Thus, tumors in the pituitary gland encroaching (as they do initially) on the crossing fibers of the optic nerve will result in degeneration of optic nerve fibers arising in the nasal halves of both retinae. This results in loss of vision in both temporal fields of vision (bitemporal hemianopia) (Fig. 14–5, *B*).

The crossed and uncrossed fibers from both optic nerves join caudal to the optic chiasma to form the optic tract. Lesions of the optic tracts, therefore, will result in degeneration of optic nerve fibers from the temporal half of the ipsilateral retina and nasal half of the contralateral retina. This produces loss of vision in the contralateral half of the visual field (homonymous hemianopia) (Fig. 14–5, *C*). The optic tracts give off collaterals to the pretectal area as part of the pupillary light reflex (see the chapter on the mesencephalon) and continue their course to project upon neurons in the lateral geniculate nucleus.

The lateral geniculate nucleus is laminated into six layers. The crossed fibers in the optic tract terminate upon neurons in laminae I, IV, and VI. The uncrossed fibers terminate upon neurons in laminae II, III, and V. Not all parts of the retina are represented equally in the lateral geniculate nucleus. There is proportionally much more of the nucleus devoted to the representation of the central area than to the periphery of the retina.

Axons of neurons in the lateral geniculate nucleus project to the visual cortex in the occipital lobe via the geniculocalcarine tract (visual radiation). Geniculocalcarine fibers from the upper halves of both retinae course directly backward around the lateral ventricle in the inferior part of the parietal lobe to reach the visual cortex. Geniculocalcarine fibers from the lower halves of the retinae course forward toward the tip of the temporal horn of the lateral ventricle and then loop backward (Meyer's loop) in the temporal lobe to reach the visual cortex. Lesions of the geniculocalcarine

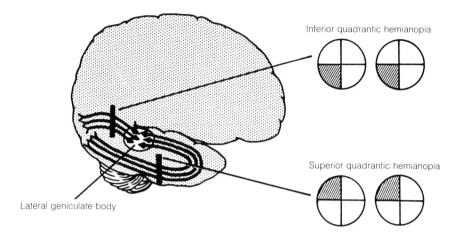

Inferior quadrantic hemianopia

Superior quadrantic hemianopia

Lateral geniculate body

14–6 Schematic diagram showing the clinical manifestations of lesions in the optic radiation in the temporal and parietal lobes.

tract give rise to a contralateral homonymous hemianopia similar to that following lesions of the optic tract (Fig. 14–5, *D*). Because of the spread of geniculocalcarine fibers in the parietal and temporal lobes, a lesion involving part of this fiber system at these sites produces a quadrantic defect (upper if the temporal fibers are affected and lower if the parietal fibers are affected) contralateral to the lesion (Fig. 14–6).

The geniculocalcarine fibers project upon neurons in the visual cortex. As described in the chapter on the cerebral cortex, fibers from the upper retina terminate in the upper calcarine gyrus, those from the lower retina in the lower calcarine gyrus, those from the macular area posteriorly, and those from the peripheral retina anteriorly in the visual cortex. Thus, a lesion destroying the whole of the visual cortex on one side produces contralateral homonymous hemianopia, whereas a lesion destroying the upper or lower calcarine gyrus will produce only a lower or an upper quadrantic hemianopia contralateral to the lesion. As stated in the chapter on the cerebral cortex, vascular lesions of the occipital cortex tend to spare the macular area, probably because this area receives a double blood supply.

In addition to the classic geniculostriate visual pathway discussed above, a second visual pathway has been described; this is the retinocolliculopulvinar-parietal lobe pathway. The classic geniculostriate pathway is concerned with the identification of objects, whereas the second visual pathway is concerned with the detection of events and their location in space. Patients with lesions of the second system become inattentive to the contralateral visual field.

Audition

Sound waves traverse the external and middle ears before reaching the inner ear, where the auditory end organ (organ of Corti) is located.

The tympanic membrane between the external and middle ears vibrates in response to pressure changes produced by the incoming sound waves. Vibrations of the tympanic membrane are transmitted to the bony ossicles of the middle ear (malleus, incus, and stapes). The handle of the malleus is attached to the tympanic membrane and the footplate of the stapes is attached to the oval window between the middle and inner ears. Vibrations of the footplate of the stapes are then transmitted to the membrane of the oval window and subsequently to the fluid medium (perilymph) of the inner ear.

The tensor tympani muscle attached to the handle of the malleus and the stapedius muscle attached to the neck of the stapes have a dampening effect on sound waves. Loud sounds will contract these muscles reflexly to prevent strong sound waves from stimulating excessively the hair cells of the organ of Corti; this is the tympanic reflex. When this dampening effect is lost, as in lesions of the facial nerve (which supplies the stapedius muscle), sound stimuli will be augmented unpleasantly (hyperacusis).

Because of the marked difference in elasticity and density between air and fluid, almost 99% of acoustic energy is reflected back at the air-fluid interface between the middle and inner ears. This is, however, counteracted by two mechanisms.

1. The ratio of the area of the tympanic membrane and footplate of the stapes is approximately 25:1. However, since the tympanic membrane is not a piston but a stretched membrane attached around its edge, its effective area is 60 to 75% of the actual area. Thus, the effective area ratio between the tympanic membrane and footplate of the stapes is 14:1.

2. The lever effect also counteracts energy lost at the air-fluid interface. The movements of the tympanic membrane are transmitted to the malleus and incus, which move as one unit. The manubrium of the malleus is a longer lever than the long process of the incus. The force exerted at the footplate of the stapes is thus greater than at the tympanic membrane, by a ratio of 1.3:1.

The total pressure amplification via the above two devices thus counteracts the energy lost at the air-fluid interface. The total gain in force/unit area achieved by conductance in the middle ear is a factor of about 18.

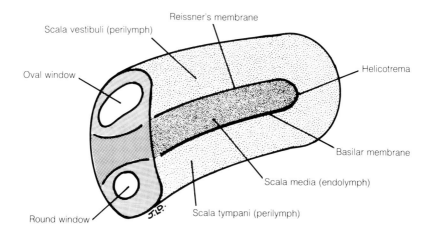

14–7 Schematic diagram showing the three compartments of the cochlea and their interrelationships.

Inner Ear (Cochlea)

The cochlea is a snail-like structure with two and one-half spirals; it is filled with fluid. It has three compartments, the 1) scala vestibuli, 2) scala tympani, and 3) scala media (cochlear duct).

The scala media separates the scala vestibuli (above) from the scala tympani (below) and contains the auditory end organ (organ of Corti). The scala vestibuli and scala tympani are continuous through the helicotrema at the apex of the coil. The oval and round windows separate, respectively, the scala vestibuli and scala tympani from the middle ear (Fig. 14–7).

Vibrations of the oval window are transmitted to the perilymph in the scala vestibuli and, subsequently, via Reissner's membrane (which separates the scala vestibuli from the scala media) to the endolymph of the scala media. Vibrations in the endolymph are then transmitted via the basilar membrane (which separates the scala media from the scala tympani) to the perilymph of the scala tympani and out through the round window.

Auditory End Organ (Organ of Corti)

The organ of Corti (Fig. 14–8) is located in the scala media (cochlear duct) and is separated from the underlying scala tympani by the basilar membrane. The organ of Corti contains the following cellular elements (Fig. 14–9).

Hair Cells   These are the auditory receptor cells and are of two types: inner hair cells, which number approximately 3,500 in a single row, and outer hair cells, which number approximately 20,000 arranged in three to four rows.

The hairs of the hair cells are in contact with the tectorial membrane which transmits to them vibrations from the endolymph. The hair cells are columnar or flask-shaped, with a basally located nucleus and about 50 to 100 hair-like projections (microvilli) emanating from their apical surface. Cochlear nerve fibers establish synapses with their basal membranes.

Supporting Cells   These are tall, slender cells extending from the basilar membrane to the free surface of the organ of Corti. They include the following cell types: pillar or rod cells (outer and inner), phalangeal (Deiters') cells (outer and inner), and cells of Hensen.

Pillar Cells   These cells are filled with tonofibrils. The apices of the inner and outer pillar cells converge at the free surface of the organ of Corti and fan out as a cuticle to form, along with a similar formation of Deiters' cells, a thin plate through which the apices of the inner and outer hair cells pass.

Phalangeal (Deiters') Cells   These are arranged in three to four outer rows and one inner row to give support to the outer and inner hair cells, respectively. Like all supporting cells, they extend from the basilar membrane to the free surface of the organ of Corti, where they contribute to the formation of the cuticular plate through which the hairs of the hair cells pass. Phalangeal cells are flask-shaped and contain tonofibrils. Some of the tonofibrils support the base of the hair cells; others extend along their sides to the free surface of the organ.

Cells of Hensen   These are columnar cells located adjacent to the outermost row of outer phalangeal cells. They constitute the outer border of the organ of Corti. They merge laterally with cuboidal cells (cells of Claudius). Similar (cuboidal) cells adjacent to the inner phalangeal cells are known as border cells and constitute the inner border of the organ.

Tectorial Membrane   This is a gelatinous structure in which are embedded filamentous elements. It extends over the free surface of the organ of Corti. The hairs of the hair cells are attached to the tectorial membrane. Vibrations in the endolymph are transmitted to the tectorial membrane and result in deformation of the hairs attached to it. Such deformation

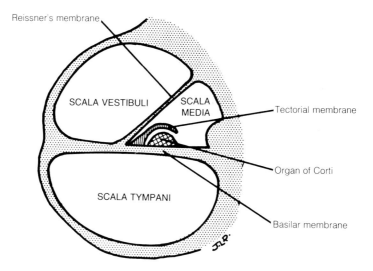

14–8 Schematic diagram of the cochlear compartments showing the organ of Corti in the scala media.

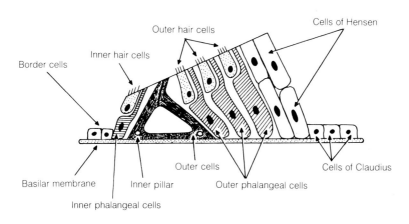

14–9 Simplified schematic diagram of the cellular components of the organ of Corti.

initiates an impulse in the afferent nerve fibers in contact with the basal part of hair cells.

Nerve Supply The hair cells of the organ of Corti receive two types of nerve supply, afferent and efferent.

The afferent fibers are peripheral processes of bipolar neurons in the spiral ganglion located in the bony core of the cochlear spiral. There are about 30,000 bipolar neurons in the spiral ganglion; 90% of them innervate the inner hair cells. Each inner hair cell receives contacts from about 10 fibers; each fiber contacts only one inner hair cell. The remaining 10% of the peripheral processes of bipolar neurons innervate the outer hair cells; each fiber diverges to innervate many outer hair cells.

The efferent fibers originate in the contralateral superior olive in the pons. These fibers form the olivocochlear bundle of Rasmussen, which leaves the brain stem via the vestibular component of the vestibulocochlear (CN VIII) nerve, joins the cochlear component (vestibulocochlear anastomosis), and terminates peripherally upon the outer hair cells and the afferent terminal boutons innervating inner hair cells. These fibers have an inhibitory effect upon auditory stimuli.

Auditory Physiology

Conduction of Sound Waves   Sound waves may reach the inner ear via three routes.

Ossicular Route   This is the route that normally conducts sound. Sound waves entering the external auditory meatus produce vibrations in the tympanic membrane which are transmitted to the bony ossicles of the middle ear and through them to the footplate of the stapes. The energy lost at the air-fluid interface in the oval window is counteracted by the factors outlined previously.

Air Route   This is an alternate route used when the orthodox ossicular route is not operative due to disease of the ossicles. In this situation, vibrations of the tympanic membrane are transmitted through air in the middle ear to the round window. This route is not effective in sound conduction.

Bone Route   Sound waves may also be conducted via the bones of the skull directly to the perilymph of the inner ear. This route plays a minor role in sound conduction in normal individuals but is made use of in deaf people who need hearing aids.

Fluid Vibration   Vibrations of the footplate of the stapes are transmitted to the perilymph of the scala vestibuli. Pressure waves in the perilymph are transmitted via Reissner's membrane to the endolymph of the scala media and, through the helicotrema, to the perilymph of the scala tympani.

Vibrations of Basilar Membrane   Pressure waves in the endolymph of the scala media produce traveling waves in the basilar membrane of the organ of Corti.

The basilar membrane varies in width and degree of stiffness in different regions. It is widest and stiffest at its base and thinnest and least stiff at its apex.

Pressure waves in the endolymph will initiate a traveling wave in the basilar membrane that proceeds from the base toward the apex of the membrane. The amplitude of the traveling waves varies at different sites on the membrane depending on the frequency of sound waves. High frequency sounds elicit waves with highest amplitude toward the base of the membrane. With low frequency sounds, the highest amplitude waves occur toward the apex of the membrane. Similarly, each sound frequency has a site of maximum amplitude wave on the basilar membrane. The frequency of the wave measured in cycles per second (cps) or hertz (Hz) determines its pitch. The amplitude of the wave is correlated with its loudness; a special scale, the decibel scale, is used to measure this aspect of sound. Thus, the basilar membrane exhibits the phenomenon of tonotopic localization seen along the central auditory pathways all the way to the cortex.

Receptor Potential   Vibrations of the basilar membrane produce displacement of the hair cells, the hairs of which are attached to the tectorial membrane. The shearing force produced on the hairs by the displacement of hair cells is the adequate stimulus for the receptor, nonpropagated potential of the hair cells. This receptor potential is also known as the cochlear microphonic potential. It can be recorded from the hair cells and their immediate neighborhood and is a faithful replica of the mechanical events of sound waves described above. The genesis of receptor potentials is not fully understood. It is believed, however, to be due to a change in membrane potential between the hair cells and the surrounding endolymph induced by the bending of hairs of hair cells.

Action Potential   The receptor potential initiates an action potential in the afferent nerves in contact with hair cells. The exact mechanism by which receptor potentials initiate action potentials is not fully understood. Records of afferent nerve activity reveal that the afferent nerves have a constant background activity (background noise) which is modified by an incoming sound stimulus. This is similar to the situation encountered in the optic system.

Increasing the intensity of sound of a particular frequency will increase the number of hair cells stimulated, the number of afferent nerve fibers activated, and the rate of discharge of impulses. A single nerve fiber will respond to a range of frequencies but is most sensitive to a particular frequency called its characteristic frequency. This is related to the region of the basilar membrane which the fiber innervates. Fibers innervating the part of the basilar membrane near the oval window have high characteristic frequencies, whereas those innervating the part of the basilar membrane near the apex of the cochlea have low characteristic frequencies.

Central Transmission The action potential generated in the afferent nerve fibers travels via the central component (axons) of the bipolar neurons in the spiral ganglion to reach the cochlear nuclei in the pons. The cochlear nuclei contain a variety of physiologic cell types. In addition to cells that respond to tone bursts in a manner similar to primary eighth nerve fibers, there are cells that respond only to the onset of the stimulus, some in which the rate of firing builds up slowly during the course of the stimulus, and others that pause, showing no response to the onset of the stimulus. The central pathways from the cochlear nuclei to the auditory cortex in the temporal lobe have been outlined previously (see the chapter on the pons).

Audiometry

The quantitative clinical assessment of hearing acuity is known as audiometry; the resulting record is the audiogram. In audiometry, pure tones of known frequency and varying intensity are presented via earphones to the individual, who is asked to push a light button whenever a tone is heard. The examiner records the audible frequencies and intensities on a chart. The record is then examined to compare the audible range of the individual with that of normal individuals.

Deafness

The range of audible frequencies in the normal adult is from 20 to 20,000 Hz. With advancing age, there is a decrease in perception of high frequencies (high frequency deafness). This is correlated with the loss of hair cells in the basal turns of the cochlea. Similar high frequency deafness is encountered in individuals intoxicated by the antibiotic streptomycin. Rock band performers, on the other hand, develop middle frequency deafness.

Deafness disorders are generally separated into two groups, conductive deafness and sensorineural deafness.

The first group includes those individuals whose deafness is due to obstruction of the external auditory meatus by wax, as well as those individuals with middle ear diseases (chronic otitis media, ossicle sclerosis, etc.).

The second group includes individuals whose hair cells are affected (elderly people, streptomycin toxicity) or who suffer from pathology of the auditory nerve, as occurs in nerve tumors (acoustic neuroma).

The two types of deafness can be identified clinically by use of the tuning fork. A vibrating tuning fork is placed in front of the ear and then on a bony prominence over the skull. A normal individual can hear the tuning fork better when it is placed in front of the ear. A patient with conductive type deafness will hear the tuning fork better when it is placed over a bony prominence, since sound waves will bypass the site of obstruction in the external auditory meatus or the middle ear and reach the auditory end organ via the round window or directly through skull bones to the perilymph.

Vestibular Sensation

The receptors of the vestibular sense organ are located in the semicircular canals, utricle, and saccule in the inner ear. The utricle and saccule are located in the main cavity of the bony labyrinth, the vestibule; the semicircular canals, three in number, are extensions from the utricle (Fig. 14–10). Vestibular sensory receptors are located in the floor of the utricle, wall of the saccule, and in dilated portions (ampullae) of each of the three semicircular canals. The optimal stimulus for receptors in the utricle and saccule is linear acceleration of the body, whereas receptors in the semicircular canals respond to angular acceleration.

The vestibular receptor in the semicircular canal (crista ampullaris) is composed of hair cells and supporting cells (Fig. 14–11). The hair cells are of two types. Type I hair cell is flask-shaped and is surrounded by a nerve terminal (calyx). Type II hair cell is cylindric in shape and is not surrounded by a calyx. Both types of hair cells show on their free surface about 40 to 100 short stereocilia (modified microvilli) and one long kinocilium attached to one border of the cell. The short stereocilia increase progressively in length toward the kinocilium. The stereocilia are nonmotile; the kinocilium is motile.

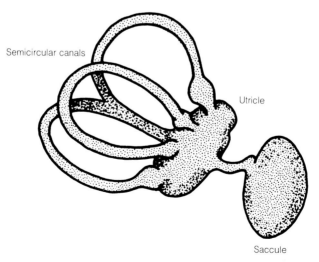

Semicircular canals

Utricle

Saccule

14–10   Schematic diagram of the vestibular end organ.

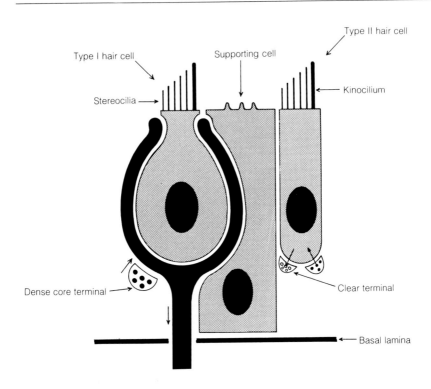

14–11 Schematic diagram of the vestibular sensory receptor.

Supporting cells are slender columnar cells that reach the basal lamina; their free surfaces are specialized into microvilli. The subapical parts of supporting cells are related to adjacent hair cells by junctional complexes.

The apical processes of hair and supporting cells are embedded in a dome-shaped, gelatinous protein-polysaccharide mass, the cupula. The cupula swings from side to side in response to currents in the endolymph which bathes the cupula.

The vestibular receptor organ of the utricle and saccule (macula) is similar in structure to that of the semicircular canals. The gelatinous mass into which the apical processes of hair and supporting cells project is the otolithic membrane. It is flat and contains numerous small crystalline bodies, the otoliths or otoconia, composed of calcium carbonate and protein.

The hair cells of the semicircular canals, utricle, and saccule receive both afferent and efferent nerve terminals (Fig. 14–11). The afferent terminals contain clear vesicles, whereas efferent terminals contain dense core vesicles. In type II hair cells, both afferent and efferent terminals are related to the cell body and are sites of neurochemical transmission. In type I hair cells, the calyx that surrounds the hair cell is regarded as the afferent nerve

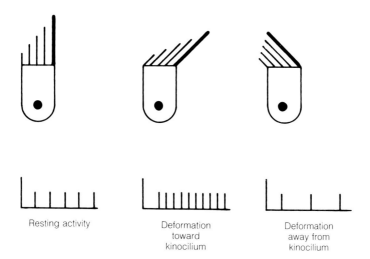

Resting activity

Deformation
toward
kinocilium

Deformation
away from
kinocilium

14–12 Schematic diagram showing the effect of deformation of stereocilia on rate of impulse discharge from the vestibular sense organ.

terminal; it has not been established whether transmission in the calyx is chemical or electrical. The efferent terminals in this type of hair cell are applied to the external surface of the calyx.

Type I hair cells receive vestibular nerve fibers that are large in diameter and fast conducting. Each vestibular nerve fiber innervates a small number of type I hair cells. Thus, type I hair cells are regarded as more discriminative than type II hair cells, which receive small diameter, slow-conducting vestibular nerve fibers projecting upon a large number of hair cells.

The adequate stimulus to discharge hair cells is movement of the cupula or otolithic membrane, which bends or deforms the stereocilia. The manner in which this deformation triggers ionic conductance in hair cells is uncertain. It is now well established that the resting vestibular end organ has a constant discharge of impulses detected in afferent vestibular nerve fibers. This resting activity is modified by mechanical deformation of the stereocilia. Bending the stereocilia toward the kinocilium increases the frequency of resting discharge, whereas bending the stereocilia away from the kinocilium lowers the frequency (Fig. 14–12). The signals emitted by hair cells of the vestibular end organ are transmitted to the central nervous system via processes of bipolar cells in Scarpa's ganglion. The course of such input in the central nervous system is discussed in Chapter 6.

Although we are normally not aware of the vestibular component of our sensory experience, this component is essential for the coordination of motor responses, eye movements, and posture.

References

Barbur, J.L.; Ruddock, K.H.; Waterfield, V.A.: Human Visual Responses in the Absence of the Geniculo-Calcarine Projection. Brain 103 (1980) 905–928.

Brown, K.T.: Physiology of the Retina. In: Medical Physiology, 14th Ed., Vol. 1, pp. 504–543, Ed. by V.B. Mountcastle. The C.V. Mosby Co., St. Louis, 1980.

Goldstein, M.H.: The Auditory Periphery. In: Medical Physiology, 14th Ed., Vol. 1, pp. 428–456, Ed. by V.B. Mountcastle, The C.V. Mosby Co., St. Louis, 1980.

Hubel, D.H.; Wiesel, T.N.: Functional Architecture of Macaque Monkey Visual Cortex. Proc R Soc Lond B Biol Sci 198 (1977) 1–59.

Hubel, D.H.; Wiesel, T.N.: Brain Mechanisms of Vision. Sci Am 241, No. 3 (1979) 150–162.

Kaneko, A.: Physiology of the Retina. Ann Rev Neurosci 2 (1979) 169–191.

Schober, W.: Zur Morphologie der funktionellen Specialisation des visuellen Systems der Säugetiere. Z Mikrosk Anat Forsch 3 (1981) 395–400.

Zeki, S.: The Representation of Colours in the Cerebral Cortex. Nature 284 (1980) 412–418.

Zihl, J.; von Cramon, D.: The Contribution of the "Second" Visual System to Directed Visual Attention in Man. Brain 102 (1979) 835–856.

15

Development, Growth, Maturation, and Aging

Development

Neurulation

The human nervous system develops from ectoderm (Fig. 15–1). The earliest development consists of a thickening of the ectoderm of the head process overlying the notochord at the 17-day stage of intrauterine life. This thickening gives rise to the neural plate. The mesoderm underlying the ectoderm in the region of the neural plate plays an important role in the determination of this change. Neuroectodermal induction is believed to be due to chemical factors released from the mesoderm. Invagination of the neural plate gives rise to the neural groove. The margins of the neural groove approximate each other in the midline and fuse to form the neural tube. A cluster of ectodermal cells originally at the margins of the neural groove separate to form the neural crest. In the human embryo, fusion of the margins of the neural groove begins on the 21st day in the region of the fourth somite (middle of the embryo, presumptive cervical region) and proceeds in both directions; it is completed by the 25th day. Two orifices delimit the completed neural tube, one at its rostral end (anterior neuropore) and the other at its posterior end (posterior neuropore). The neural tube gives rise to the central nervous system; the neural crest gives rise to the dorsal root, autonomic and cranial nerve ganglia, cells of Schwann, and capsule cells of the dorsal root ganglia.

Vesicle Formation

About the 25th day of intrauterine development, the rostral, larger portion of the neural tube subdivides into three vesicles (Fig. 15–2). These are the prosencephalon (forebrain), mesencephalon (midbrain), and rhombencephalon (hindbrain).

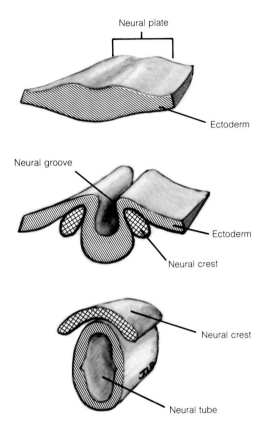

Neural plate

Ectoderm

Neural groove

Ectoderm

Neural crest

Neural crest

Neural tube

15–1 Schematic diagram showing the stages of formation of the neural tube.

About the 32nd day, the prosencephalon and rhombencephalon subdivide further into two parts each, while the mesencephalon remains undivided. The prosencephalon divides into an anterior telencephalon and a posterior diencephalon. From the diencephalon, two secondary bulges (the optic vesicles) appear, one on each side. These later differentiate to form the optic nerves and retinae. The telencephalon differentiates further into two telencephalic vesicles which extend beyond the anterior limit of the original neural tube (lamina terminalis) and eventually become the cerebral hemispheres. The rhombencephalon divides into an anterior metencephalon and a posterior myelencephalon. The metencephalon eventually becomes the pons and cerebellum and the myelencephalon differentiates into the medulla oblongata.

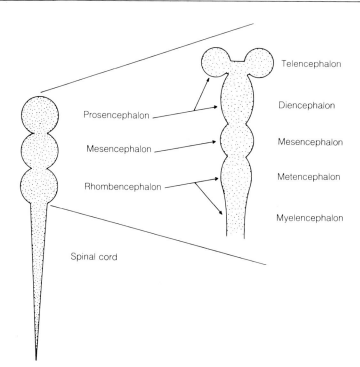

Telencephalon

Diencephalon

Prosencephalon

Mesencephalon

Mesencephalon

Metencephalon

Rhombencephalon

Myelencephalon

Spinal cord

15–2   Schematic diagram showing the vesicle stages of brain development.

Table 15–1   Developmental Sequence of Brain Regions

Three-vesicle stage	Five-vesicle stage	Brain region
Prosencephalon	Telencephalon	Cerebral hemisphere
	Diencephalon	Diencephalon
		Optic nerve and retina
Mesencephalon	Mesencephalon	Mesencephalon
Rhombencephalon	Metencephalon	Pons
		Cerebellum
	Myelencephalon	Medulla oblongata

Thus, the five vesicles that develop from the rostral part of the neural tube eventually give rise to the whole brain. Table 15–1 is a summary of the sequence of events that leads to the development of the various regions of the brain.

As a result of the unequal growth of the different parts of the developing brain, three flexures appear (Fig. 15–3).

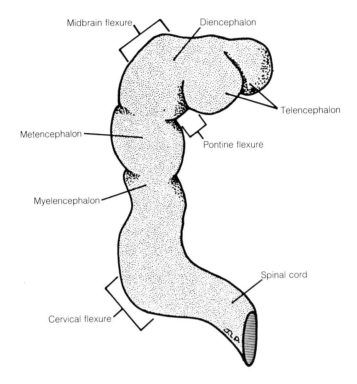

Midbrain flexure

Diencephalon

Telencephalon

Metencephalon

Pontine flexure

Myelencephalon

Spinal cord

Cervical flexure

15–3   Schematic diagram showing the formation of flexures in brain development.

Midbrain Flexure   This flexure develops in the region of the midbrain; as a result, the forebrain (prosencephalon) bends ventrally until its floor lies almost parallel to the floor of the hindbrain (rhombencephalon).

Cervical Flexure   This flexure appears at the junction of the hindbrain (rhombencephalon) and spinal cord.

Pontine Flexure   This flexure appears in the region of the developing pons.

The midbrain and cervical flexures are concave ventrally, whereas the pontine flexure is convex ventrally.

Ventricular System

With the appearance of the three vesicles in the rostral part of the neural tube, cavities develop within the vesicles. Initially, three cavities are visible, corresponding with the three vesicles: 1) prosocele, the cavity of the prosencephalon; 2) mesocele, the cavity of the mesencephalon; and 3) rhombocele, the cavity of the rhombencephalon.

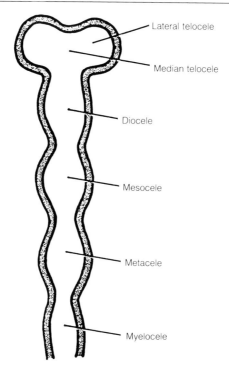

15-4 Schematic diagram showing the formation of brain cavities.

Simultaneous with the division of the prosencephalon into the two telencephalic vesicles and the diencephalic vesicle, the prosocele undergoes
corresponding divisions (Fig. 15-4) resulting in the following.

1. Two telencephalic cavities, one on each side (lateral teloceles)
2. Midline cavity between the telencephalic vesicles (median telocele)
3. Diencephalic cavity (diocele)

The two lateral teloceles develop into the two lateral ventricles. The
median telocele and the diocele develop into the third ventricle. The cavity
of the mesencephalon (mesocele) remains undivided (Fig. 15-4) and eventually becomes the aqueduct of Sylvius.

With the division of the rhombencephalon into a metencephalon and a
myelencephalon, its cavity (rhombocele) divides into the metacele, the
cavity of the metencephalon, and myelocele, the cavity of the myelencephalon (Fig. 15-4). The metacele and myelocele become the fourth
ventricle.

As the different parts of the brain change in shape, the corresponding
changes in the cavities follow. The connections between the lateral ventricles and the third ventricle become smaller and constitute the interventricular foramina of Monro. The median aperture (of Magendie) in the

Table 15-2 Developmental Sequence of Ventricular Cavities

Three-vesicle stage	Five-vesicle stage	Adult structure
Prosocele	Lateral telocele	Lateral ventricle
	Median telocele	Third ventricle
	Diocele	
Mesocele	Mesocele	Aqueduct of Sylvius
Rhombocele	Metacele	Fourth ventricle
	Myelocele	

roof of the fourth ventricle appears during the 3rd month of intrauterine life, followed by the appearance of the lateral apertures (of Luschka). Table 15–2 summarizes the sequence of events that leads to the formation of the various ventricles.

Spinal Cord

The spinal cord retains the original shape of the neural tube. Early in development, the spinal cord and vertebral column grow at the same rate; thus, the spinal cord occupies the entire length of the vertebral column and the spinal nerves emerge between the corresponding vertebral bodies. In the 4th month, however, the growth of the spinal cord slows down in comparison with that of the vertebral column. Eventually, the end of the spinal cord will lie at the level of the second lumbar vertebra. As a result, the spinal roots, which originally were horizontal, become oblique, being dragged down by the growth of the vertebral column; the degree of obliquity increases toward the lower half of the spinal cord, particularly in the lumbar and sacral segments, where the roots form the cauda equina extending well below the end of the cord.

Cellular Differentiation

Once it has been determined that a region will become part of the nervous system, its cells begin to differentiate. Differentiation involves three phases: cellular proliferation, migration of cells to characteristic positions, and maturation of cells with specific interconnections.

When the neural tube is formed, the cells of the germinating epithelium proliferate actively to form an ependymal layer of columnar cells lining the cavity of the neural tube. Some of these cells migrate peripherally to form the mantle layer. Processes of cells in the mantle layer extend to the periphery to form the marginal layer. As development continues, the central cavity diminishes in size, mitotic activity of the ependymal cells decreases, and three distinct layers become established (Fig. 15–5). These are the ependymal, mantle, and marginal. The mantle and marginal layers are the primordia of the future gray and white matter, respectively.

15-5   Schematic diagram of the three basic layers of the neural tube.

All cells of the nervous system develop from the neural tube; thus, the full term fetus is born with a full complement of neurons. Glial elements grow rapidly after birth. It is estimated that roughly 20,000 neurons are formed each minute during the period of prenatal development. The rate varies in different growth periods. In general, there are two periods of growth spurts in the human embryo. The first extends from the 10th to the 18th week of gestation. The second begins in the 30th week of gestation and extends through the 2nd year of life. The first growth spurt is vulnerable to irradiation, chromosomal anomalies, and viral infections; such factors may leave the fetus with serious defects. The second growth spurt is sensitive to such factors as malnutrition. Within any given neural region, different cell types are generated during specific periods of time. In general, large nerve cells develop before small cells, motor neurons develop before sensory neurons, and interneurons are the last to develop. Glial cells proliferate after the neurons.

Cellular Maturation

Neuronal maturation consists of four stages: 1) outgrowth and elongation of axons, 2) elaboration of dendritic processes, 3) expression of appropriate biochemical properties, and 4) formation of synaptic connections.

Alar and Basal Plates (Fig 15-6)

During the formation of the neural tube, a longitudinal groove appears on each side of the lumen. This groove, known as the sulcus limitans, divides the neural tube into a dorsal area, the alar plate, and a ventral area, the

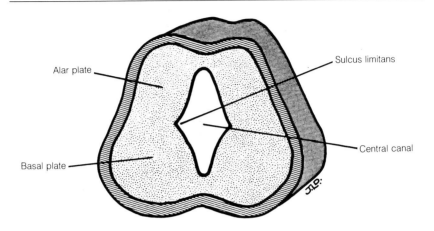

15-6 Schematic diagram showing the stage of plate formation in central nervous system development.

basal plate. Alar and basal plates give rise to all the elements destined to comprise the spinal cord, medulla oblongata, pons, and mesencephalon. The regions of the brain rostral to the mesencephalon (diencephalon and cerebral cortex) develop from the alar plate, as does the cerebellum. The mantle layer of the alar plate gives rise generally to sensory neurons and interneurons, whereas that of the basal plate gives rise to motor neurons and interneurons.

At the junction of the spinal cord and medulla oblongata, the alar plate stretches laterally to form a thin single cell layer of ependyma (roof plate) supported by a richly vascularized mesenchymal tissue (tela chorioidea) and thickened lateral walls that contain the sensory neurons of the medulla oblongata. Thus, the sensory neurons come to lie lateral or dorsolateral to the motor neuron derivatives of the basal plate (Fig. 15-7). The same pattern of organization occurs in the pons. The cerebellum develops from the thickened roof plate (rhombic lip). The alar and basal plate pattern seen in the spinal cord is again seen in the mesencephalon.

In the diencephalon, which develops solely from the alar plate, the hypothalamic sulcus (comparable to the sulcus limitans) divides the diencephalon into a dorsal thalamus and a ventral hypothalamus.

Prenatal Brain Performance

The cardiovascular and nervous systems are the first to function in the embryo. The heart begins to beat 3 weeks after conception. The earliest detectable reflex in the nervous system appears in about the 8th week of intrauterine life. If a stimulus is applied to the lip region at this time, the

15–7 Schematic diagram showing reorganization of basal and alar plate derivatives induced by formation of the fourth ventricle.

hand region exhibits a withdrawal reflex. Touching the lips at 11 weeks of gestation elicits swallowing movements. At 14 weeks of gestation, the reflexogenic zones spread so that touching the face of the embryo results in a complex sequence of movements consisting of head rotation, grimacing, stretching of the body, and extension of the extremities. At 22 weeks of gestation, the embryo manifests stretching out movements and pursing of the lips; at 29 weeks sucking movements become apparent. At birth almost all reflexes are of brain stem origin; cortical control of such reflexes is minimal.

Postnatal Growth and Structural Development

The brain of the human newborn weighs 350 gm, which is approximately 10% of body weight; in contrast, the brain of the adult weighs about 1,400 gm (roughly 2% of body weight). This difference in weight between the adult and newborn brain is accounted for by the laying down of myelin, which occurs mainly in the first 2 years of life, as well as an increase in the size of neurons, in the number of glial elements, and in the complexity of neuronal processes. Virtually no neurons are added after birth, since the human newborn has the full complement of neurons. Structurally, the brain of the newborn has all the lobes clearly distinguishable. The central lobe (island of Reil) is not covered by the frontal and temporal opercula. The color of the cortex at birth is pale, approximating that of white matter. Histologically, the newborn brain shows the six-layered cytoarchitectonic lamination of the adult cerebral cortex. In contrast to the adult cortex, however, the cells of the newborn cortex are tightly packed together with few if any processes to separate them. Nissl substance is sparse in cortical neurons and abundant in brain stem and spinal cord neurons. Dendritic development in the newborn cortex is poor, which correlates with the absence of alpha activity in the electroencephalogram of the newborn. At birth, most of the synapses are of the axodendritic variety; axosomatic synapses develop later.

At 3 months of age, the brain weighs approximately 500 gm. The island of Reil is completely covered by the frontal and temporal opercula. Although the gray and white matter remain poorly demarcated and the cortical Nissl substance remains scanty, the neurons are not as closely packed as in the newborn brain.

At 6 months of age, the brain weighs approximately 660 gm. The cytoplasm of neurons is more abundant. Nissl material is more prominent and the distinction between gray and white matter can be easily made.

At 1 year of age, the brain weighs approximately 925 gm. The density of cortical neurons is reduced as a result of an increase in neuronal and glial processes between neuronal perikarya; Nissl substance within the cell bodies is well developed.

Functional Maturation

Cerebral Oxygen Consumption

Oxygen consumption of the newborn brain is relatively low and increases gradually with maturation. It reaches approximately 5 ml/100 gm of brain tissue per min, which is equivalent to about 50% of the child's total oxygen consumption. With further development, cerebral oxygen consumption decreases to reach the adult level of 3.5 ml/100 gm of tissue per min. The low cerebral oxygen consumption of the brain at birth explains the ability of the newborn brain to tolerate states of anoxia. This tolerance to anoxia may also be explained by the dependence of the brain prior to birth on anaerobic glycolysis as a source of energy. Just prior to birth, the level of enzymes needed for aerobic glycolysis (succinodehydrogenase, succinooxidase, adenyl phosphatase, etc.) increases in preparation for the change in brain metabolism from anaerobic to aerobic processes.

Cerebral Blood Flow

The cerebral flow in the newborn brain is low. It increases with age to reach a maximum of 105 ml/100 gm per min between the ages of 3 and 5 years. It then decreases to reach the adult rate of 54 ml/100 gm per min.

Postnatal Brain Performance

Brain performance after birth proceeds through the following stages of increasing complexity.

The first stage spans the first 2 years of life. During this stage, the infant changes from a baby with no awareness of the environment to a child who is aware of the environment and is able to discriminate among varying environmental stimuli.

The second stage occupies the period between 2 and 5 years of age. This is a stage of preconceptual representation in which the child develops picture images as symbols and begins to use language as a system of symbol signs.

The third stage is noted between 5 and 8 years of age. This is a stage of conditional representation in which the child becomes aware that he is not alone in the universe and begins to interact with other features and forces of the universe.

The fourth stage, which extends from 7 to 12 years of age, is a stage of operational thinking in which the child begins to recognize the relationship between objects and appreciate their relative values, such as more or less, heavier or lighter, longer or shorter, etc.

Along with these stages of behavioral development, the child proceeds through stages of motor and sensory development of increasing complexity. In general, motor development precedes sensory development. From a subcortical creature at 1 month of age, the child proceeds to grasp, raise its head, smile, focus its eyes, hear, roll over, crawl, pick up small objects, stand, and walk.

As the above behavioral, motor, and sensory development is proceeding, the central nervous system is developing nerve processes, synapses, and myelinated pathways. It is difficult, however, to match each of the above developmental stages with a definitive structural change.

Aging

Aging in the nervous system is associated with characteristic morphologic and functional alterations.

Morphologic Alterations

The following structural alterations have been described in the aging nervous system.

1. Cortical atrophy manifested by broadening of sulci, decrease in size of gyri, and widening of ventricular cavities

2. Reduction in number and size of neurons. This is best seen in larger neurons such as the pyramidal cells of Betz and Purkinje neurons.
3. Reduction in the amount of Nissl material
4. Thickening and clumping together of neurofibrils
5. Increase in number of amyloid bodies (corpora amylacea), particularly around the ventricular surface. The origin of amyloid bodies is not established with certainty, but they are believed to represent products of neuronal degeneration.
6. Increase in lipofuscin pigment in both neurons and glia. Among the glia, the astrocytes are particularly affected, whereas the oligodendroglia and microglia are relatively spared. The predominant involvement of astrocytes in this aging process has a deleterious effect on neuronal function.
7. Thickening of walls of cerebral blood vessels

Functional Alterations

The following functional alterations are believed to contribute to some of the above structural alterations or else are the result of such structural modifications.

1. Decrease in cerebral blood flow. The reduction in cerebral blood flow can be the end product of the thickening in blood vessel walls, which in turn can lead to ischemia and dropout of neuronal elements.
2. Reduction in oxygen utilization by cerebral tissues
3. Reduction in glucose utlization by cerebral tissues
4. Increase in cerebrovascular resistance

Congenital Malformations

Congenital malformations occur in approximately 0.5% of live births and 3% of stillbirths. They are generally attributed to one of two causes. The first is exogenous causes, which include nutritional factors, radiation, viral infections, chemicals, and medications. As mentioned previously, these different etiologic factors affect the embryo adversely in a specific period of development. Endogenous causes, which are mainly hereditary, also cause congenital malformations.

The following congenital malformations are cited to illustrate the consequences of defects in brain development.

1. Anencephaly is an anomaly which occurs in early embryogenesis and results from a failure of closure of the neural groove in the brain region. In this condition, the skull is absent; the brain stem is covered instead by fibrous connective tissue. The cerebral hemispheres do not develop.

Anencephalic infants usually die in utero or shortly after birth.

2. Cranial meningocele is an anomaly which is due to partial failure of closure of the neural groove. The anomaly is usually in the midline of the occipital or frontal region. As a result of this anomaly, the meninges herniate through a bony defect and are covered only by skin. In many such cases, however, the brain is also malformed, resulting in mental retardation and convulsions.

3. Meningoencephalocele is an anomaly in which both the meninges and the brain herniate through the bony defect. Such children usually die early from infection of the meninges and brain tissue.

4. Meningomyelocele is a condition similar to meningoencephalocele, except that the herniated elements include meninges and spinal cord.

5. Diastematomyelia is an anomaly which results from a bony spicule that extends from the vertebral bodies into the spinal canal, splitting the spinal cord into two halves. It occurs usually in the lower thoracic or lumbar region.

6. Agyri (lissencephaly) is an anomaly which is due to arrest of brain growth in the 3rd or 4th month. The brain is devoid of most fissures and sulci and consists of cellular masses which are not arranged in distinct layers.

   small brain inside a small skull. Arrest of development usually occurs late in gestation. The anomaly may be the result of genetic abnormalities, X-ray exposure during pregnancy, or fetal infection, especially from the disease toxoplasmosis. Infants and children afflicted with this anomaly are usually mentally retarded.

8. Agenesis of the corpus callosum is a condition in which the development of the corpus callosum is partially or completely arrested. Infants and children with agenesis of the corpus callosum may develop normally or may show signs of mental deficiency and convulsions.

References

Cowan, W.M.: The Development of the Brain. Sci Am 241, No. 3 (1979) 112–133.

Crelin, E.S.: Development of the Nervous System. Ciba Clin Symp 26, No. 2 (1974).

Hayflick, L.: The Cell Biology of Human Aging. Sci Am 242 (1980) 58–65.

Rockstein, M.: Development and Aging in the Nervous System. Academic Press, New York, 1973.

16

Control of Posture
and Movement

The story of the neural control of posture and movement is one of the most fascinating chapters in the study of the nervous system. A proper understanding of neural control is essential not only to the comprehension of the mechanisms underlying normal posture and movement, but also to an appreciation of functional disturbances in those who have developed a disease of the system of control and who therefore have lost the ability either to execute or to coordinate movement.

In studying this system, one is often inclined to overemphasize the role of one component of the system, the corticospinal tract. Although no one denies the importance of this tract, one should not underemphasize the roles of less voluminous but otherwise important tracts such as the reticulospinal, vestibulospinal, and rubrospinal. In the same vein, one should not underestimate the role of modifying inputs from the cerebellum and basal ganglia. Last but not least, one should add to the schema the input into this system from peripheral organs, the muscle fibers without which movement could not be executed.

It is obvious from the above that the story of the neural control of posture and movement is multifaceted. In the final analysis, all levels of control work in unison to produce coordinated and integrated movement; however, for didactic purposes, the individual contributions of each of the different levels of control of posture and movement will be dealt with separately.

Spinal Cord

The spinal cord contains, in its anterior horn, motor neurons with axons which supply somatic body musculature. Activation of groups of motor neurons will give rise to contraction of groups of skeletal muscle and hence movement. Motor neurons of the spinal cord are activated by 1) impulses from the periphery as part of reflex mechanisms and 2) impulses from higher levels with descending fibers which exert a modifying influence on reflex mechanisms.

In order to study the role of spinal reflex mechanisms in posture and movement, experimentalists had to resort to artificial preparations in which the spinal cord was disconnected from higher levels by transection. Such an animal preparation is known as a spinal animal.

The reflexes elicited in such an animal include the following.

1. Stretch (myotatic) reflex
2. Inverse myotatic reflex
3. Flexor reflex
4. Crossed extension reflex
5. Other reflexes

Stretch (Myotatic) Reflex (Fig. 16–1)

Stretching a muscle (by tapping its tendon) will activate the muscle spindle of the intrafusal muscle fiber (primary annulospiral endings). Impulses from the activated muscle spindle will activate monosynaptically via Ia fibers the homonymous (corresponding, ipsilateral) alpha motor neurons in the anterior horn of the spinal cord. This type of excitation is known as autogenic. Impulses traveling via the axons of such alpha motor neurons will then reach the stretched skeletal muscle and result in contraction of the muscle. Ia afferents will also make direct monosynaptic excitatory connections with alpha motor neurons which innervate muscles that are synergistic in action to the muscle from which the Ia fiber originated. The activity in the Ia fibers will, in addition, inhibit disynaptically the motor neurons that supply the antagonistic muscle (reciprocal inhibition). This obviously facilitates contraction of the homonymous muscle.

In the human, myotatic stretch reflexes can be elicited in the following sites and are part of a neurologic examination.

Biceps Jerk   This reflex is elicited by tapping the tendon of the biceps muscle. The biceps muscle will contract, resulting in flexion at the elbow.

Triceps Jerk   This reflex is elicited by tapping the tendon of the triceps muscle. As a result, the triceps will contract and extend the elbow joint.

Radial Jerk   Tapping the tendon of the brachioradialis muscle at the wrist will contract the brachioradialis muscle and flex the wrist joint.

Knee Jerk (Quadriceps Myotatic Reflex)   This reflex is elicited by tapping the tendon of the quadriceps femoris muscle at the patella. The quadriceps muscle contraction will extend the knee joint.

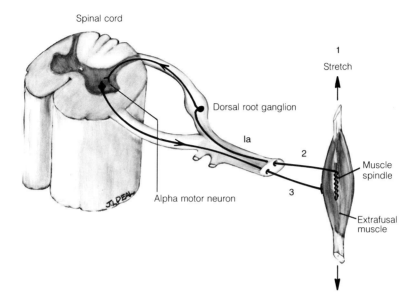

16–1 Schematic diagram of the components of the stretch reflex. Muscle stretch (*1*) will activate Ia sensory nerve fibers (*2*) which will monosynaptically activate motor neurons. Axons of activated motor neurons (*3*) will synapse on skeletal muscle fibers and produce contraction.

Ankle Jerk Tapping the tendon of the gastrocnemius muscle at the Achilles tendon will contract the gastrocnemius and plantar flex the ankle.

Pathology anywhere in the path of the reflex arc from the receptor to the effector site will interfere with these reflexes. Reduction or absence of myotatic reflexes reflects pathology in the receptor site (the muscle spindle), the afferent or efferent nerve fibers (peripheral neuropathy), or the central neurons (anterior horn cells), as in poliomyelitis.

Myotatic reflexes may be exaggerated (hyperactive) in diseases interfering with the descending modifying influences. Such a condition occurs in upper motor neuron disorders (stroke, multiple sclerosis, spinal cord tumors, etc.).

The above technique of eliciting a muscle contraction, namely stretching the muscle by tapping its tendon, is the clinical method. There is, however, another way by which muscle can be made to contract; this is by eliciting a contraction of the muscle spindle without stretching the muscle. Activity in gamma neurons within the anterior horn of the spinal cord will send impulses via the gamma efferent fibers to both poles of the muscle spindle. Contraction of the poles of the muscle spindle will activate the primary (annulospiral) endings. Consequently, impulses will travel via the Ia nerve

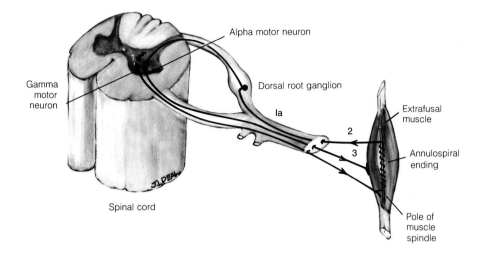

16-2 Schematic diagram of the components of the gamma loop. Activation of gamma motor neurons (*1*) results in contraction of the poles of the muscle spindle and activation of the annulospiral ending. Impulses travel via the Ia afferents (*2*) and activate alpha motor neurons. Axons (*3*) of the alpha motor neurons will contract the skeletal muscle fiber.

fibers to activate monosynaptically alpha motor neurons, resulting in contraction of the extrafusal muscle fibers. This type of muscle contraction is elicited through activity in the gamma loop system (Fig. 16-2).

Thus, under normal conditions, the cerebral cortex can trigger muscle contraction and initiate postural changes and movement via two mechanisms: by activating the alpha motor neuron directly and by activating the alpha motor neuron indirectly via the gamma system loop.

Voluntary, precise, and sensitive movements are executed by the simultaneous activation of both systems. In general, activation of the alpha system predominates when a quick response is desired, whereas activation of the gamma system predominates when a smooth and precise movement is desired. The two systems are complementary.

The importance of and rationale for the described role of the gamma loop can be illustrated in the mechanism of standing posture. Upon assuming a standing posture, the stretch of the quadriceps tendon will activate the muscle spindle and the alpha motor neuron, thus producing muscle contraction. As soon as muscle contraction occurs, tension on the muscle spindle will cease, rate of discharge upon the alpha motor neuron diminishes, and subsequently the muscle will relax. The gamma system, however, will correct this and the tension of the spindle necessary for posture will

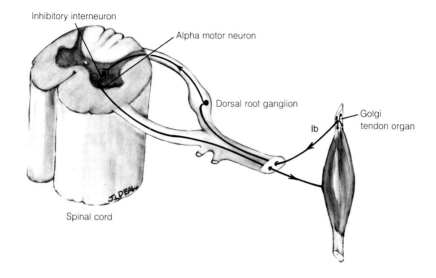

Inhibitory interneuron

Alpha motor neuron

Dorsal root ganglion

Ib

Golgi tendon organ

Spinal cord

16–3 Schematic diagram of the components of the inverse myotatic reflex.

be maintained. The gamma neuron will be activated by descending influences from the cortex, cerebellum, etc. This will maintain activity in the muscle spindle and secure constant firing of Ia nerve fibers and the alpha motor neuron. As a result, muscle contraction necessary for standing posture will be maintained.

Inverse Myotatic Reflex (Fig. 16–3)

Severe tension in a muscle produced by stretch or contraction will stimulate nerve endings in its tendon (Golgi tendon organ). Impulses from Golgi tendon organs travel via Ib nerve fibers. In the spinal cord, they project upon inhibitory neurons, which in turn will inhibit alpha motor neurons supplying the muscle under tension (homonymous motor neurons). The result is relaxation of the muscle (lengthening reaction, autogenic inhibition). At the same time, the Ib activity will facilitate motor neurons that supply the antagonistic muscle. It was originally believed that the primary role of the Ib afferents was protective (*i.e.*, they prevented the muscle from being torn under great tension). This reflex was also thought to underlie the mechanism of the "clasp knife" phenomenon noted in spastic muscles. In such situations, passive stretching of the spastic muscle will be met with great resistance up to a point, after which the muscle gives way suddenly. The phenomenon has been termed "clasp knife" by Sherrington because of its similarity to the action of a jackknife or a switchblade knife.

While it is still believed that Ib afferents play a protective role in the clasp knife phenomenon, they are not considered to be the sole mechanism. Recent studies assign the major role to the inhibitory action of group II afferents. Furthermore, these studies have elucidated other roles for the Ib afferents. It has been shown that the Golgi tendon organs (source of Ib afferents) are sensitive to active muscle contraction and that the Ib afferents act as a tension feedback system. Increases in muscle tension beyond a desired point produce negative feedback from Golgi tendon organs, thus inhibiting further development of tension. Alternately, decreases in muscle tension, as when a muscle begins to fatigue, have the opposite effect of reducing activation of Golgi tendon organs, producing less inhibition of homonymous and synergist motor neurons and more tension, thus compensating for the muscle fatigue. Other recent studies have shown that interneurons in the reflex pathways of Ib afferents receive short-latency excitation from low threshold cutaneous afferents and from joint afferents. If a limb movement is initiated and suddenly meets an obstacle, inputs from cutaneous and joint receptors will trigger the Ib afferent inhibitory system, with the result that tension in the limb will be reduced, preventing further force against the obstacle.

In reviewing the myotatic and inverse reflexes and their role in muscular activity, it becomes evident that there are three controlling mechanisms.

One is a length-controlling mechanism subserved by the annulospiral endings of the intrafusal fiber. This mechanism is sensitive to changes in length and mediates its effects via the Ia nerve fibers.

A second is a tension-controlling mechanism subserved by the Golgi tendon organ. This mechanism is sensitive to tension in the muscle developed by either stretch or contraction of the muscle and is mediated via the Ib nerve fibers.

A third is a follow-up control system in which extrafusal muscle fiber length follows intrafusal muscle fiber length and is mediated via the gamma loop.

Flexor Reflex (Fig. 16–4)

The proper stimulus for eliciting this reflex is a nociceptive or painful one, such as pin prick, or one that inflicts injury or damage to the skin or deeper tissues. The primary receptors for this reflex are the pain (free nerve endings) receptors, although light touch receptors elicit a weaker and less sustained flexor reflex. The purpose of this reflex is withdrawal of the injured part from the stimulus, hence the reflex is also called the withdrawal reflex.

From the stimulated receptors, impulses travel via group III nerve fibers to the spinal cord where they establish polysynaptic relations (at least three to four interneurons) with a number of motor neurons. The net effect of

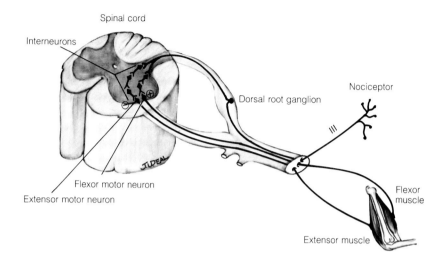

16–4 Schematic diagram of the components of the flexor reflex.

this circuitry is twofold: 1) facilitation of ipsilateral flexor motor neurons and 2) inhibition of ipsilateral extensor motor neurons.

Efferent outflow of the activated motor neurons will effect contraction of flexor muscles (flexion) and relaxation of antagonist extensor muscles in the stimulated part of the body.

Crossed Extension Reflex (Fig. 16–5)

This reflex is actually a byproduct of the flexion reflex. The incoming impulses from a nociceptive stimulus will cross in the anterior commissure of the spinal cord and establish multisynaptic relationships with both flexor and extensor motor neurons. Their effect on these motor neurons, however, is the reverse of that described ipsilaterally: 1) facilitation of extensor motor neurons and 2) inhibition of flexor motor neurons. As a result, the limb contralateral to the stimulated part of the body will be extended.

Thus, in response to a nociceptive stimulus, the ipsilateral limb will be flexed and the contralateral limb will be extended in preparation for withdrawal. Very strong nociceptive stimuli will spread activity in the spinal cord through intersegmental reflexes to involve all four extremities. In response to a stimulus applied to one extremity (hindlimb), a spinal cat will withdraw the stimulated limb, extend the opposite hindlimb and ipsilateral forelimb, and flex the contralateral forelimb.

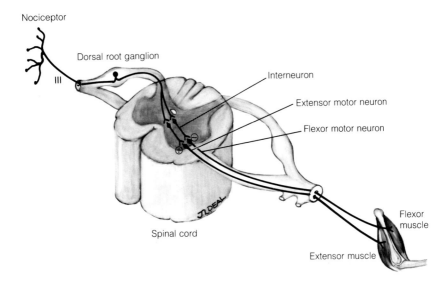

Nociceptor

Dorsal root ganglion

Interneuron

Extensor motor neuron

Flexor motor neuron

III

Spinal cord

Flexor muscle

Extensor muscle

16–5   Schematic diagram of the components of the crossed extensor reflex.

Other Reflexes

An animal in which the spinal cord has been disconnected from higher levels (spinal animal) can still perform the following activities related to posture and movement.

Positive Supporting Reaction   Pressure on the foot pad of a spinal animal will stiffen the limb sufficiently to support the body.

Stepping   Rhythmic flexion and extension movements of limbs, as if stepping, are seen in the spinal animal.

It is obvious from the above that the spinal cord contains the basic neural mechanisms necessary for reflex actions. The local spinal mechanisms, however, are constantly modulated by descending influences (facilitatory and inhibitory) from higher brain regions.

Brain Stem

Contribution of brain stem structures to posture and movement can be studied in two types of experimental preparations, the decerebrate animal and the midbrain animal.

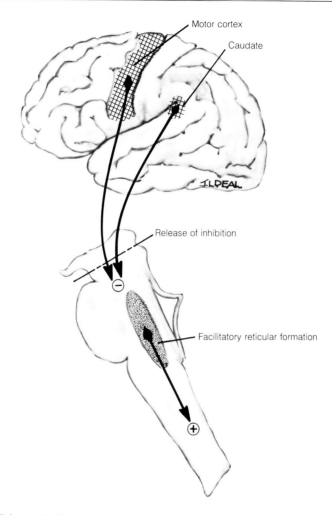

16-6 Schematic diagram showing the mechanism of decerebrate rigidity.

Decerebrate Animal

In the decerebrate animal, the disconnection between lower and upper levels for control of posture and movement is made at the midcollicular level between the superior and inferior colliculi. In addition to the spinal cord, the medulla oblongata and pons are intact in such an animal. The facilitatory part of the reticular formation at the level of the pons is released from the inhibitory effect of the caudate nucleus and cerebral cortex (Fig. 16–6).

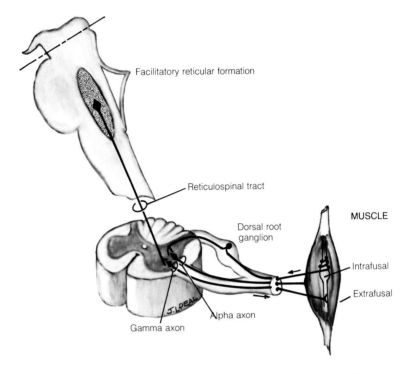

Facilitatory reticular formation

Reticulospinal tract

MUSCLE

Dorsal root
ganglion

Intrafusal

Extrafusal

Gamma axon

Alpha axon

16–7 Schematic diagram showing the mechanism of decerebrate rigidity.

The reticular formation thus released tonically activates gamma motor neurons in the spinal cord (Fig. 16–7). The activated gamma motor neurons stimulate the annulospiral endings of the intrafusal muscle fibers through the gamma loop. Activation of the latter generates impulses via the Ia nerve fibers, which discharge the alpha motor neurons monosynaptically (myotatic reflex). As a result, skeletal muscles are tonically activated and rigidity sets in. Decerebrate rigidity involves predominantly antigravity muscles. Animals in which the extensor muscles are the antigravity muscles maintain a rigid posture, holding all four extremities in the extended position while the head and tail are maximally extended backward. Although the reticulospinal system plays the major role in decerebrate rigidity, the vestibulospinal system is also important. The lateral vestibular nucleus has a powerful descending excitatory influence on alpha and gamma extensor motor neurons. Ablation of the lateral vestibular nucleus in a decerebrate preparation will greatly reduce the rigidity. In contrast, lesions in the anterior lobe of the cerebellum will increase the rigidity in decerebrate animals. This is due to the fact that such cerebellar lesions will eliminate tonic cerebellar inhibition of the lateral vestibular nucleus, releasing the powerful extensor excitation of the nucleus.

Tonic neck reflexes and tonic labyrinthine reflexes can be elicited in the decerebrate animal.

Tonic Neck Reflexes   In the decerebrate animal in which the labyrinth and cerebellum have been removed, upward extension of the head will trigger further extension of the forelimbs and flexion of the hindlimbs. Downward flexion of the head, on the other hand, triggers a reduction in extensor tone of the forelimbs. Rotation of the head to the right side produces extension of the limbs on the right side and flexion of the contralateral limbs. The observed changes in the extensor tone of the limbs in response to head movements are mediated via receptors in neck muscles and in the joints of cervical vertebrae.

Tonic Labyrinthine Reflexes   Tonic labyrinthine reflexes are best studied in a decerebrate animal in which the head has been immobilized to eliminate the effect of tonic neck reflexes. In such an animal, the extremities are maximally extended when the animal is in the supine position and minimally extended when the animal is in the prone position. The receptors for the tonic labyrinthine reflexes are in the semicircular canals which sense position of head in space. Impulses are mediated via the vestibular nerve, the vestibular nuclei, and the vestibulospinal pathways to initiate corrective action in body musculature in response to changes in position of the head in space.

From the above, it becomes clear that in the brain stem animal the reticular formation maintains the rigid extension posture while the reflexes from receptors in the muscles of the neck, joints of the cervical vertebral column, and vestibular end organ (semicircular canals) trigger the necessary corrective posture to maintain equilibrium.

Midbrain Animal

As the name indicates, the midbrain animal has the whole brain stem (through the mesencephalon) intact. The cut is rostral to the midbrain, thus disconnecting the brain stem from the diencephalon, basal ganglia, and cerebral cortex. Such an animal is not able to initiate spontaneous movement, but is able to right itself and stand spontaneously. The reflexes elicited in such an animal are thus called righting reflexes. Their purpose is to maintain the upright posture. Receptors for righting reflexes are located in the neck muscles (neck righting reflexes) and labyrinth (labyrinthine righting reflexes), as well as in the body surface (body righting reflexes).

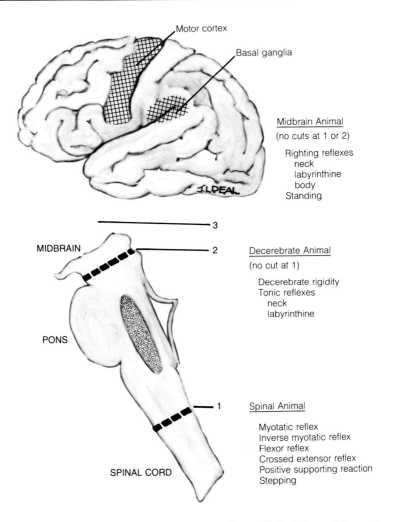

Motor cortex

Basal ganglia

Midbrain Animal
(no cuts at 1 or 2)

   Righting reflexes
    neck
    labyrinthine
    body
   Standing

MIDBRAIN

3

2

Decerebrate Animal
(no cut at 1)

   Decerebrate rigidity
   Tonic reflexes
    neck
    labyrinthine

PONS

1

Spinal Animal

   Myotatic reflex
   Inverse myotatic reflex
   Flexor reflex
   Crossed extensor reflex
   Positive supporting reaction
   Stepping

SPINAL CORD

16–8 Schematic diagram showing postural reflexes elicited from different levels of the neuraxis.

Thus, if such an animal is turned on one side, it will right itself. If the animal is dropped blindfolded from a height, it will extend its legs and land in the upright position.

Figure 16–8 is a schematic diagram summarizing the spinal and brain stem preparations discussed so far and the postural mechanisms operative in each preparation.

Cerebellum

The cerebellum is intimately related to all regions involved in motor activity. Thus, it is related to the peripheral organ (muscle) as well as to all the central levels concerned with movement (spinal cord, brain stem, thalamus, cerebral cortex). It is perfectly suited, therefore, to play the role of coordinator and integrator of motor activity. The cerebellum plays this role in both voluntary and involuntary motor activities. Although it is generally acknowledged that the cerebellum exerts its effect on movement that has already been initiated elsewhere (*i.e.*, cerebral cortex), recent evidence suggests that the cerebellum is involved in the planning and initiation of movement, as well as in the moment-to-moment control of movement. Electrophysiologic recordings from the cerebellum have shown that the Purkinje neurons discharge prior to the start of movement. It is believed that the intent to perform a movement involves the activation of the motor association areas of the cerebral cortex, which act in cooperation with the lateral portions of the cerebellar hemispheres in the planning of movement.

It is generally agreed that the cerebellum plays a role in regulating the following parameters of voluntary movement: 1) rate, 2) range, 3) force, and 4) direction.

The cerebellum is able to execute this role via the multitude of feedback mechanisms that exist between it and the various motor centers (Fig. 16–9). Through these feedback circuits, the cerebellum can detect errors in movement and institute corrective measures. If a moving limb appears to be moving too fast (rate), to the degree of overshooting the intended target, the cerebellum will detect this and institute inhibitory impulses through the cerebral cortex to slow down the movement and prevent the overshoot (range). It is obvious that in order to do this the cerebellum must exert its influence both on the agonist group of muscles moving the part and on the antagonist group. By inhibiting the agonists and facilitating the antagonist motor neurons at the calculated time, movement can be brought to a halt at the appropriate time and place. In cerebellar disease, this ability to control the rate and range of movement is defective. As a result, the patient tends to move the limb farther than intended. This is referred to as dysmetria. In clinical practice, this phenomenon can be shown by asking the patient to touch a fingertip to the tip of the nose. A patient with cerebellar disease tends to overshoot the nose and reach the cheek or ear.

In the smooth execution of movement, proper timing of the initiation and termination of sequential steps in movement is extremely important. A delay in the initiation of each successive movement will lead to a failure of proper progression. In clinical medicine, this is demonstrated by asking the patient to perform repetitive movements with the hand or tongue. Failure to do this in orderly succession is referred to as dysdiadochokinesia.

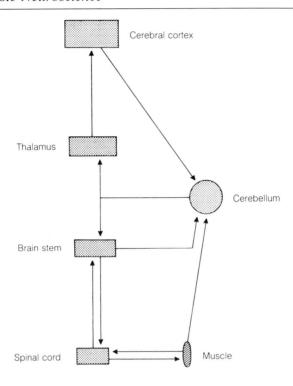

16–9 Schematic diagram showing the feedback mechanisms between the cerebellum and other motor centers.

Also important in the smooth execution of movement is the force of movement. In diseases of the cerebellum, the normal steady increase and decrease in the force of movement are affected. Such patients, therefore, execute movement in a jerky, irregular manner. This phenomenon is known as dyssynergia. In clinical situations, dyssynergia can be manifested in the irregular, jerky movements of the patient's finger as it is moving toward the finger of the examiner.

The defective feedback mechanisms for the control of the force and timing of movement in cerebellar disease are responsible for volitional tremor. This type of tremor is characteristically absent when the limb is at rest but becomes manifest when the patient attempts to move the limb.

In addition to its role in control of movement, the cerebellum plays an equally important role in maintenance of body equilibrium. Lesions in the flocculonodular lobe of the cerebellum (archicerebellum) are associated with disturbances in body equilibrium. Such patients manifest unsteadiness of gait. This unsteadiness results from the inability of the diseased cerebellum to detect changes in direction of motion as signaled by the semicircular canals and to institute corrective action to maintain a steady gait.

Basal Ganglia

Although the key role of the basal ganglia in motor control is undisputed, the exact mechanism by which the basal ganglia exert this control remains incompletely explored in spite of the voluminous experimental work and published literature on the subject. A decorticate primate, an animal in which the cortex has been removed leaving the rest of the nervous system including the basal ganglia intact, is capable of maintaining almost normal posture and movement, except for fine and precise types of movements that require an intact motor cortex. In man, the decorticate state is characterized by flexor rigidity in the upper limbs. The reason for this is not known, although some speculate that flexor muscles in the upper limbs of man are antigravity muscles.

Like the cerebellum, the basal ganglia exert a modifying and coordinating effect on already initiated movement. As in the cerebellum, recent evidence suggests that the basal ganglia may play a role in the initiation of motor activity. Recordings of unit activity in the globus pallidus and putamen have revealed activity in their neurons prior to the onset of movement.

Both anatomic and physiologic data suggest that the basal ganglia exert their modifying effect on movement via two systems (Fig. 16–10).

1. Feedback circuit from the motor cortex to the basal ganglia, thalamus, and back to the motor cortex and spinal cord
2. Descending pathway from the basal ganglia to motor centers of the brain stem and from there to the spinal cord

It is evident that the basal ganglia do not exert direct influence on motor activity in the spinal cord.

The thalamus is the central meeting place for inputs from the cerebellum and basal ganglia. The significance of this in the coordination of cerebellar and basal ganglia roles in motor activity is obvious. The relief of basal ganglia and cerebellar involuntary movement by lesions in the thalamus attests to this important focal role of the thalamus.

Most knowledge about the role of basal ganglia in motor control has been derived from clinical material. Unfortunately, most of the clinical syndromes of basal ganglia diseases cannot be reproduced in experimental animals, a fact that is at the core of the scarcity of information about the exact pathophysiologic mechanisms.

In man, disturbances in basal ganglia function are manifested in disturbances in muscle tone and involuntary movements.

Different nuclei of the basal ganglia may have varying effects on muscle tone, whereas the sum total effect of the basal ganglia is inhibitory on muscle tone. This effect is mediated via the reticular formation of the brain stem. Thus, in lesions of basal ganglia, the tone of muscle is increased leading to a state of rigidity, as in Parkinson's disease. This rigidity, unlike

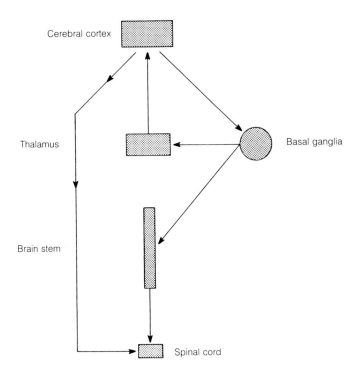

Cerebral cortex

Thalamus

Basal ganglia

Brain stem

Spinal cord

16–10 Schematic diagram showing the feedback mechanisms between the basal ganglia and other motor centers.

that of decerebrate or gamma type rigidity, is an alpha type rigidity exerted via the alpha motor neuron.

Disorders of movement in basal ganglia dysfunction are generally of two types, hyperkinetic and hypokinetic. The hyperkinetic variety includes such involuntary movements as chorea, athetosis, hemiballismus, and the rhythmic tremor of Parkinson's disease. The hypokinetic variety is exemplified by the akinesia of Parkinson's disease. The description of each of these involuntary movements is detailed in the chapter on basal ganglia. In contrast to cerebellar tremor, the involuntary movements of basal ganglia disorders are manifest in repose or in the absence of motion; hence, they are known as rest tremor or postural tremor.

Although complete correlation of the type of involuntary movement with a specific nucleus of the basal ganglia has not been achieved, it is generally accepted that hemiballism is associated with lesions in the subthalamic nucleus, parkinsonism with lesions of the nigrostriatal axis, and chorea with caudate nucleus lesions.

Furthermore, in the last decade, significant advances have been made in our understanding of the neurochemical basis of basal ganglia disorders.

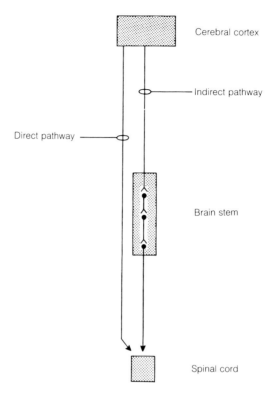

16-11   Schematic diagram showing the direct and indirect corticospinal pathways.

The relationship of parkinsonism to the cholinergic-dopaminergic system is such an example and has been outlined in the chapter on basal ganglia.

Cerebral Cortex

The cerebral cortex role in control of movement assumes more importance as one ascends in the phylogenetic tree. The areas of the cerebral cortex that are involved in the control of movement and posture have been described in the chapter on the cerebral cortex. They include the primary motor cortex, the premotor area, the supplementary motor cortex, and part of the primary sensory cortex.

The cerebral cortex exerts its effects on movement and posture via two pathways (Fig. 16–11): 1) the direct, oligosynaptic pathway (direct corticospinal) and 2) the indirect, multisynaptic pathway (indirect corticospinal).

The role of the direct pathway is mainly in the control of rapid, voluntary, and fine skilled movements. The role of the indirect pathway is in the control of slow postural type movements. The two pathways have been referred to as the pyramidal and extrapyramidal pathways, respectively. The pyramidal pathway exerts a facilitatory effect on motor neurons, whereas the sum total effect of the extrapyramidal pathway is inhibitory.

In the execution of voluntary motor activity, the descending influences from the cortex and subcortical structures via these two pathways most likely act simultaneously on alpha and gamma motor neurons of the spinal cord. Alpha activation, however, predominates in the case of rapid movements, whereas gamma activation predominates in the case of slow, graduated movements.

Selective lesions in the two pathways in man are difficult to produce and both are usually affected together to varying degrees. Lesions of the motor areas of the cortex or of their axons along the neuraxis give rise generally to a clinical picture known collectively as upper motor neuron syndrome. It is usually seen in stroke patients and is characterized by the following signs.

1. Paresis (weakness) or paralysis (loss of movement), particularly affecting distal muscles controlling fine skilled movements
2. Hyperactive deep tendon reflexes
3. Babinski sign
4. Spasticity
5. Clonus

Careful observation and analysis of these different signs, however, allow their division into two groups.

Immediately after onset of the lesion, there is paresis or paralysis, hypotonia, and reduction or absence of deep tendon reflexes (hypo- or areflexia). These early signs are attributable to the affection of the pyramidal pathway.

Later on, the following signs appear: 1) spasticity, 2) hyperactive deep tendon reflexes (hyperreflexia), 3) Babinski sign, and 4) clonus. These later signs are attributed to the affection of the extrapyramidal pathway. The mechanism of the Babinski sign, however, remains uncertain. It is believed to be due to involvement of the supplementary motor area or its outflow fibers.

The further course of this clinical picture is characterized by the reappearance of gross postural movements, usually in proximal muscles. This return of postural function is attributed to the part of the extrapyramidal areas or pathways not involved in the lesion.

The cerebral cortex has long been recognized as the initiator of movement. Electrophysiologic studies confirm this concept and show that the motor neurons in the cerebral cortex begin to discharge prior to the onset of movement. The cerebral cortex also plays a central role in the execution

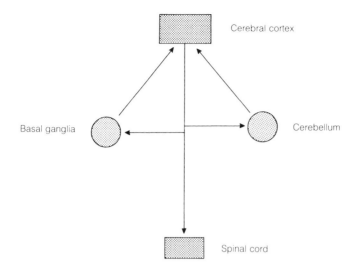

16–12 Schematic diagram showing the feedback circuits between the cortex, cerebellum, and basal ganglia.

of appropriate movement. It can accomplish this by virtue of the feedback it receives from the cerebellum and basal ganglia, which supply the cerebral cortex with continuous information regarding the progress of movement so that corrective action can be taken. In turn, the cerebral cortex, by virtue of collaterals to the cerebellum and basal ganglia, keeps these two structures informed of ongoing activity (Fig. 16–12).

Blood flow studies have improved our knowledge about the part the cerebral cortex plays in motor control. Such studies identify the role of the supplementary motor cortex in programming movement, the premotor area in initiating new programs and in introducing changes in programs in progress, and the primary motor cortex in executing the program of movement. These studies have also shown that the supplementary motor, premotor, and primary sensory motor cortices are bilaterally active during movement in intrapersonal space, whereas the superior and inferior parietal lobules are bilaterally active during movement in extrapersonal space. The parietal lobe is visualized as providing information to the programmer about the direction and progress of movement.

Locomotion

The older concept of locomotion as a set of chain reflexes in which the sensory input from a given part of a step cycle triggers the next part of the cycle by reflex action has been challenged and found incorrect. The present concept suggests that locomotion is not reflex in nature but is generated by neurons located exclusively in the spinal cord. Although, according to this concept, afferent inputs are not essential, they are nevertheless important in grading the individual component movements.

The spinal cord neurons concerned with programming locomotion not only produce alternate flexor and extensor activation, they also correctly time the contraction of appropriate muscles at the right moment for normal locomotion. Such neurons have been termed pattern generators or neural oscillators. It has been shown that there are individual pattern generators for each limb; however, when all limbs are active, as in normal walking, the pattern generators of the different limbs are coupled to one another.

As in posture and movement, spinal mechanisms for locomotion are under the influence of modulatory descending inputs from supraspinal centers. Rubrospinal, vestibulospinal, and reticulospinal tracts are rhythmically active in phase with locomotor movements. In addition, it has been shown that locomotion can be triggered by stimulation of a midbrain region, the mesencephalic locomotor region. Recent attention has focused on noradrenergic neurons of the locus ceruleus as possibly mediating the effect of the mesencephalic locomotor region.

It has also been shown that both dorsal and ventral spinocerebellar tract neurons in the spinal cord are active during locomotion. The two tracts have been shown to convey different information to the cerebellum; the dorsal tract ordinarily informs the cerebellum about the state of muscle activity in the periphery, whereas the ventral tract conveys information about the active processes within the spinal cord and pattern generation for locomotion.

Experimental Models for Dyskinesias

Experimental models have been developed for the tremor of cerebellar disease and for hemiballismus. These models have contributed significantly to an understanding of the underlying pathophysiologic mechanisms and rationale for available methods of treatment.

Attempts to produce parkinsonian tremor, chorea, or athetosis experimentally have met with failure.

Cerebellar Tremor

Lesions placed in the deep cerebellar nuclei or in the brachium conjunctivum of experimental animals have produced a volitional tremor indistinguishable from that seen in humans with lesions in the cerebellar hemispheres. In such animals, subsequent lesions placed in the ventrolateral (VL) nucleus of the thalamus, motor cortex, or corticospinal tract have abolished the tremor.

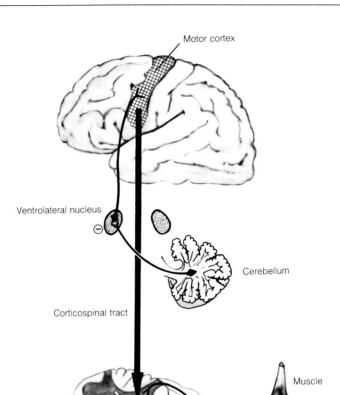

16-13   Schematic diagram showing the mechanism of tremor in cerebellar lesions.

Obviously, when the second lesion was placed in the motor cortex or corticospinal tract, paresis or paralysis usually developed. Since the sum total output from the cerebellum is inhibitory, the tremor that ensues from cerebellar lesions is attributed to the release of the thalamus (VL nucleus) from the inhibitory and regulatory effects of cerebellar input. In this situation, the VL nucleus of the thalamus acts as a tremorogenic center, exciting the motor cortex, which in turn will transmit this effect to the spinal cord and thence to the muscles (Fig. 16-13). Lesions in the VL nucleus of the thalamus, therefore, relieve the tremor by removing the driving force of the tremor. Ablation of the motor cortex or corticospinal tract relieves the tremor by abolishing all voluntary movements (paralysis).

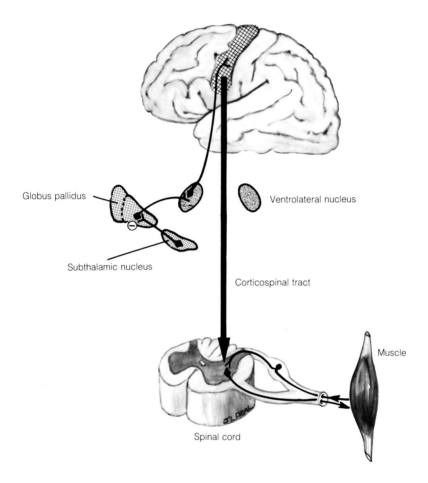

Globus pallidus

Subthalamic nucleus

Ventrolateral nucleus

Corticospinal tract

Muscle

Spinal cord

16–14 Schematic diagram showing the mechanism of tremor in lesions of the subthalamic nucleus.

Hemiballismus

Lesions placed in the subthalamic nucleus in monkeys have produced an abnormal movement in the contralateral part of the body indistinguishable from hemiballismus in man. The mechanism of this type of abnormal movement is similar to that described for cerebellar tremor. The subthalamic nucleus exerts inhibitory and regulatory effects on the globus pallidus.

Lesions of the subthalamic nucleus, therefore, release the globus pallidus, which is connected to the motor cortex via the thalamus. The motor cortex conveys this activity to the spinal cord via the corticospinal tract (Fig. 16–14).

Parkinsonism

Although no experimental model has been developed for Parkinson's disease, insight into the pathophysiologic mechanisms underlying the abnormal movements of parkinsonism has been developed from the available neuroanatomic, neurophysiologic, and neurochemical data. It is well established now that neurons of the substantia nigra contain the catecholamine dopamine. This dopamine is transmitted via axons of the substantia nigra to the neostriatum, where it is stored in the nerve endings of nigral axons. The substantia nigra and neostriatum form a closely related system (nigrostriatal system) with afferent and efferent connections. Dopamine is known to be an inhibitory transmitter at this site. The neostriatum projects to the globus pallidus, which in turn projects to the thalamus. The latter projects to the motor cortex. Activity in the motor cortex is then relayed to the spinal cord and thence to muscles (Fig. 16–15). The depletion of dopamine in Parkinson's disease, therefore, releases the globus pallidus from the inhibitory and regulatory effects of the neostriatum. This release from inhibition wili be reflected in the VL nucleus of the thalamus. Recordings in the VL nucleus in patients undergoing surgery for relief of tremor have revealed rhythmic activity similar in rate to that of parkinsonian tremor. The rhythmic activity in the VL nucleus is transmitted to the periphery via the motor cortex, corticospinal tract, and motor neuron axons.

Relief of parkinsonian tremor can therefore be achieved by the following methods.

1. Depleted dopamine stores are replaced in the neostriatum. This is achieved by administration of L-dopa, which is metabolized into dopamine.
2. Lesions are placed in the thalamus (VL nucleus) to silence the tremorogenic center.
3. Lesions are placed in the motor cortex or corticospinal tract. Although this method is neither desirable nor practiced because of the accompanying paralysis, it is observed in those parkinsonian patients who develop a stroke. In such patients, the tremor that was prominent prior to the stroke disappears following the stroke.

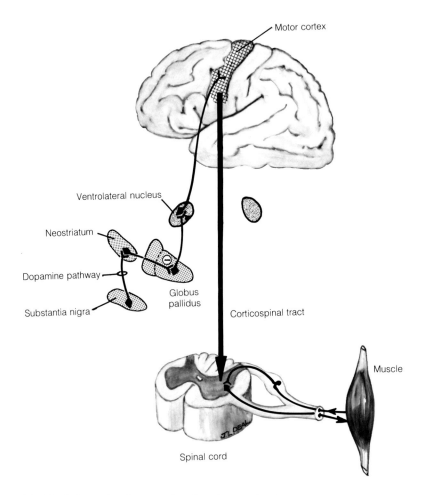

16–15 Schematic diagram showing the mechanism of tremor in lesions of the substantia nigra.

Overview

It is evident from the preceding presentation that normal posture and movement is the product of interaction among a number of neural structures. In the final analysis, spinal motor neurons have to be activated to move the muscles. The spinal motor neurons are in turn controlled by suprasegmental influences originating from cortical and subcortical motor centers. The latter are also under cortical control. Superimposed upon this vertical axis (represented by the direct and indirect corticospinal pathways) are modifying influences from the basal ganglia and the cerebellum (Fig. 16–16).

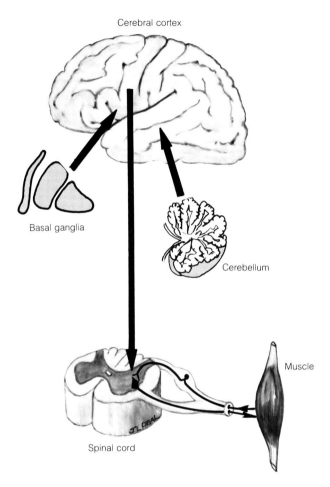

16–16 Simplified diagram showing the interaction of motor centers concerned with posture and movement.

Lesions along the vertical axis (whether in the cerebral cortex, corticospinal tract, or spinal cord) will produce a partial or total loss of movement. Lesions of the modifying motor centers (basal ganglia, cerebellum), on the other hand, will result in disorganized, abnormal movement. The disorganized movement of cerebellar lesions is manifest on volition, whereas that of basal ganglia lesions is manifest in repose.

Figure 16–17 is a simplified schematic diagram showing the loci of pathology commonly encountered in clinical practice, with a listing of the major motor deficits accruing from such lesions.

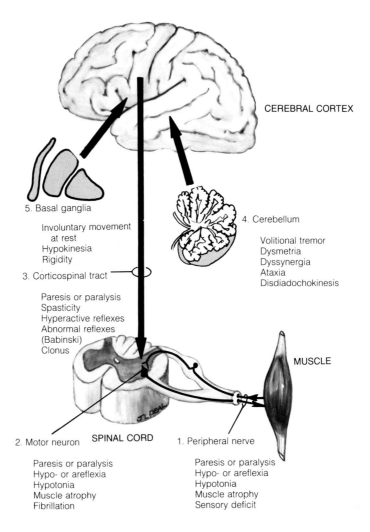

CEREBRAL CORTEX

5. Basal ganglia

Involuntary movement
at rest
Hypokinesia
Rigidity

3. Corticospinal tract

Paresis or paralysis
Spasticity
Hyperactive reflexes
Abnormal reflexes
(Babinski)
Clonus

4. Cerebellum

Volitional tremor
Dysmetria
Dyssynergia
Ataxia
Disdiadochokinesis

MUSCLE

2. Motor neuron   SPINAL CORD   1. Peripheral nerve

Paresis or paralysis
Hypo- or areflexia
Hypotonia
Muscle atrophy
Fibrillation

Paresis or paralysis
Hypo- or areflexia
Hypotonia
Muscle atrophy
Sensory deficit

16–17 Simplified diagram showing the motor deficits that result from lesions in different loci concerned with movement and posture.

1. Lesions interrupting the axons of motor neurons to the muscle (as in peripheral neuropathy or severance of the axons) produce weakness (paresis) or paralysis in the group of muscles supplied by the affected nerve or nerves. Because such a lesion will interrupt the reflex arc of myotatic reflexes, such reflexes will be depressed (hyporeflexia) or lost (areflexia) and the muscles will be hypotonic. Since the majority of peripheral nerves are mixed (containing both motor and sensory fibers), such lesions will also be manifested by sensory loss.

2. Lesions of the motor neurons in the spinal cord (as in poliomyelitis) produce paresis or paralysis of all muscles supplied by the affected spinal cord segments. Because of the interruption of the reflex arc, the muscles will be hypotonic and myotatic reflexes will be either reduced or lost. Loss of the trophic influence of motor neurons on the muscle fibers leads to atrophy of these fibers, which also exhibit spontaneous movements at rest (fibrillation) attributed to denervation hypersensitivity at the motor endplate.

3. Lesions of the corticospinal tract anywhere along its path, from its origin in the cerebral cortex to its termination in the spinal cord (as in stroke, hemorrhage, tumor, or trauma), produce the upper motor neuron syndrome characterized by paresis, spasticity, hyperactive myotatic reflexes, abnormal reflexes (Babinski reflex), and clonus.

4. Lesions of the cerebellum produce a disorganized and erratic type of movement characterized by volitional tremor on movement, ataxia of gait, dysmetria, disturbances in alternate motion rate (dysdiadochokinesia), and dyssynergia.

5. Lesions of the basal ganglia produce involuntary movements in repose, as seen in the tremor of Parkinson's disease, chorea, athetosis, and hemiballismus. Such lesions also produce rigidity of muscles and, in some cases, reduction in movement (hypokinesia).

References

Arshavsky, Y.I.; Berkinblit, M.B.; Fukson, O.I.; Gelfand, I.M.; Orlovsky, G.N.: Recordings of Neurones of the Dorsal Spinocerebellar Tract during Evoked Locomotion. Brain Res 43 (1972) 272–275.

Asanuma, H.: Cerebral Cortical Control of Movement. Physiologist 16 (1973) 143–166.

Evarts, E.V.; Bizzi, E.; Burke, R.E.; DeLong, M.; Thach, W.T.: Central Control of Movements. Neurosci Res Program Bull 9 (1971) 1–170.

Grillner, S.; Shik, M.L.: On the Descending Control of the Lumbosacral Spinal Cord from the "Mesencephalic Locomotor Region." Acta Physiol Scand 87 (1973) 320–333.

Henneman, E.: Motor Functions of the Brain Stem and Basal Ganglia. In: Medical Physiology, 14th Ed., Vol. 1, pp. 787–812, Ed. by V.B. Mountcastle. The C.V. Mosby Co., St. Louis, 1980.

Henneman, E.: Organization of the Spinal Cord and Its Reflexes. In: Medical Physiology, 14th Ed., Vol. 1, pp. 762–786, Ed. by V.B. Mountcastle. The C.V. Mosby Co., St. Louis, 1980.

Lance, J.W.: The Control of Muscle Tone, Reflexes, and Movement: Robert Wartenberg Lecture. Neurology 30 (1980) 1303–1313.

17

Cerebral
Circulation

The constantly active brain requires a rich blood supply to sustain its
ongoing activity. Irreversible brain damage results if the blood supply to
the brain is interrupted for more than a few minutes; consciousness is lost
if the blood supply is interrupted for about 5 sec. Lesions of the nervous
system due to interruption of blood supply constitute the commonest type
of central nervous system disorders.

It is estimated that about 15% of cardiac output reaches the brain; about
20% of oxygen utilization of the body is consumed by the adult brain and
as much as 50% by the infant brain. The blood flow through the human
brain is estimated to be 800 ml per min or approximately 50 ml/100 gm of
brain tissue per min. This average value increases with an increase in
functional activity of the brain or regions within it. The blood flow is
markedly increased in the sensory motor area upon vigorous exercise of
the contralateral limb. Cerebral blood flow is faster in gray matter (70 to
80 ml/100 gm per min) than in white matter (30 ml/100 gm per min).
Irreversible brain damage will occur if the cerebral blood flow is less than
15 ml/100 gm per min.

Sources of Supply

The brain receives its blood supply from four arterial trunks; these are two
internal carotid arteries and two vertebral arteries.

Internal Carotid Artery

The internal carotid arteries arise at the bifurcation of the common carotid
arteries in the neck, ascend in front of the transverse processes of the upper
three cervical vertebrae, and enter the base of the skull through the carotid
canal. Within the cranium, the internal carotid artery lies in the cavernous

sinus. It then pierces the dura to begin its subarachnoid course. The internal carotid gives rise to the ophthalmic, anterior choroidal, anterior cerebral, middle cerebral, and posterior communicating branches.

Ophthalmic Artery　The ophthalmic artery is the first intracranial branch of the internal carotid as it courses through the cavernous sinus. The ophthalmic artery gives rise to the central artery of the retina. Thus, interruption of the blood supply from the internal carotid system may result in disturbances in visual acuity. The ophthalmic artery is also of importance because of its anastomotic connections with branches of the external carotid system; this anastomotic relationship is essential in establishing collateral circulation when the internal carotid system is occluded in the neck.

Anterior Choroidal Artery　The anterior choroidal artery arises from the internal carotid artery after it emerges from the cavernous sinus. It passes ventral to the optic tract and supplies the optic tract, cerebral peduncles, lateral geniculate body, posterior part of the posterior limb of the internal capsule, tail of the caudate nucleus, uncus, amygdala, anterior hippocampus, choroid plexus of the temporal horn, and sometimes the globus pallidus. The anterior choroidal artery is prone to occlusion by thrombus because of its small caliber.

Anterior Cerebral Artery　The anterior cerebral artery (Fig. 17–1) originates from the internal carotid lateral to the optic chiasm and courses dorsal to the optic nerve to reach the interhemispheric fissure, where it curves around the genu of the corpus callosum and continues as the pericallosal artery dorsal to the corpus callosum. As the two anterior cerebral arteries approach the interhemispheric fissure, they are joined by the anterior communicating artery. The anterior cerebral artery supplies the medial aspect of the cerebral hemisphere as far back as the parieto-occipital fissure. The following are among its major branches.

　Recurrent Artery of Heubner (Medial Striate Artery)　This artery arises from the anterior cerebral as the latter approaches the interhemispheric fissure caudal to the anterior communicating artery. It supplies the anterior limb and genu of the internal capsule and parts of the head of the caudate, rostral putamen and globus pallidus.

　Orbitofrontal Artery　This branch arises distal to the anterior communicating artery and supplies the orbital gyri at the base of the frontal lobe and part of the septal area. The orbitofrontal artery or its branches may be displaced by subfrontal tumors, thus providing a clue, in cerebral angiograms, to the extracerebral location of the tumor (*e.g.*, subfrontal meningioma).

　Frontopolar Artery　Arising at the level of the genu of the corpus callosum, this artery supplies most of the pole of the frontal lobe.

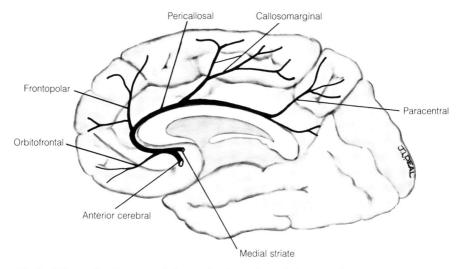

17-1   Schematic diagram of the major branches of the anterior cerebral artery and the areas they supply.

Callosomarginal Artery   This is the major branch of the anterior cerebral artery. It passes backward and upward and gives off internal frontal branches before terminating in the paracentral branch around the paracentral lobule.

Pericallosal Artery   This is the terminal branch of the anterior cerebral artery. It courses fairly close to the corpus callosum. It ordinarily gives rise to the paracentral artery, which may also be derived from the callosomarginal artery. The pericallosal artery terminates as the precuneal branch, which supplies the precuneus gyrus of the parietal lobe.

Occlusion of the anterior cerebral artery, in the absence of collateral circulation, will result in paralysis and sensory loss of the contralateral leg due to interruption of the blood supply to the leg area of the sensory motor cortex on the medial aspect of the hemisphere.

Middle Cerebral Artery   The middle cerebral artery (Fig. 17–2) is a continuation or the main branch of the internal carotid artery. It courses within the lateral (sylvian) fissure and divides into a number of branches that supply most of the lateral surface of the hemisphere. The following are some of the more important branches.

Cortical Branches   These include the rolandic (which supplies the primary sensory motor cortex), frontal, temporal, and parietal branches. The most rostral cortical division of the middle cerebral artery is known as the candelabra branch because of its division into two segments, simulating a candelabra.

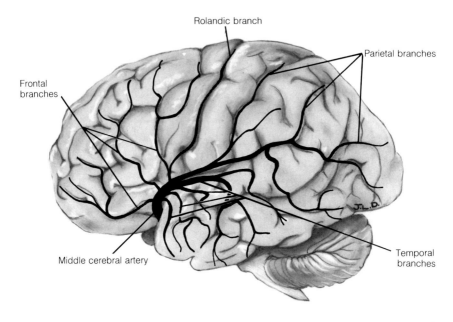

Rolandic branch

Parietal branches

Frontal
branches

Middle cerebral artery

Temporal
branches

17–2 Schematic diagram of the major branches of the middle cerebral artery and the areas they supply.

Central Branches   These include the lenticulostriate arteries which supply the major parts of the caudate, putamen, globus pallidus, internal capsule, and thalamus.

Posterior Communicating Artery   The posterior communicating artery connects the internal carotid artery with the posterior cerebral artery. Some anatomists consider the posterior cerebral artery as the continuation of the posterior communicating artery. Branches of the posterior communicating artery supply the genu and anterior part of the posterior limb of the internal capsule, the anterior part of the thalamus, and parts of the hypothalamus and subthalamus.

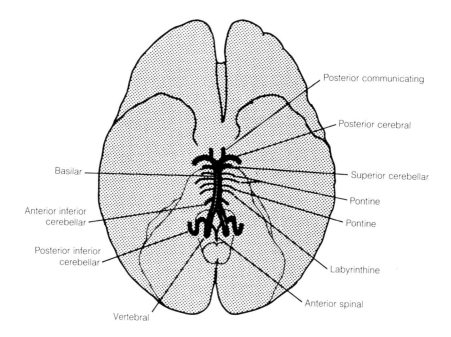

Posterior communicating

Posterior cerebral

Basilar

Superior cerebellar

Pontine

Anterior inferior
cerebellar

Pontine

Posterior inferior
cerebellar

Labyrinthine

Anterior spinal

Vertebral

17–3 Schematic diagram of the major branches of the vertebral and basilar arteries.

Vertebral Artery

The vertebral arteries arise from the subclavian arteries and ascend within the foramina of the transverse processes of the upper six cervical vertebrae, curve backward around the lateral mass of the atlas, and enter the cranium through the foramen magnum. Within the cranium, the vertebral arteries lie on the inferior surface of the medulla oblongata. The two vertebral arteries join at the caudal end of the pons to form the basilar artery. The vertebral artery gives rise to the posterior spinal, anterior spinal, and posterior inferior cerebellar branches (Fig. 17–3). Meningeal branches supply the meninges of the posterior fossa, including the falx cerebelli.

Posterior Spinal Artery The two posterior spinal arteries pass caudally over the medulla and the posterior surface of the spinal cord. They supply the posterior aspect of the medulla below the obex, as well as the posterior column and posterior horns of the spinal cord. One or both posterior spinal arteries may arise from the posterior inferior cerebellar arteries.

Anterior Spinal Artery The anterior spinal artery starts as two vessels that join to form a single artery which descends on the ventral aspect of the medulla and into the anterior median fissure of the spinal cord. It supplies the medullary pyramids and the paramedian medullary structures, as well as the anterior two-thirds of the spinal cord. Occlusion of this artery in the spinal cord results in sudden onset of paralysis below the occlusion.

Posterior Inferior Cerebellar Artery   Asymmetric in level of origin and diameter, these arteries follow an S-shaped course over the olive and inferior cerebellar peduncle to supply the inferior surface of the cerebellum, dorsolateral surface of the medulla oblongata, choroid plexus of the fourth ventricle, and part of the deep cerebellar nuclei. Occlusion of this artery gives rise to a characteristic group of signs and symptoms comprising the lateral medullary syndrome (Wallenberg's syndrome).

Basilar Artery

Formed by the union of the two vertebral arteries at the caudal end of the pons, the basilar artery (Fig. 17–3) runs in the pontine groove on the ventral aspect of the pons and terminates at the rostral end by dividing into the two posterior cerebral arteries. Branches include a series of median (penetrating) arteries which supply the median zone of the basilar portion of the pons (basis pontis) and a series of short and long circumferential arteries.

Median Penetrating Arteries   These branches travel for variable distances caudally before penetrating the brain stem; hence, a lesion in the brain stem may appear at levels more caudal than that of the occluded vessel.

Short Circumferential Arteries   These branches supply the anterolateral and posterolateral parts of the pons.

Long Circumferential Arteries.   There are three long circumferential arteries.

Auditory (Labyrinthine) Artery   This artery accompanies the facial (CN VII) and vestibulocochlear (CN VIII) cranial nerves and supplies the inner ear and the root fibers of the facial nerve. Occlusion of this artery gives rise to deafness.

Anterior Inferior Cerebellar Artery   This artery supplies the inferior surface of the cerebellum, the brachium pontis and the restiform body, as well as the tegmentum of the lower pons and upper medulla. It may arise from a common stem with the auditory artery.

Superior Cerebellar Artery   This is the last branch of the basilar artery before its terminal bifurcation into the two posterior cerebral arteries, from which it is separated by the rootlets of the oculomotor nerve. It supplies the superior surface of the cerebellum, part of the dentate nucleus, the brachia pontis and conjunctivum, tegmentum of the upper pons, and the inferior colliculus.

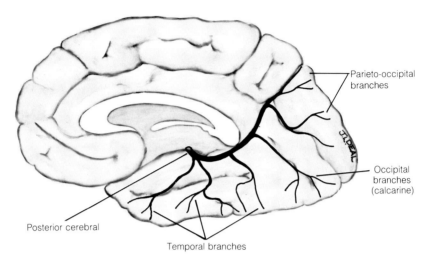

17–4   Schematic diagram of the major branches of the posterior cerebral artery and the areas they supply.

Posterior Cerebral Arteries   These constitute the terminal branches of the basilar artery. They pass around the cerebral peduncle and supply the medial surface of the occipital lobe, including the primary and association visual cortices, temporal lobe, and caudal parietal lobe (Fig. 17–4). Perforating branches supply the cerebral peduncle and the mesencephalon. Other branches include the thalamogeniculate artery, which supplies the lateral geniculate body and posterior thalamus, and the posterior choroidal artery, which supplies the choroid plexus of the third and lateral ventricles. Posterior cerebral artery branches also pass over the dorsal edge of the cerebral hemisphere to supply a small part of the lateral surface of the caudal parietal lobe and occipital lobe. The posterior cerebral artery may be compressed by the herniation of the uncus in cases of increased intracranial pressure. As a consequence, the circulation of the visual cortex is impaired, resulting in cortical blindness.

Circle of Willis

The proximal portions of the anterior, middle, and posterior cerebral arteries connected by the anterior and posterior communicating arteries form a circle, the circle of Willis (Fig. 17–5), around the infundibulum of the pituitary and the optic chiasm. The circle constitutes an important anastomotic channel between the internal carotid and the vertebral basilar systems. The circle of Willis is complete in only 20% of individuals. In the majority of individuals, variation in size and/or origin of vessels is the rule.

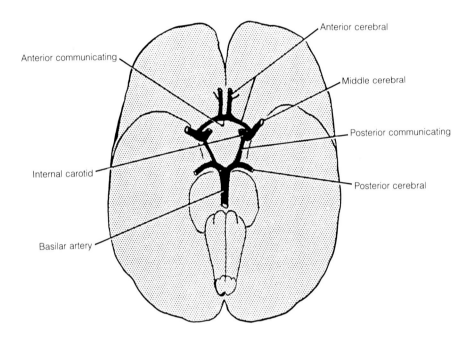

Anterior cerebral

Anterior communicating

Middle cerebral

Posterior communicating

Internal carotid

Posterior cerebral

Basilar artery

17–5 Schematic diagram of the circle of Willis and arteries that contribute to the formation of the circle.

Conducting and Penetrating Vessels

The arteries of the brain fall into two general types. The conducting or superficial arteries are those that run in the pia arachnoid and include the internal carotid and vertebral basilar systems and their branches. These vessels receive autonomic nerves and function as pressure equalization reservoirs to maintain an adequate perfusion pressure for the penetrating arteries. It is estimated that the drop in the pressure head from large vessels to the penetrating arterioles does not exceed 10 to 15%. The penetrating arterioles supply the cortex and white matter and are organized in vertical and horizontal patterns. These are presumed to be the primary sites of regional autoregulation and do not receive a significant neural supply.

Histology of Cerebral Vessels

Cerebral arteries differ from arteries elsewhere in the body in the following features.

1. Thinner walls
2. Absent external elastic laminae
3. Presence of astrocytic processes
4. Presence of a perivascular reticular sheath consisting of arachnoid trabeculae. The latter acquire an outer pial membrane when the vessel penetrates the brain substance.

Cerebral capillaries are structurally similar to capillaries elsewhere, except for being surrounded by perivascular glial (astrocytic) processes.

Cerebral veins have thinner walls and are devoid of valves and muscle fibers. The absence of valves allows reversal of blood flow when occlusion of the lumen occurs in disease.

Collateral Circulation

Anastomotic channels are present in all parts of both the arterial and venous circulation. Their main purpose is to ensure a continuing blood flow to the brain in case of a major occlusion of a feeding vessel. Some of these channels, however, are not very effective in collateral circulation because of their small caliber. The following are the major sites of collateral circulation.

1. Extracranial anastomoses are found between cervical vessels, such as the vertebral and external carotids of the same side.
2. Extracranial-intracranial anastomoses occur between branches of the external carotid and the ophthalmic artery. This is a major site of communication between extracranial and intracranial circulation. Thus, when the internal carotid is obstructed proximal to the origin of the ophthalmic, flow is reversed in the ophthalmic artery. Another site of extracranial-intracranial anastomoses is through the rete mirabile, a group of small vessels which connect meningeal and ethmoidal branches of external carotid arteries with leptomeningeal branches of cerebral arteries.
3. Intracranial anastomoses occur in the circle of Willis. Under normal conditions, there is very little side flow or flow from posterior to anterior segments in the circle of Willis. In the presence of major occlusion, however, the communications across the anterior or posterior communicating artery become a very important channel for collateral circulation. Other sites of intracranial anastomoses include those among the superior cerebellar, anterior inferior cerebellar, and posterior inferior cerebellar in the cerebellum.

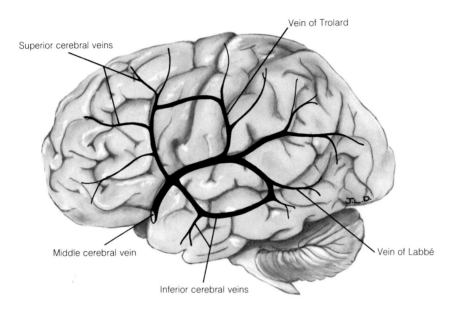

Vein of Trolard

Superior cerebral veins

Middle cerebral vein

Inferior cerebral veins

Vein of Labbé

17–6 Schematic diagram of the superficial system of venous drainage of the brain.

Cerebral Venous Drainage

Cerebral venous drainage occurs through two systems, the superficial and the deep.

Superficial Venous System

The superficial system of veins (Fig. 17–6) is divided into three groups.

Superior Cerebral Group These veins drain the dorsolateral and dorsomedial surfaces of the hemisphere and enter the superior sagittal sinus at a forward angle against the flow of blood. Conventionally, the most prominent of these veins in the central sulcus is called the superior anastomotic vein of Trolard, which interconnects the superior and middle groups of veins.

Middle Cerebral Group These veins run along the sylvian fissure, drain the inferolateral surface of the hemisphere and open into the cavernous sinus.

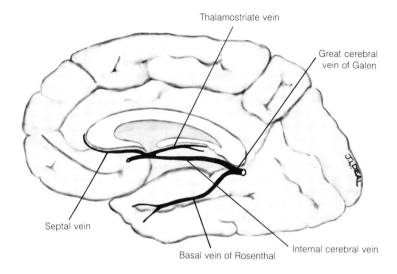

Thalamostriate vein

Great cerebral vein of Galen

Septal vein

Basal vein of Rosenthal

Internal cerebral vein

17–7   Schematic diagram of the deep system of venous drainage of the brain.

Inferior Cerebral Group   These veins drain the inferior surface and open into the cavernous and transverse sinuses. The middle and inferior groups are interconnected by the inferior anastomotic vein of Labbé. The medial surface of the hemisphere is drained by a number of veins which open into the superior and inferior sagittal sinuses, as well as into the basal vein and the great cerebral vein of Galen.

Deep Venous System

The deep venous system (Fig. 17–7) consists of a number of veins which drain into two main tributaries; these are the internal cerebral vein and the basal vein. The two join beneath the splenium of the corpus callosum to form the great cerebral vein of Galen, which opens into the straight sinus.

Internal Cerebral Vein   This vein receives two tributaries.
Terminal Vein (Thalamostriate)   Draining the caudate nucleus and possibly the thalamus, this vein passes forward in a groove between the caudate nucleus and thalamus in the body of the lateral ventricle and empties into the internal cerebral vein at the interventricular foramen of Monro.
Septal Vein   This vein drains the septum pellucidum, the anterior end of the corpus callosum, and the head of the caudate nucleus and passes backward from the anterior column of the fornix to open at the interventricular foramen into the internal vein. The internal cerebral vein of each

side runs along the roof of the third ventricle in the velum interpositum and passes caudally between the pineal body (below) and the splenium of the corpus callosum (above). The two internal cerebral veins join below the splenium of the corpus callosum to form the great vein of Galen.

Basal Vein of Rosenthal   This vein begins under the anterior perforated substance and runs backward to empty into the great cerebral vein. It drains blood from the base of the brain.

Visualization of the cerebral veins, particularly the deep group, is used during cerebral angiography in the localization of deep brain lesions.

Cerebellar Venous Drainage

The cerebellum is drained by three groups of veins; these are the superior, anterior, and posterior groups.

1. The superior group drains the entire superior surface of the cerebellum and empties into the great cerebral vein or the straight sinus.
2. The anterior cerebellar vein (known to neurosurgeons as the petrosal vein) is a constant vein, draining the inferior anterior surface of the cerebellum and the pontine venous plexus. It opens into the superior petrosal sinus.
3. The posterior cerebellar vein empties into either the straight or transverse sinus.

Factors Regulating Cerebral Circulation

Cerebral blood flow is a function of the pressure gradient and cerebral vascular resistance. The pressure gradient is determined primarily by arterial pressure. Resistance is a function of blood viscosity and size of cerebral vessels.

Extrinsic Factors

Systemic Blood Pressure   Arterial pressure is regulated by several circulatory reflexes, the most important of which are the baroreceptor reflexes. Baroreceptors in the aortic arch and carotid sinus are tonically active when arterial pressure is normal and vary their impulse frequency directly with fluctuations in blood pressure. An increase in arterial pressure increases impulses from baroreceptors, with inhibition of sympathetic efferents to the cardiovascular system and stimulation of the cardiac vagus nerve, leading to a decrease in arterial pressure. The reverse occurs if the arterial pressure is decreased. Baroreceptor regulation of arterial pressure ceases when arterial pressure falls below 50 to 60 mm Hg.

Fluctuations in systemic arterial blood pressure in the healthy young individual have very little if any effect on cerebral blood flow. Cerebral blood flow will be maintained with fluctuations in systolic blood pressure between 200 and 50 mm Hg. A fall in systolic blood pressure below 50 mm Hg may be accompanied by a reduction in cerebral blood flow; however, because more O_2 is extracted, consciousness is usually not impaired. Cerebral blood flow may also decrease if systolic pressure rises above 200 mm Hg or diastolic pressure rises above 110 to 120 mm Hg. The range of blood pressure fluctuations beyond which cerebral blood flow is affected is narrower in individuals with arteriosclerosis of cerebral vessels.

Blood Viscosity   Cerebral blood flow is inversely proportional to blood viscosity in man. A major factor controlling blood viscosity is the concentration of red blood cells. A reduction in blood viscosity, as occurs in anemia, will increase cerebral blood flow. On the other hand, an increase in viscosity, as occurs in polycythemia, will decrease cerebral blood flow.

Vessel Lumen   Minor reductions in the lumina of carotid and vertebral arteries are without effect on cerebral circulation. The vessel lumen must be reduced by 70 to 90% before a reduction in cerebral circulation occurs.

Intrinsic Factors

Autoregulation   The single most important factor controlling cerebral circulation is the phenomenon of autoregulation, by which smooth muscles in small cerebral arteries and arterioles can change their tension in response to intramural pressure to maintain a constant flow despite alterations in perfusion pressure. Thus, cerebral blood vessels constrict in response to an increase in intraluminal pressure and dilate in response to a reduction in intraluminal pressure. This phenomenon is particularly useful in shunting blood from healthy regions where intraluminal pressure is higher to ischemic regions where a reduction in blood flow has occurred, resulting in a reduction in intraluminal pressure. Autoregulation operates independently of, but synergistically with, other intrinsic factors such as biochemical changes. The mechanism of autoregulation is poorly understood. In general, three theories have been proposed; these are the neurogenic, myogenic, and metabolic theories.

Biochemical Factors   Several biochemical factors regulate cerebral circulation.

Carbon Dioxide Arterial PCO_2 is a major factor in the regulation of cerebral blood flow. Hypercapnia (high PCO_2)produces marked vasodilatation and an increase in cerebral blood flow. The reverse occurs in hypocapnia (low PCO_2). Thus, inhalation of CO_2 increases cerebral blood flow, whereas hyperventilation decreases cerebral blood flow. Under normal conditions, it is estimated that a change of 1 mm Hg in PCO_2 will induce a 5% change in cerebral blood flow.

The control of cerebral blood flow by CO_2 is mediated via the cerebrospinal fluid bathing cerebral arterioles. The pH of the cerebrospinal fluid (CSF) reflects the arterial PCO_2 and is also influenced by the level of bicarbonate in the CSF.

The effect of CO_2 on cerebral blood flow is important in dampening the effects of tissue PCO_2 in areas of brain ischemia. The increase in cerebral blood flow in such areas helps to wash out metabolically produced CO_2 and thus re-establishes homeostasis of brain pH.

Oxygen Moderate changes in arterial PO_2 do not alter cerebral blood flow. However, more marked changes in arterial PO_2 alter cerebral blood flow in a manner which is the reverse of that described for PCO_2. Thus, low PO_2 will increase cerebral blood flow and high PO_2 will decrease cerebral blood flow. Although the exact mechanism of this effect is not known, it is believed to be independent of changes in PCO_2.

pH Cerebral blood flow increases with the lowering of the pH and decreases in alkalosis.

Neural Factors

Sympathetic Supply Sympathetic innervation of conducting vessels is amply documented from the cervical sympathetic chain. In contrast, very few if any penetrating vessels receive adrenergic nerves. Both myelinated preganglionic and unmyelinated postganglionic nerve plexuses have been demonstrated in the periadventitial tissue. Synaptic terminals have also been traced to the outer part of the muscular media. The number of nerve plexuses and terminals decreases with reduction in the caliber of the conducting vessel. Stimulation of the sympathetic system produces vasoconstriction and a decrease in cerebral blood flow. The effect is greater in the internal carotid artery system than in the vertebral basilar system.

Parasympathetic Supply Although parasympathetic nerve fibers have been demonstrated in cerebral vessels of the conducting variety, a physiologic role for this system in the regulation of cerebral circulation is yet to be found.

The vasoactive effects of sympathetic stimulation are counteracted by a minor change in pH. Thus, neural factors in the regulation of cerebral blood flow are believed to be of minor importance when compared with the biochemical factors.

Mean and Regional Cerebral Blood Flow

Mean cerebral blood flow is rather constant during the performance of daily physiologic activities, such as muscular exercise, changes in posture, mental activity, and sleep. It is altered, however, in some pathologic conditions such as convulsions (increased), coma (decreased), anemia (increased), and cerebral vessel sclerosis (decreased). In contrast, regional cerebral blood flow is altered during the performance of physiologic activities; thus, the regional blood flow in the occipital cortex is increased with visual activity and in the motor cortex during limb movement. Studies of regional cerebral blood flow in normal individuals have contributed significantly to a better understanding of the role of different brain regions in the performance of physiologic activities, such as reading, speaking, hearing, and movement. Determinations of regional cerebral blood flow have also elucidated regional derangements of distribution of blood flow in disease states, such as cerebral stroke.

Clinical Correlates

Steal Syndrome

Ischemia of brain tissue, in which cerebral blood flow is below 20 ml/100 gm per min, results in accumulation of lactic acid and secondary loss of tone of the regional blood vessels. These vessels are not capable of responding normally, in view of vasomotor paralysis, to factors that alter cerebral blood flow, such as CO_2 and O_2. In such patients, administration of a vasodilator drug or induction of a state of hypercapnia dilates the normal vessels and increases blood flow in the brain regions supplied by such vessels at the expense of the ischemic region (steal syndrome). These agents should be used with great caution in such patients to avoid a serious and possibly fatal reduction in cerebral blood flow in the already ischemic region.

Autoregulation and Hypertension

Cerebral blood flow is normal in patients with moderate hypertension. Such patients, therefore, do not have cerebral symptoms. It has been found that the autoregulatory mechanism in such patients is set at a higher threshold than that in normal individuals. However, if the blood pressure is increased acutely, then autoregulatory mechanisms break down and cerebral symptoms appear.

Cerebral Blood Flow in Epilepsy

During an epileptic attack, mean cerebral blood flow increases two- to threefold. This is probably a response to the increased metabolic demands of brain tissues during such attacks.

Cerebral Blood Flow in Coma

The mean cerebral blood flow is severely reduced in states of unconsciousness. Attempts to correlate the degree of reduction of cerebral blood flow with the chances of recovery from the comatose state have not been successful.

References

Ingvar, D.H.; Schwartz, M.S.: Blood Flow Patterns Induced in the Dominant Hemisphere by Speech and Reading. Brain 97 (1974) 273–288.

Lassen, N.A.: Control of Cerebral Circulation in Health and Disease. Circ Res 34 (1974) 749–760.

Kuschinsky, W.; Wahl, M.: Local Chemical and Neurogenic Regulation of Cerebral Vascular Resistance. Physiol Rev 58(1978) 656–689.

Soh, K.; Larsen, B.; Skinhøj, E.; Lassen, N.A.: Regional Cerebral Blood Flow in Aphasia. Arch Neurol 35(1978) 625–632.

Waddington, M.M.: Atlas of Cerebral Angiography with Anatomic Correlation. Little, Brown and Co., Boston, 1974.

18

Cerebrospinal Fluid and the Barrier System

Anatomy of the Ventricular System

The brain contains four ependyma-lined cavities known as cerebral ventricles; these are the right and left lateral ventricles, the third ventricle, and the fourth ventricle (Fig. 18–1). The four cavities communicate with each other and with the subarachnoid space: the lateral and third ventricles through the foramen of Monro, the third and fourth ventricles through the aqueduct of Sylvius (cerebral aqueduct or iter), and the fourth ventricle and the subarachnoid space through the foramina of Magendie and Luschka. The term "fifth ventricle" is sometimes used to refer to the cavity (Fig. 18–2) that develops within the septum pellucidum (the cavum septum pellucidum). This, however, is a misnomer because the cavity does not have the epithelial lining characteristic of ventricular cavities, nor does it contain cerebrospinal fluid.

Ventricular cavities are lined by ependymal epithelium. In some specific sites, the ependymal lining is invaginated by a vascular pial fold known as the choroid plexus. Such choroid plexus sites are encountered in the body of the lateral ventricle, the inferior horn of the lateral ventricle, the roof of the third ventricle, and the posterior part of the roof of the fourth ventricle (Fig. 18–1).

The lateral ventricles have an arch-like configuration corresponding to the shape of the hemisphere. Each lateral ventricle is subdivided into five segments (Fig. 18–1).

1. Frontal (anterior) horn
2. Body
3. Atrium
4. Occipital (posterior) horn
5. Temporal (inferior) horn

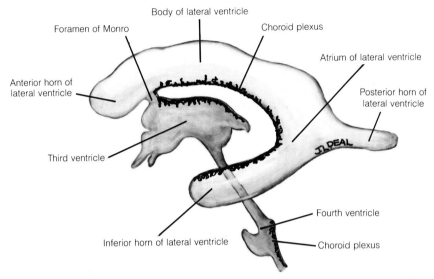

18–1   Schematic diagram showing the ventricular system of the brain in a composite sagittal view.

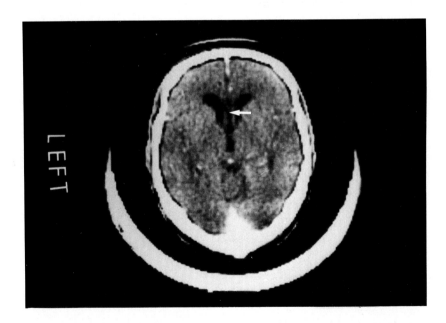

18–2   Computerized tomography (CT) scan showing the cavum septum pellucidum (*arrow*).

The frontal horn is the part of the lateral ventricle rostral to the foramen of Monro. In coronal sections, this part of the ventricle has a butterfly configuration with the corpus callosum forming its roof, the septum pellucidum and fornix its medial wall, and the caudate nucleus bulging into the lateral wall. This characteristic bulge of the caudate nucleus into the lateral wall disappears in degenerative diseases of the brain involving the caudate nucleus.

The body of the lateral ventricle extends from the foramen of Monro posteriorly to the region of the splenium of the corpus callosum (Fig. 18–1).

The atrium or trigone is the area of confluence of the posterior part of the body with the occipital and temporal horns. The atrium is the most expanded subdivision of the ventricle and the site of early ventricular enlargement in degenerative diseases of the brain.

The occipital horn extends from the atrium backward toward the occipital pole. It is the most variable subdivision in shape and size and may be rudimentary or altogether absent. The calcarine fissure produces an impression in the medial wall of the occipital horn known as the calcar avis.

The temporal horn extends from the atrium downward and forward into the temporal lobe and ends approximately 3 cm behind the temporal tip.

The lateral ventricles communicate with the third ventricle through the interventricular foramen of Monro. The cavity of the third ventricle is enclosed between the two diencephalons. It is bounded anteriorly by the lamina terminalis and the anterior commissure, superiorly by ependyma attached to the stria medullaris thalami, and inferiorly by hypothalamic structures.

The third ventricle has a number of recesses that are important in localizing lesions in the region of the third ventricle. These recesses include the suprapineal recess above the pineal gland, the optic recess above the optic chiasma, and the infundibular recess into the infundibulum (Fig. 18–3).

The aqueduct of Sylvius (cerebral aqueduct or iter) is a narrow canal that connects the third and fourth ventricles through the midbrain. It is about 1.5 to 2.0 cm long and 1 to 2 mm in diameter. Stenosis (narrowing) or complete obstruction of the aqueduct, which may occur congenitally or as the consequence of inflammatory processes, results in accumulation of cerebrospinal fluid, an increase in cerebrospinal pressure, and ventricular dilatation rostral to the site of obstruction.

The fourth ventricle lies between the anterior surface of the cerebellum and the posterior (dorsal) surfaces of the pons and medulla oblongata. The fourth ventricle boundaries are discussed in the chapter on the medulla oblongata. The fourth ventricle communicates with the subarachnoid space

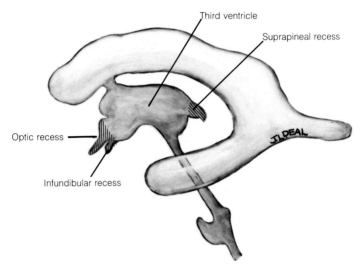

18–3   Schematic diagram of the ventricular system showing the recesses of the third ventricle (*stippled areas*).

through three foramina in its roof. These are a central foramen of Magendie and two lateral foramina of Luschka, which drain the lateral recesses of the fourth ventricle.

Subarachnoid Cisterns

The subarachnoid cisterns are dilatations in the subarachnoid spaces located principally at the base of the brain. Radiologic visualization of the subarachnoid cisterns is important in localization of pathologic processes, especially those due to tumors in the base of the brain. The clinically relevant subarachnoid cisterns include the following.

1. The cisterna magna (cisterna cerebellomedullaris), largest of the subarachnoid cisterns, is located between the medulla oblongata, the cerebellum, and the occipital bone (Fig. 18–4). Cerebrospinal fluid from the fourth ventricle reaches the cisterna magna via the foramina of Magendie and Luschka. The cisterna magna is continuous anteriorly with the cisterna pontis.

2. The cisterna pontis is located between the basis pontis and the clivus. It has a midline segment and two lateral extensions. The midline segment is important in localizing pathologic processes in the pontine area, whereas the lateral extensions are useful in localization of pathologic processes in the cerebellopontine angle.

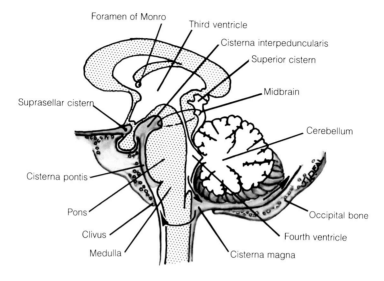

18–4 Schematic diagram showing the major subarachnoid cisternae.

3. The cisterna interpeduncularis extends between the cerebral peduncles and is helpful in localization of pathology in that region.
4. The suprasellar cistern is located dorsal to the sella turcica and communicates with the cisterna interpeduncularis. Some authors divide the suprasellar cistern into prechiasmatic and postchiasmatic parts. The former is located anterior to and above the optic chiasma, whereas the latter is located behind and below the optic chiasma. The suprasellar cistern is thus useful in localizing pathologic processes in or around the sella turcica and optic chiasma.
5. The superior cistern (cisterna ambiens) is located dorsal and lateral to the midbrain.

Cerebrospinal Fluid

The classic concepts of formation, circulation, and absorption of cerebrospinal fluid (CSF) elaborated early in this century have undergone major modifications in the last 25 years.

Classic Concepts

According to the classic concepts elaborated by Cushing, Weed, and Dandy, the cerebrospinal fluid is formed by the choroid plexus and circulates in the lateral ventricles, the foramen of Monro, the third ventricle, the aqueduct of Sylvius, and the fourth ventricle. It flows via the foramina of Magendie and Luschka to the cisterna magna and subarachnoid spaces, where it is finally absorbed through the arachnoid granulations in the superior sagittal sinus into the venous circulation.

Present Concepts

Formation   Although the choroid plexus remains one of the sites of CSF formation, CSF production can be maintained up to 75% in the absence of the choroid plexus. Alternate sites of formation include 1) the ependyma, 2) the cerebral pial surface, 3) the cerebral extracellular spaces, and 4) the subarachnoid space. It is estimated that approximately 60% of CSF is formed in the lateral, third, and fourth ventricles and 40% is formed in the subarachnoid space. Approximately half of the CSF formed in the ventricles comes from the choroid plexus; the rest comes from the ependymal lining. In man, CSF is formed at the rate of 0.35 ml per min. Its average volume in the adult is 130 ml, with 30 ml distributed in the ventricles and 100 ml in the subarachnoid space. It is estimated that the turnover rate of CSF is four to five times per day.

The rate of CSF formation is rather constant and is not generally affected by alterations in CSF pressure below 200 mm of CSF. There is evidence, however, to suggest a decrease in CSF formation rate in chronic, experimentally produced, or human hydrocephalus. CSF formation from the choroid plexus is also decreased with local arteriolar vasoconstriction or hypotension. Almost total cessation of CSF formation from the choroid plexus may result following vasoconstriction induced by low PCO_2 during hyperventilation. On the other hand, vasodilatation induced by CO_2 inhalation has been shown to result in a substantial increase in CSF formation. Drugs acting on enzyme systems may influence CSF formation by interfering with active transport mechanisms. Drugs that inhibit carbonic anhydrase, such as Diamox, can partially or completely inhibit CSF formation. Ouabain, an ATPase inhibitor, can produce effects similar to those of Diamox. Glucocorticoids have been shown to exert an inhibitory effect on the rate of CSF formation. Several diuretic agents have also been shown to reduce the rate of CSF formation. Although both respiratory and metabolic alkalosis have been shown to depress the rate of CSF formation, the former is more effective than the latter. CSF formation is known to increase with maturation; this may reflect the maturation of the enzyme systems involved in the secretory process.

CSF was considered to be an ultrafiltrate of plasma. Recent evidence seems to suggest, however, that CSF is formed by the following mechanisms.

Diffusion   The rate of diffusion depends upon particle size and the lipid solubility of the compound.

Active Transport   Major cations that pass through the choroid plexus into the CSF are sodium and potassium. The concentration of sodium is higher in CSF than in plasma, whereas that of potassium is lower. Of all the cations in CSF, sodium is found in the greatest amount and is used to stabilize the pH and total cation concentration in CSF. Most of the sodium in CSF enters via the choroid plexus and only a very small fraction traverses the brain capillaries and brain substance. The concentration of potassium in CSF is very stable and is not affected by fluctuations in blood or CSF pH. A proper balance between intracellular and extracellular potassium is critical to nerve cell function. Excess CSF potassium is quickly incorporated by neural tissue, whereas reduction in CSF potassium is compensated by movement of potassium from neural tissue to CSF. Chloride constitutes the major anion in CSF and seems to diffuse passively through the choroid plexus, although this passage is closely regulated by sodium and potassium transport.

Certain metabolic substances of low lipid solubility, such as glucose and some amino acids, reach CSF by means of specific carrier transport systems. The carrier systems for amino acids are independent from the glucose carriers.

Free Passage of Water   Water moves freely across the barrier. Large molecules, such as plasma proteins, are almost completely blocked by the choroid plexus from entering CSF, although water movement is unrestricted. Studies utilizing perfusion techniques have shown that albumin transfer from blood to CSF is only partially dependent on bulk flow; a portion of the albumin probably enters CSF from surrounding neural tissue.

Circulation   CSF flows from the lateral ventricles through the foramen of Monro to the third ventricle, and then through the aqueduct of Sylvius to the fourth ventricle, where it reaches the subarachnoid space through the foramina of Magendie and Luschka.

Using isotope cisternography, CSF circulation can be followed from the lateral ventricles to the superior sagittal sinus, where it is resorbed. CSF reaches the basal cisterns in a few minutes, flowing from there into the rostral subarachnoid space and sylvian fissure and finally into the convexity of the brain. Isotope injected into the lumbar subarachnoid space can be detected in basal cisterns within 1 hour.

Three factors seem to facilitate CSF circulation.

Drift   The drift of CSF from areas of positive balance to areas of negative balance facilitates circulation. Although CSF production and absorption are in almost perfect balance when the total CSF space is considered, any one point in the system may be at positive or negative balance. CSF will therefore drift from areas of positive balance to those of negative balance. This drift will contribute to CSF flow.

Oscillation CSF is also in a continuous state of oscillation, with a to and fro movement the amplitude of which increases as the fluid approaches the fourth ventricle. This oscillation contributes to the flow of CSF and the increase in amplitude in the fourth ventricle facilitates the flow of CSF into the cisterna magna.

Pulsatile Movement Rhythmic movements synchronous with arterial pulse have been described in CSF. These pulsatile oscillations assume an upward and downward movement in the fourth ventricle and basal cisterns. The origin of these oscillations is believed to be the expansion of the cerebrum and its arteries during systole, rather than choroid plexus pulsations as previously assumed.

Resorption The classic concept of CSF resorption states that the fluid is resorbed through the arachnoid granulations into the venous system of the superior sagittal sinus. This concept was based on experiments in which CSF flow was studied after Prussian blue was injected intrathecally. Earlier studies on CSF resorption were hampered by the use of substances foreign to CSF, such as trypan blue and phenosulfophthaline, which do not occur naturally and to which the subarachnoid space is highly sensitive. With the advent of radioisotopic techniques, it was possible to study the behavior of substances which normally occur in CSF. Such studies have yielded the following observations.

1. Electrolytes are resorbed more slowly than water.
2. Electrolytes are resorbed more readily in the ventricles than in the subarachnoid space.
3. Albumin leaves the subarachnoid space more readily than it leaves the ventricles.
4. Albumin disappears more slowly than water or electrolytes.
5. Resorption occurs not only in arachnoid granulations but also in the ependyma of the ventricles.
6. Resorption in the subarachnoid space occurs by a fast component through the leptomeningeal vascular route and by a slow component into the perineural spaces.

Thus, the present concepts of CSF resorption point to the following resorption sites.

1. Arachnoid granulations
2. Cerebral and spinal vessels
3. Perineural spaces
4. Ependyma

The controversy over reconciling the behavior of CSF outflow with its structural basis remains unresolved. Earlier studies suggest that substances varying widely in molecular weight and lipid solubility pass readily from CSF pathways to the blood. Such studies are at variance with ultrastructural observations of the arachnoid granulations, which show the presence of intact endothelium with tight junctions effectively separating CSF and blood compartments. More recent studies, however, may have resolved this controversy by suggesting a mechanism for CSF resorption in the arachnoid granulations similar to that described for drainage of ocular fluid in the canal of Schlemm. According to this hypothesis, endothelial cells of the arachnoid villus undergo vacuolation on the CSF side. Vacuoles increase in size because of the differential pressure gradient between CSF and blood compartments and ultimately reach the blood side of the endothelial cells, where they rupture and create a patent channel between CSF and blood. Such a hypothesis has been confirmed by electron microscopic observations of the behavior of arachnoid granulations.

In addition to this filtration route, it is believed that substances are resorbed by the two other routes of diffusion and active transport.

Function

CSF serves three principal functions.

1. It supports the weight of the brain within the skull. This function is disturbed when CSF is withdrawn, resulting in headache.
2. It acts as a buffer between the brain and adjacent dura and skull; it protects the brain from physical trauma during injury to the skull by dampening the effects of trauma.
3. It provides a stable chemical environment for the central nervous system. The chemical composition of CSF is rather stable even in the presence of major changes in the chemical composition of plasma.

Composition

CSF is composed of the following substances and elements.

Water Water is the major constituent of CSF.

Protein The value of protein in normal CSF is approximately 15 to 45 mg%. This value increases in various disease states of the nervous system (infection, tumor, hemorrhage), as well as after obstruction of CSF pathways.

Sugar The amount of glucose in normal CSF is approximately two-thirds that of the blood. This ratio is higher in newborns and premature infants, probably because of the immaturity of the blood-CSF barrier. The value decreases in meningitis and after meningeal infiltration by tumors.

Cells   A normal sample of CSF contains up to three lymphocytes per mm³. An increase in the number of white cells in CSF occurs in meningitis. Normal CSF contains no red blood cells (RBC). The presence of RBC in CSF occurs as a result of hemorrhage into the CSF.

Electrolytes   CSF contains sodium, potassium, chloride, magnesium, and calcium. Sodium and potassium constitute the major cations, whereas chloride constitutes the major anion. The concentration of sodium, chloride, and magnesium ions is higher in CSF than in plasma, whereas the concentration of potassium and calcium ions is lower.

Physical Properties

Specific Gravity   The specific gravity of normal CSF varies between 1.006 and 1.009. An increase in the protein content of the CSF raises its specific gravity.

Pressure   Normal CSF pressure varies between 50 and 200 mm of CSF (up to 8 mm Hg), measured with the patient in the lateral recumbent position and relaxed. The normal pressure range is higher when measured in the upright position. CSF pressure is increased in central nervous system infections (meningitis), tumors, hemorrhage, thrombosis, and hydrocephalus.

Clinical Application

The examination of CSF is of major value in neurologic diagnosis. Access to CSF for diagnosis dates back to 1891 when Quinke introduced the lumbar puncture. CSF can be obtained from three sites; these are 1) the spinal subarachnoid space (spinal or lumbar puncture), 2) the cisterna magna (cisternal puncture), and 3) the lateral ventricles (ventricular puncture). The first route is the most commonly used. In this procedure (spinal or lumbar tap), a special needle is introduced using sterile techniques and local anesthesia in the L_2-L_3, L_3-L_4, or L_4-L_5 vertebral space. It is gently eased into the subarachnoid space and CSF is withdrawn. Since the conus medullaris of the spinal cord ends at the L_1 or L_2 vertebral level and the meninges extend to the S_1 or S_2 vertebral level, the space between L_2 and S_2 vertebrae constitutes a safe area into which to introduce the lumbar tap needle, without the danger of injuring the spinal cord. The subarachnoid space, the cisternal space and the ventricles are entered not only to obtain CSF for examination but also to inject air (Fig. 18–5), contrast material (Fig. 18–6), or drugs for either diagnosis or treatment of neurologic disorders.

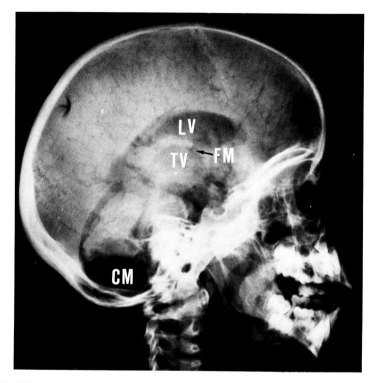

18–5 The lateral ventricle (*LV*), foramen of Monro (*FM*), third ventricle (*TV*), and a spacious cisterna magna (*CM*) are shown in a pneumoencephalogram obtained by injection of air into the subarachnoid space.

Blood-Brain Barrier

The concept of a barrier system between blood and brain dates back to 1885, when it was found that intravenously injected acidic dyes stained all organs of the body except the brain. It was later observed that when these acidic dyes were injected into the CSF, the brain was stained. Thus, a barrier was assumed to be located at the blood-brain interface that prevented entry of acidic dyes into the brain. It has since been discovered that these acidic dyes bind themselves to serum albumin and that the barrier to their entry to the brain is the low permeability of brain capillaries to the albumin to which the dyes are bound.

Although earlier studies conceived of only one barrier, at the blood-brain interface, studies dating back to the thirties have elucidated the existence of other brain barrier sites. Consequently, the term "blood-brain barrier" has been replaced by the more useful term of "brain barrier

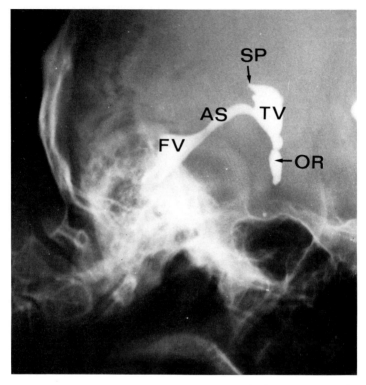

18–6 The third ventricle (*TV*), suprapineal recess (*SP*), optic recess (*OR*), aqueduct of Sylvius (*AS*), and fourth ventricle (*FV*) are shown in a ventriculogram obtained by injection of radiopaque material into the ventricles.

system." The sites of this barrier system include 1) blood-brain, located at the interface between the capillary wall and brain substance; 2) blood-CSF, located in the choroid plexus; 3) CSF-brain, handling the transfer of materials from CSF into brain substance through the ventricular lining; and 4) CSF-blood, dealing with exchanges from CSF directly into the blood vessels of the subarachnoid spaces or via the arachnoid granulations into the venous system of the superior sagittal sinus.

Studies on the mechanisms of the barrier system have identified the following anatomic substrates: 1) vascular endothelium, 2) capillary basement membrane, 3) perivascular glial processes, and 4) intercellular brain substance. None of these sites, however, can account for all the observed phenomena of the barrier system. It is thus conceivable that several factors are operative in the barrier system. These factors include the following.

1. The anatomic substrate as defined above.
2. Protein binding. Brain capillaries are essentially impermeable to albumin. Substances in plasma that are bound to protein will therefore have no access to the brain.
3. Lipid solubility. Substances with high lipid solubility enter the brain rather rapidly, whereas substances with low or no lipid solubility enter the brain very slowly or not at all.
4. Blood flow. This factor is operative in the entry to the brain of substances of high lipid solubility. The rate of blood flow to a brain region will determine the amount of entry of such substances.
5. Metabolic requirement. The rate of entry of some substances into the brain seems to be dependent on the metabolic requirement of that region of the brain for the particular substance. Cholesterol, for example, is accumulated in the brain during myelin formation and decreases when myelination is completed.

Thus, factors that determine the brain barrier system are both anatomic and physiologic. They are 1) transported substance (protein binding, lipid solubility), 2) capillary wall (endothelial lining, basement membrane), and 3) brain substance (glial membranes, metabolic requirements, regional blood flow, extracellular space).

The brain barrier system is more permeable in newborn infants and young laboratory animals than in adults and older animals. As the brain matures with age, the barrier system becomes less permeable. The brain of the newborn, for example, is permeable to bilirubin; excessive rise in serum bilirubin in the adult does not affect the brain.

Certain areas of the brain are devoid of a barrier system. These areas include the area postrema of the medulla oblongata, hypophysis, pineal body, hypothalamic regions, and subfornical organ. All these areas are characterized by rich vascularity and some are secretory in function. Unlike vessels elsewhere in the brain, the endothelial lining of vessels in these areas is fenestrated.

References

Alami, S.Y.; Afifi, A.K.: Cerebrospinal Fluid Examination. In: Laboratory Medicine, Vol. 4, Chap. 2, pp. 1–26, Ed. by G.J. Race. Harper & Row, Hagerstown, 1973.

Vastola, E.F.: CSF Formation and Absorption Estimates by Constant Flow Infusion Method. Arch Neurol 37 (1980) 150–154.

19

Reticular Formation, Wakefulness, and Sleep

Reticular Formation

The term reticular formation refers to a mass of neurons and nerve fibers extending from the caudal medulla to the rostral midbrain and continuous with the zona incerta and reticular nuclei of the diencephalon. Although older accounts of the reticular formation described it as a mass of inter-meshed, poorly organized neurons and nerve fibers, it has now been established that the reticular formation is organized into definite nuclear groups with known afferent and efferent connections. As a whole, the reticular formation comprises a nonspecific neural system with multiple inputs and a multisynaptic system of impulse conduction. Current methodologies such as histo- and immunofluorescent techniques, the new generation of orthograde and retrograde fiber tracing methods, and intra- as well as extracellular microphysiology have enriched our knowledge of the organizational precision and complexity of this system.

Nomenclature

There is no entirely satisfactory term to designate the complex of cell pools, neuropil fields and associated fiber systems which make up the reticular core of the brain stem. The term reticular formation was used by early neuroscientists to describe the reticulated appearance of the core formed by the unpatterned mixture of neurons and myelinated fibers. A more recent designation, the nonspecific system, differentiates it from the specific system represented by the medial lemniscus and the spinothalamic tracts. The nonspecific system is turning out to be, in many respects, more highly ordered and more complex than the specific system. A term that gained popularity in the fifties and sixties is the ascending reticular activating system, which focused attention on the core's role in wakeful and alert states. It is now known that the functions of this system transcend this behavioral role. In the absence of a fully satisfactory term, the term "brain stem reticular core" remains in common use.

Nuclei

In general, the reticular formation is divided into three nuclear groups. The medial group includes the following nuclei.

1. Nucleus reticularis magnocellularis of the medulla oblongata
2. Nucleus reticularis ventralis of the medulla oblongata
3. Nucleus reticularis pontis oralis
4. Nucleus reticularis pontis caudalis
5. Mesencephalic reticular nucleus

The lateral group includes the following nuclei.

1. Lateral reticular nucleus of the medulla oblongata
2. Parvicellular nucleus of the medulla oblongata
3. Parvicellular nucleus of the pons

The raphe group includes the following nuclei, all of which produce the transmitter serotonin.

1. Caudal nucleus of the raphe in the medulla oblongata (raphe magnus)
2. Rostral nucleus of the raphe in the pons
3. Raphe nucleus of the midbrain

Functional Subdivisions

Based on physiologic studies, the brain stem reticular core has been divided into five zones. Zone I includes the nucleus reticularis pontis caudalis and part of the nucleus reticularis magnocellularis and is concerned with control of whole body postural adjustments (*e.g.*, the orienting response). Zone II includes the nucleus reticularis gigantocellularis and part of the nucleus reticularis ventralis of the medulla oblongata and is concerned in a more specialized way with the axial component of whole body postural adjustments. Zone III includes the bulk of the nucleus reticularis ventralis of the medulla oblongata and probably plays a role in the postural atonia associated with the REM (rapid eye movement) stage of sleep. Zone IV is dorsal to zones I and II and is concerned with control of head and neck movements in relation to shifts of gaze. Zone V corresponds to the nucleus reticularis pontis oralis and is concerned with events occurring during sleep cycles.

Connections

Afferent Connections   The reticular formation receives fibers from the following sources.

Sensory Systems   Most sensory systems (somatic and visceral) project fibers upon the reticular formation. The medial lemniscus is the exception. As a rule, sensory projections upon reticular nuclei are from second order neurons.

Spinal Cord   Spinoreticular fibers project mainly upon the medial group of reticular neurons in the medulla and pons bilaterally.

Cerebral Cortex   Cortical projections to the reticular formation arise from wide areas of the cerebral cortex (motor and sensory areas). These fibers comprise the corticoreticular tract.

Cerebellum   Cerebellar projections to the reticular formation arise mainly from the nucleus fastigi.

Brain Stem   Projections to the reticular formation are reported from the lateral hypothalamus and the superior colliculus.

Basal Ganglia   Pallidal projections to the reticular formation have been described.

Efferent Connections   The reticular formation projects fibers both rostrally (ascending) and caudally (descending). The efferent connections arise primarily from the medial and raphe groups.

Ascending Connections   The reticular formation projects rostrally to the following structures.

Diencephalon   Reticular fibers reaching the thalamus terminate upon the nonspecific thalamic nuclei and reticular nucleus.

Cerebral cortex   Reticular fibers reach the cortex after relays in the diencephalon (thalamus, hypothalamus and subthalamus), particularly in the intralaminar nuclei of the thalamus. Some reticular efferents may reach the cerebral cortex directly.

The ascending projections to the diencephalon and cortex comprise the ascending reticular activating system, which plays a role in arousal and wakefulness.

Cerebellum   The lateral reticular nucleus projects to both sides of the cerebellum but mainly to the ipsilateral side.

Locus Ceruleus   The reticular connection with the locus ceruleus plays a role in sleep mechanisms.

Descending Connections   The reticular formation projects caudally to the spinal cord via the following tracts.

Medial reticulospinal tract
Lateral reticulospinal tract

These tracts originate in the pontine and medullary reticular formation (medial and raphe groups), respectively. Their sites of termination and functions have been described in the chapter on the spinal cord.

Connections with Cranial Nerve Nuclei   The reticular formation projects to practically all nuclei of cranial nerves. This is a part of the corticoreticulobulbar pathway which brings cortical influences to cranial nerve nuclei.

Local Connections   In addition to the afferent and efferent connections of the reticular formation, there are local connections between the different groups of reticular nuclei. These are from the lateral to the medial group and from the raphe to the medial group.

Chemically Specified Systems

Two chemically specified systems have been identified among the rich ensemble of reticular neurons; these are the cholinergic and monoaminergic systems.

Cholinergic System   The cholinergic system courses in two bundles within the tegmentum of the brain stem. The dorsal tegmental bundle originates in the midbrain and spreads widely through the tectum, pretectal area, geniculate bodies, and into the nonspecific as well as the specific thalamic nuclei. Some fibers of this bundle reach the globus pallidus and cerebral cortex. The ventral tegmental bundle arises from the pons and midbrain and projects upon the globus pallidus and anterior thalamus.

Monoaminergic System   Four types of monoamine neurons have been identified within the brain stem reticular core: dopaminergic, noradrenergic, adrenergic, and serotonergic.

Dopaminergic neurons form small clusters at several brain loci. Many of these neurons are found in the ventral tegmentum of the midbrain and the adjacent substantia nigra. Axons of these cells are directed toward the basal ganglia, hypothalamus, limbic system, and neocortex. A component of this system, the nigrostriatal system, provides the dopaminergic innervation to the neostriatum. A second component, the mesocortical system, projects upon the telencephalon.

Noradrenergic neurons of the brain stem are divided into two major components. The first is the norepinephrine system of the locus ceruleus (catecholamine neuron cell group A6). The second is the lateral tegmental norepinephrine system, comprising another series of noradrenergic cell groups scattered in the pons and medulla (groups A1 to A7). Axons of these neurons are directed to the spinal cord, brain stem, cerebellum, diencephalon, and telencephalon.

Adrenergic neurons are located in the same regions of the caudal medulla as the noradrenergic neurons. They project to the spinal cord, brain stem, thalamus, and hypothalamus. This system is small in comparison with the dopaminergic and noradrenergic systems and represents a minor component of the monoaminergic system.

Serotonergic neurons comprise nine cell groups designated B1 to B9. More recently, it has become apparent that the vast majority of serotonergic neurons lie within the raphe nuclei of the midbrain, pons and medulla oblongata. Axons of these neurons project to the spinal cord, brain stem, cerebellum, striatum, diencephalon, and cerebral cortex. The mesencephalic serotonergic neurons project mainly to the forebrain, whereas the pontine and medullary serotonergic neurons project mainly caudally. The projection from the nucleus raphe magnus of the medulla oblongata to the spinal cord has received much attention. This projection has been shown to inhibit dorsal horn neurons that give rise to the spinothalamic tract.

The dopaminergic system neurons have a discrete topography and restricted area of terminal distribution, whereas the noradrenergic, adrenergic, and serotonergic neuron systems have a more diffuse and widespread projection, with little evidence of topography. Thus, the reticular formation contributes to selective transmission of sensory impulses.

Function

The reticular formation has somatic motor, somatic sensory, visceral motor, and arousal and sleep functions.

Somatic Motor Function   The somatic motor function is mediated via reticular connections to cranial nerve nuclei and motor neurons of the spinal cord. These effects are triggered by activities in the cerebral cortex and cerebellum. The role of the reticulospinal tracts in control of somatic motor activity has been outlined in the chapter on posture and movement.

Descending reticulospinal pathways modify both alpha and gamma motor neuron activity, exerting facilitatory as well as inhibitory effects on both reflex and cortically induced motor activity. In general, the pontine reticular formation exerts facilitatory influences, whereas the medullary reticular formation exerts inhibitory influences. Interruption of the reticular connections to nuclei of cranial nerves results in a deficit in function (pseudoparalysis) of muscles supplied by these cranial nerves.

Somatic Sensory Function   The reticular formaton also exerts an effect on the transmission of sensory impulses. As in the case of somatic motor function, the effect of the reticular formation on sensory transmission is triggered by cortical activity. This effect is both facilitatory and inhibitory and is exerted on sensory nuclei of the spinal cord and brain stem, including cranial nerve nuclei. The modulation of activity in the posterior column nuclei by the reticular formation is one such example. The role of the nucleus raphe magnus of the medulla oblongata in the inhibition of pain transmission at the spinal cord level has been well established.

Visceral Motor Function   Physiologic data are available to suggest the presence of centers in the reticular formation for the control and regulation of several visceral functions.

Stimulation of the medial group of reticular nuclei in the medulla oblongata elicits an inspiratory response and depressor effect on the circulatory system (slowing of the heart rate and reduction in blood pressure).

Stimulation of the lateral group of reticular nuclei elicits the opposite effect, namely an expiratory response and pressor circulatory effect (acceleration of the heart rate and elevation in blood pressure).

A pontine reticular center (pneumotaxic center) which regulates respiratory rhythm has been identified. Direct connections from the pontine respiratory center to the medullary respiratory centers have been recently demonstrated.

Arousal and Sleep   The ascending efferent connections to the diencephalon and cortex play a role in arousal of the organism. The connections with the nucleus ceruleus are important in sleep mechanisms. These will be discussed later in this chapter.

Ascending Reticular Activating System

The multisynaptic pathways from the medial reticular formation to the diencephalon and subsequently to the cortex play a major role in arousal and in sharpening the attentiveness of the cortex to incoming sensory stimuli. This phenomenon of cortical arousal is associated with a characteristic electroencephalographic (EEG) pattern consisting of low voltage, high frequency waves known as a desynchronization pattern.

Stimulation of the ascending reticular activating system produces a state of arousal, alertness, and attentiveness. Experiments have shown that learning is greatly improved during stimulation of the reticular activating system. Destruction of this system, on the other hand, produces a state of somnolence or coma.

Activity in the ascending reticular activating system is a tonic one maintained by incoming afferent stimuli. Although the reticular activating system responds in a nonspecific fashion to all incoming sensory stimuli, some stimuli are more effective than others. Auditory stimuli are more effective than visual stimuli. Impulses from pain receptors are more effective than those from other receptors. Trigeminal stimuli are particularly effective. Animals in which the brain stem has been sectioned below the level of the trigeminal nerve in the pons retain the arousal response. However, if a cut is made at the level of the trigeminal nerve, such animals lose the arousal response and become stuporous.

The conversion of various sensory inputs on the reticular formation, its multisynaptic connections and the diversion of its projections to wide areas of the cerebral cortex make this system best suited for the arousal phenomenon.

It should be emphasized, however, that the reticular activating system receives constant feedback from the cerebral cortex and the peripheral receptors. These feedback mechanisms help maintain the state of arousal. The depression in the state of consciousness seen in degenerative brain disease is due in part to interruption of the feedback from the cortex to the reticular formation.

The reticular activating system is particularly sensitive to general anesthetics and tranquilizing drugs. These drugs may either suppress or attenuate transmission in this system, thus producing sleep or tranquilization. They do not, however, suppress transmission along the specific lemniscal system.

Recent interest in the reticular activating system has been focused on the substrate for selective awareness (how attention is selectively focused toward one sensory stream to the exclusion of other inputs). Anatomic and physiologic evidence suggests that the nucleus reticularis thalami plays a central role in selective awareness. The nucleus reticularis thalami, activated by volleys ascending along thalamocortical axons, in turn projects back upon thalamic nuclei and the mesencephalic tegmentum, exerting tonic and/or phasic inhibition of cell groups in the thalamus and mesencephalic tegmentum. Recent physiologic studies have also demonstrated facilitatory influences of the frontal cortex upon units in the nucleus reticularis thalami. Thus, a concept is emerging of a reticularis complex selectively gating interactions between the specific thalamic nuclei and the cerebral cortex under the control of the brain stem reticular formation and frontal cortex. This gating mechanism seems highly selective: depending on the nature of the alerting stimulus or locus of central stimulation, only that portion of the nucleus reticularis thalami which controls the appropriate thalamic sensory field will open.

Sleep and Wakefulness

Sleep is an altered state of consciousness necessary for the well-being of the organism. Humans deprived of sleep for long periods of time become emotionally disturbed and may even manifest psychotic behavior. It is estimated that humans spend approximately one-third of their lives asleep.

Stages of Sleep

There are two recognized stages of sleep; these are slow wave sleep and paradoxical sleep.

Slow wave sleep is also known as synchronized sleep, light sleep, slow sleep, and non-REM (rapid eye movement) sleep. It constitutes 75% of the sleeping period in adults and is characterized by the following somatic, behavioral, and electroencephalographic manifestations.

1. Reduced muscle tone
2. Decline in blood pressure, heart rate, and respiratory rate
3. Synchronized slow electroencephalographic activity of high voltage; hence the name slow wave sleep

Slow wave sleep can be divided into four stages: drowsiness (stage I), light sleep (stage II), moderately deep sleep (stage III), and deep sleep (stage IV).

Paradoxical sleep is also known as desynchronized sleep, dreaming sleep, REM sleep, fast wave sleep, and deep sleep. It constitutes 25% of sleeping time in adults and is characterized by the following manifestations.

1. Marked hypotonia, especially in neck muscles, hence head drop in people entering this stage while sitting up in a chair
2. Increase in blood pressure and heart rate; irregular and rapid respiration
3. Erection in males
4. Teeth grinding
5. Dreaming, hence the name dreaming sleep
6. Rapid eye movements (50 to 60 movements per min), hence the name REM sleep
7. High voltage potentials in the pons, lateral geniculate nucleus, and occipital cortex (PGO for pons, geniculate, and occipital activity)
8. Rapid, low voltage, irregular electroencephalographic activity resembling the waking pattern (desynchronization pattern)
9. Increased threshold of arousal, hence deep sleep

The coexistence of rapid, low voltage cortical activity (active state) and deep sleep justifies calling this stage the paradoxical stage of sleep.

During sleep, one alternates between stages III and IV of slow wave sleep and paradoxical sleep. The cycle repeats itself roughly every 90 min. Thus, one passes through 4 to 6 cycles of paradoxical sleep every night, each lasting from 5 min to 1 hour.

In general, there is more paradoxical sleep toward the morning and more of the slow wave sleep early at night. Furthermore, paradoxical sleep constitutes almost all sleeping time in the fetus and about 50% of sleeping time in the infant. As the brain matures, slow wave sleep increases, constituting 75% of sleeping time in the adult.

Drugs affect the stages of sleep differentially. Barbiturates and alcohol suppress REM sleep but have little effect on stage IV of non-REM (slow wave) sleep. On the other hand, benzodiazepines (Valium, Librium) suppress stage IV non-REM sleep and have less effect on REM sleep.

Theories of Sleep

Theories of sleep implicate one of two processes, either the passive or the active. According to the passive theory, sleep is merely absence of wakefulness. This theory has now been replaced by the active process theory. According to the active theory, sleep is actively triggered by known brain stem structures and through known chemical transmitters. Recent studies on the mechanisms of sleep have added significantly to present knowledge. Although some of the concepts which have developed from these studies remain controversial, there is strong evidence to support others. The following is a summary of some of these concepts.

Slow wave sleep is related to the raphe nuclei and to the transmitter serotonin [5-hydroxytryptamine (5HT)] produced in these nuclei. Serotonin is believed to act on cortical neurons to induce sleep. Destruction of the raphe nuclei or depletion of serotonin results in insomnia (lack of sleep). An increase in cerebral serotonin leads to hypersomnia (excessive sleep).

Serotonin seems to have another role in sleep, as a "priming" mechanism that leads to paradoxical sleep.

The locus ceruleus and norepinephrine seem to be responsible for paradoxical sleep.

Catecholamine neurons of the brain stem (locus ceruleus, reticular neurons, substantia nigra) which produce norepinephrine and dopamine seem to be responsible for cortical arousal. Inhibition of catecholamine synthesis produces sedation in animals with insomnia.

Catecholamines produced in the locus ceruleus are responsible for the marked hypotonia, rapid eye movements, and PGO activity of paradoxical sleep.

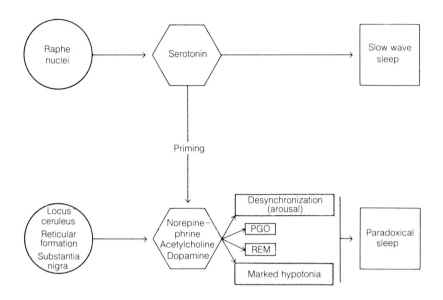

19–1 Schematic diagram of the loci in the brain that contribute to sleep and the proposed neurotransmitters that play a role in the different stages of sleep.

Cholinergic mechanisms of the brain stem play a role in cortical arousal and in PGO activity. The latter can be blocked by atropine.

In summary, the above model proposes that serotonin produced in the raphe nuclei is responsible for slow wave sleep and for priming catecholinergic and cholinergic mechanisms that contribute to the manifestations of paradoxical sleep. The locus ceruleus is a key structure in the genesis of paradoxical sleep (Fig. 19–1).

Finally, the rostral hypothalamus and basal forebrain seem to play a role in sleep. Lesions in these sites produce insomnia, whereas their stimulation induces sleep.

The above cholinergic and monoaminergic models of sleep have been challenged by some researchers in the field. These researchers propose that there are probably other transmitters and brain regions involved in sleep. A number of sleep-promoting peptides have been reported in blood and cerebrospinal fluid. A nona-peptide, the delta sleep-inducing peptide (DSIP), has been localized in the thalamus and has been shown to induce delta waves and spindle patterns in the EEG associated with reduced motor activity. Another peptide, the sleep-promoting substance (SPS), acts by increasing the duration of slow wave sleep and by decreasing locomotor activity. A third factor, the precise structure of which is not known, produces an increase in both REM and non-REM sleep.

Coma

Coma is a state of loss of consciousness characterized by impairment in the motor and sensory responses of the individual. A patient in coma cannot vocalize, has no spontaneous eye movements, and responds reflexly or not at all to painful stimuli. The electroencephalogram is characterized by slow activity in the delta range (about 3 cps).

There are grades of loss of consciousness. These vary from a state of lethargy (also called obtundation), in which wakefulness is barely maintained (drowsiness), responses to stimuli are sluggish or delayed, and vocalization is slow, slurred and spontaneous, to a state of stupor (semi-coma), in which there are some spontaneous eye movements, motor responses only to painful stimuli, and no spontaneous vocalization.

Coma can result from different causes. These include diseases of the central nervous system (infection, tumor, trauma, hemorrhage, thrombosis, etc.), metabolic disorders (acidosis, hypoglycemia, etc.), and drug overdosage (barbiturates, tranquilizers, etc.).

In coma secondary to central nervous system affection, involvement of the brain stem reticular formation (ascending reticular activating system) is pivotal in the genesis of coma. Coma, however, can result from extensive cortical disease without significant involvement of the brain stem reticular formation.

A special variety of altered state of consciousness in which the patient lies immobile and is unable to vocalize, but responds to verbal stimuli by eye movements, is known as akinetic mutism or coma vigile. The lesion in this condition has been described in the brain stem, orbital surface of the frontal lobe, cingulate gyrus, and septal area.

Another special variety of altered state of consciousness is the "locked-in" syndrome. This condition is similar to the state of akinetic mutism except that the locked-in patient gives signs of being aware of himself and of the environment. Locked-in states have been described in lesions of the pontine tegmentum and cerebral peduncle.

Brain Death

Brain death is a state of irreversible brain damage so severe that normal respiration and cardiovascular function can no longer be maintained. Such patients are in deep coma, remain unresponsive to external stimuli, and their respiration and cardiovascular functions are maintained by external means (respirators, pressor drugs, etc.). In modern clinical medicine, cessation of life is equated with brain death rather than with cessation of heart beat.

Several criteria have to be present before a state of brain death is declared. These criteria include the following.

1. Unresponsiveness to external stimuli
2. Absence of spontaneous breathing
3. Dilated fixed pupils
4. Absence of reflexes
5. No recognizable reversible cause for the coma
6. Flat electroencephalogram (absence of electrical activity) on two records run 24 hours apart
7. Nonfilling of cerebral vessels in arteriography or radioisotope angiography

Comatose patients who fulfill the above criteria are considered dead; heroic measures to save life are futile.

References

Bystrzycka, E.K.: Afferent Projections to the Dorsal and Ventral Respiratory Nuclei in the Medulla Oblongata of the Cat Studied by the Horseradish Peroxidase Technique. Brain Res 185 (1980) 59–66.

Corvaja, N.; Grofová, I.; Pompeiano, O.; Walberg, F.: The Lateral Reticular Nucleus in the Cat. I. An Experimental Anatomical Study of Its Spinal and Supraspinal Afferent Connections. Neuroscience 2 (1977) 537–553.

Hobson, J.A.; Scheibel, A.B.: The Brainstem Core: Sensorimotor Integration and Behavioral State Control. Neurosci Res Program Bull 18, No. 1(1980).

Kastin, A.J.; Olson, G.A.: Schally, A.V.; Coy, D.H.: DSIP–More Than a Sleep Peptide? Trends Neurosci 3 (1980) 163–165.

Künzle, M.: Autoradiographic Tracing of the Cerebellar Projections from the Lateral Reticular Nucleus in the Cat. Exp Brain Res 22 (1975) 255–266.

Moore, R.Y.: The Reticular Formation: Monoamine Neuron Systems. In: The Reticular Formation Revisited: Specifying Function for a Nonspecific System, International Brain Research Organization Monograph Series, Vol. 6, pp. 67–81, Ed. by J.A. Hobson and M.A.B. Brazier. Raven Press, New York, 1980.

Scheibel, A.B.: Anatomical and Physiological Substrates of Arousal: A View from the Bridge. In: The Reticular Formation Revisited: Specifying Function for a Nonspecific System, International Brain Research Organization Monograph Series, Vol. 6, pp. 55–66, Ed. by J.A. Hobson and M.A.B. Brazier. Raven Press, New York, 1980.

Zemlan, F.P.; Pfaff, D.W.: Topographical Organization in Medullary Reticulospinal Systems as Demonstrated by the Horseradish Peroxidase Technique. Brain Res 174 (1979) 161–166.

20

Pain

Pain is both a blessing and a curse to mankind. It is a blessing because it alerts one to impending danger. An individual born with congenital absence of pain may be severely mutilated from repeated injuries and die young. On the other hand, suffering from pain can be one of the most distressing of human experiences. Because of this, man over the centuries has persistently endeavored to discover the mechanisms of pain and ways of alleviating it. In spite of all these efforts, our present understanding of pain and its mechanisms remains incomplete.

Pain Receptors

Pain impulses arise from the surface of the skin, deep tissues, and viscera. The receptors that respond to painful stimuli are the free nerve endings. However, they are not specific for pain, since they also respond to touch and thermal stimuli. They receive both myelinated and unmyelinated nerve fibers. Free nerve endings are not the only pain receptors. Intense stimulation of most receptors will elicit pain.

Cutaneous Pain

The pain elicited from stimulation of cutaneous receptors has two components. The quick component is instantaneous, momentary, and sharp in nature and disappears when the stimulus ceases (*e.g.*, superficial penetration of the skin by a sharp needle). The second component, elicited by pushing the needle deeper into the skin, is dull, aching and stinging, outlasts the stimulus, and is poorly localized. These two components of pain are referred to as the fast and slow components, respectively. They are conducted via two types of fibers. The fast component is conducted via the A-delta fibers, whereas the slow component is conducted via the thinly myelinated or nonmyelinated C-fibers.

Deep Somatic Tissue Pain

Pain elicited from deep somatic tissues is dull and poorly localized. Sensitivity to painful stimuli varies from one structure to another. The periosteum, joint capsules, nerve sheaths, and blood vessels are highly sensitive to painful stimuli; muscle is less sensitive. Sensitivity of deep structures to painful stimuli is probably a reflection of the distribution of nerve endings in each structure.

Visceral Pain

Pain elicited from viscera is similar in quality to that elicited from deep somatic tissues. It is often associated with overlying muscle rigidity. The rigidity of lower right quadrant abdominal muscles associated with an inflamed appendix is such an example. The viscera are not sensitive to cutting, heat, or cold. The pain receptors are usually stimulated by stretching, distention, spasm, or ischemia of a visceral organ. A peculiar quality of deep tissue and visceral pain is its referral to distant cutaneous areas. These cutaneous areas are supplied by the same dorsal root as the affected organ or deep somatic tissue. The referral of cardiac pain to the left shoulder and upper extremity and that of the diaphragm to the right shoulder are examples of such referred pain. This is explained by the fact that the affected organ or deep tissue and the cutaneous area to which pain is referred share a common neuronal pool in the spinal cord.

Pain Stimulus

The pain receptors are stimulated by tissue damage from varying causes. Heat, physical injury, or vascular injury damages tissues, thereby releasing proteolytic enzymes. These enzymes then act on tissue globulins to release chemical substances (potassium, histamine, bradykinin, substance P or a similar peptide, or prostaglandin) which are believed to depolarize nerve endings. Attempts to demonstrate such chemical substances in adequate concentrations in skin have not been successful except for substance P, which has been demonstrated in significant amounts in the skin and the central nervous system. Further evidence in support of the release of chemical substances at cutaneous receptors is the presence of enzymes around such receptors. Nonspecific and specific cholinesterases have been demonstrated around somatic and visceral endings, respectively. Most people feel pain when their skin temperature reaches 45 to 47°C. This is also the temperature at which tissue damage occurs. Tissue ischemia (reduction of blood supply to a tissue) from vascular occlusion or stenosis (narrowing) also causes pain. The mechanism of pain associated with vascular ischemia is attributed to tissue damage and release of bradykinin and histamine.

Furthermore, the accumulation of lactic acid in such tissues may play a role in the genesis of pain. Pain is also frequently associated with muscle spasm. The mechanism of such pain is probably due to two factors: 1) muscle spasm (contraction) produces a relative ischemia to the muscle because of the increase in the metabolic rate of contracting muscle and 2) muscle contraction squeezes the intramuscular blood vessels, thus reducing the blood supply to the muscle (ischemia).

Pain-Conducting Nerves

There are no specific nerve fibers purely for pain conduction. Peripheral nerves that conduct pain impulses also conduct other sensory modalities. However, it is generally agreed that somatic pain impulses travel via two types of peripheral nerve fibers; these are myelinated A-delta fibers and nonmyelinated or thinly myelinated C-fibers. The former conduct impulses faster (6 to 30 m/sec) than the latter (0.5 to 2.0 m/sec). As stated previously, A-delta fibers conduct the fast component of cutaneous pain and the C-fibers conduct the slow component. In man, almost 100% of C-fibers are nociceptive.

Pain impulses traveling via the A-delta fibers are intermittent in character, whereas those traveling via the C-fibers have a continuous constant quality.

Visceral pain impulses are conducted via small myelinated and unmyelinated nerve fibers that accompany the autonomic peripheral nerve fibers or the autonomic fibers in some cranial nerves, such as the facial, glossopharyngeal, and vagus, which conduct pain impulses from the pharynx, trachea, esophagus, external ear, and tympanic membrane. There is no evidence to suggest convergence of somatic and visceral activity on single neurons in deep layers of the dorsal horn of the spinal cord.

Pain Pathways

Classic Pathways

Lateral Spinothalamic Tract   The spinothalamic tract is located in the lateral funiculus of the spinal cord. From neurons of origin in the dorsal root ganglia, thinly myelinated root fibers travel in the dorsal root (occupying its ventrolateral area) and establish synapses in Rexed laminae I to VI in the dorsal horn of the spinal cord. Axons of neurons in these laminae, in turn, establish synapses with neurons in Rexed laminae V to VIII. Dorsal horn neurons are divided into three classes. Class I neurons are excited by cutaneous mechanoreceptors, class II are excited by both mechano- and nociceptors, and class III respond only to noxious stimuli. Class III neurons are subdivided into those that receive A-delta input (IIIa neurons) and those that receive both A-delta and C-fibers (IIIb neurons). Substance P is now well established as the neurotransmitter for nociceptive neurons in the dorsal horn, especially in the marginal and substantia gelatinosa zones. Fibers arising from neurons in laminae V to VIII cross to the other side in the anterior white commissure, roughly one to two segments above their level of entry into the spinal cord. They gather in the contralateral lateral funiculus as the lateral spinothalamic tract. The tract shows a pattern of somatotopic organization in which sacral fibers are located most laterally and those of cervical origin more medially. In addition to this segmental lamination, the spinothalamic tract shows an incomplete pattern of modality organization whereby fibers carrying pain sensibility are anteriorly located and those carrying thermal sensibility are more posteriorly placed. Once formed, this tract ascends throughout the length of the neuraxis to reach the thalamus, where it synapses upon neurons in the posteroventral lateral nucleus and the posterior thalamic nuclear group (PO). From the thalamus, fibers project in the internal capsule to the primary somesthetic cortex in the parietal lobe.

Trigeminal Lemniscus Pain sensibility from the face, oral mucosa, and anterior aspect of the head travels via the sensory root of the trigeminal nerve. From neurons of origin in the trigeminal (Gasserian) ganglion, root fibers enter the brain stem at the level of the pons. They descend in the pons, medulla, and the upper cervical segments as the descending (spinal) tract of the trigeminal nerve. Throughout their course, they send collaterals to neurons in the adjacent nucleus of the descending tract of the trigeminal nerve (spinal trigeminal nucleus). Axons of neurons in the spinal trigeminal nucleus cross to the contralateral side and ascend as the ventral secondary ascending trigeminal tract, which reaches the thalamus and projects upon neurons of the posteroventral medial nucleus and the intralaminar thalamic nuclei. From these nuclei axons travel via the internal capsule to reach the primary somesthetic cortex in the parietal lobe.

Other Pathways

The persistent search for modes of transmission of painful impulses has revealed that the lateral spinothalamic tract and trigeminal lemniscus are not the only pathways for pain. Other pathways conveying this modality include a multisynaptic reticular pathway and the spinotectal tract.

Spinoreticular Pathway This is a multisynaptic pathway with spinospinal and spinoreticular relays. It passes through the reticular formation of the brain stem and projects upon neurons in the intralaminar nuclei of the thalamus. From the thalamus, fibers project to the frontal and limbic lobes of the cerebral cortex. By the nature of its projection, this pathway is concerned primarily with affective reaction to pain and with the determination of intensity and awareness of sensory perception of pain.

Spinotectal Pathway   This pathway occupies a position in the lateral funiculus of the spinal cord close to the lateral spinothalamic pathway. There is some doubt about the separate identity of this pathway, since there is evidence to suggest that it is composed of collaterals from the spinothalamic tract. Fibers in the spinotectal pathway project upon neurons in the midbrain and possibly upon reticular neurons in the medulla and pons.

Discriminative versus Nondiscriminative Pain Pathways

The above pathways can be grouped functionally into two categories, the discriminative and nondiscriminative pain pathways. The discriminative pain pathways include the lateral spinothalamic tract and trigeminal lemniscus. They are direct (compared with multisynaptic) pathways that project to specific thalamic and cortical areas and are concerned with the sharp, well-localized type of pain perception. The nondiscriminative pain pathways (spinoreticular) are multisynaptic and project to the nonspecific thalamic nuclei and the frontal and limbic lobes of the cerebral cortex. They are concerned with the affective, unpleasant, poorly localized, emotional reaction to pain.

Posterior Column and Pain

It is now established that the posterior column plays a role in pain mechanisms. Fibers leave the posterior column and project upon Rexed laminae II and III. These fibers exert an inhibitory influence on pain mechanisms. This fact has been used in clinical situations to relieve states of intractable pain by stimulation of the posterior column system.

Medulla Oblongata and Pain

Attention has recently been focused on the role of the nucleus reticularis gigantocellularis in pain mechanisms. The nucleus receives input from the periaqueductal gray region (concerned with pain modulation) and projects upon posterior horn neurons. Ablation of the nucleus renders opiate receptor agonists ineffective in pain relief. Whether the nucleus serves as a nociceptive relay in the pathway to the cortex or whether it mediates reflex activity (vasomotor, respiratory) associated with nociceptive activation or both is not yet settled.

Pulvinar Nucleus and Pain

During the past 10 years, increasing evidence has accumulated to suggest that the pulvinar nucleus has a role in pain mechanisms. The pulvinar has been shown to receive a projection from the paleospinothalamic system and to be activated by noxious stimuli applied to somatosensory pathways. Clinical studies have shown that lesions in the pulvinar result in pain relief. The pathways by which the pulvinar influences pain mechanisms include its projection to the intralaminar and reticular nuclei of the thalamus, as well as its projections to the cerebral cortex.

Central Appreciation of Pain

Centrally, pain is perceived primarily at three levels. These are the thalamus, cortex, and midbrain.

Thalamus

Pain impulses project upon neurons in the posteroventral lateral, posteroventral medial, posterior group, and intralaminar nuclei of the thalamus. The thalamus plays a role in the crude perception of pain. The thalamus is also believed to have a filtering effect on the unpleasant component of pain sensation. Thus, lesions of the thalamus may be associated with an unpleasant and spontaneous type of pain sensation referred to as central pain. Such pain is precipitated by the slightest, even nonpainful, stimulus and usually outlasts the stimulus. This pain sensation has a long latency period and is the most difficult to treat.

Cortex

The cerebral cortex, particularly the primary somesthetic cortex in the parietal lobe, is concerned with the perception of the discrete, well-localized type of pain. However, it is not essential for pain perception, since pain can be perceived after ablation of the somesthetic cortex. Thus, the primary somesthetic cortex serves an important spatiotemporal discriminative function but is not essential for the perception of impending tissue damage in man.

Other cortical areas concerned with pain are the prefrontal cortex and the temporal lobe. The former determines intellectual alertness to pain, whereas the latter plays a role in the memory of painful experience, as well as the affective alertness to pain. The prefrontal lobe or its connection to subcortical structures may be ablated to relieve the suffering from intractable pain.

Midbrain

The periaqueductal gray region of the midbrain has been shown to play an important role in pain mechanisms. The neuropeptide enkephalin has been identified in this region. Stimulation of certain sites within the periaqueductal gray releases enkephalins, which act on serotonergic neurons in the medulla oblongata, which in turn project on primary afferent axons concerned with pain conduction within the dorsal horn of the spinal cord to produce analgesia. Stimulus-produced analgesia has been achieved by stimulation of the caudal and medial region of the periaqueductal gray. In contrast, stimulation of the rostral and lateral periaqueductal gray facilitates pain conduction. The injection of morphine into the periaqueductal gray has been shown to be more effective in pain relief than similar injections into any other part of the brain.

Modulation of Pain

Modulating effects on pain mechanisms arise from several levels of the central nervous system. These effects may be facilitatory or inhibitory to the ongoing activity in Rexed laminae II and III. The major modulating impulses arise from the cerebral cortex, thalamus, periaqueductal gray, and posterior column.

Psychology of Pain

The reaction of the individual to painful stimuli is controlled by several environmental factors. These include cultural habits, past experience, and meaning of the situation.

Anthropologic studies have reported cultures in which labor pains are felt not by the delivering woman but by her husband, who goes to bed groaning and moaning while his wife is giving birth painlessly.

The individual's past experience seems to play a role in reaction to pain. Children whose parents react to wounds and bruises in an exaggerated way tend to react more strongly to painful stimuli as they become adults.

The situation in which the painful stimulus is applied is also important. War experience has shown that soldiers feel little pain when severely wounded in combat but feel pain more strongly when transferred away from the battle zone.

Pharmacology of Pain

Monoamines

It has been known for over two decades that monoamine levels modulate morphine analgesia. Recently, it has been shown that stimulus-produced analgesia is markedly depressed by substances that deplete the monoamines. Blockade of dopamine receptors has been shown to impair stimulus-produced analgesia, whereas stimulation of dopamine receptors increases stimulus-produced analgesia. In humans, L-dopa administration increases the threshold of and tolerance to chronic pain.

Enkephalins and Endorphins

The term "enkephalin" was originally used to describe substances with opiate-like properties extracted from brains of animals. These substances were later found to be pentapeptides, of which the two most prevalent in the brain are methionine-enkephalins and leucine-enkephalins. The methionine-enkephalins are the more active forms. The enkephalins are found in many regions of the brain and spinal cord, particularly in the periaqueductal gray of the midbrain, hypothalamus, basal ganglia, limbic system, and the dorsal horn of the spinal cord. These areas contain high concentrations of receptors for the enkephalins. In rats, microinjection of enkephalins into the periaqueductal gray blocks the behavioral response to pain. In patients with intractable pain, electrical stimulation of the periaqueductal gray induces analgesia. The endorphins are a broader group of endogenous opiate-like molecules. Enkephalins are endorphins, but not all endorphins are enkephalins. There are many endorphins, the most common of which are the alpha, beta, and gamma. The major type in the brain is the beta endorphin. Most endorphin neurons are located in the hypothalamus. Their projections are restricted to the diencephalon, periaqueductal gray, locus ceruleus, and raphe nuclei. High concentrations of beta endorphins are also found in the pituitary gland. Beta endorphins have a very high affinity for opiate receptors and are highly analgesic. It is more potent than morphine when injected intraventricularly or intravenously. Endorphins are more potent and have a longer lasting analgesic effect than the enkephalins.

Opiate Receptors

Opiate receptors are widely distributed in the brain. A high concentration of such receptors has been found in the limbic system, basal ganglia, hypothalamus, periaqueductal gray, and thalamus. Opiate receptors in the spinal cord are concentrated in laminae I to III of Rexed.

Substance P

There is evidence to indicate that substance P has a role in pain mechanisms. Substance P is present in the central terminals of nociceptive afferents in laminae I to III of the dorsal horn; iontophoretic or systemic administration of substance P causes a selective excitation of nociceptive neurons. Intrathecal administration of substance P or its analogue decreases the pain threshold; reduction of spinal levels of substance P increases the pain threshold.

Theories of Pain

Prior to the "gate control theory of pain" proposed by Melzack and Wall in 1965, there were two main theories to explain pain mechanisms.

Specificity Theory

According to this theory, pain is a specific modality with its own specific receptors, peripheral fibers, and central pathways. Since its introduction, there has been mounting evidence against this theory.

Pattern Theory

The pattern theory proposes that receptor stimulation elicits a certain pattern of responses which reflects the quality, intensity, and duration of the stimulus. These complicated patterns are fed into the central nervous system, which deciphers them and initiates the appropriate response.

Gate Control Theory

According to this theory, there is a gating mechanism in the posterior horn of the spinal cord (lamina III of Rexed). This gating mechanism modulates activity in spinal cord neurons that give rise to the central tracts for pain (T-cells) and thus increases or decreases the flow of impulses from the periphery into the central nervous system. The gating mechanism in the posterior horn is influenced by two types of inputs from the periphery.

One input is via a small (A-delta or C) fiber system which is continuously active, thus keeping the gate open. This system has a facilitatory role in pain mechanisms and acts to enhance the effect of incoming impulses. The second input is via a large (A-beta), thickly myelinated fiber system which fires in response to a stimulus. Both systems project upon neurons in lamina III of Rexed, which is considered to be the modular center for pain in the spinal cord. The thin fibers inhibit and the thick fibers facilitate neurons in this lamina. Both fiber systems also project upon neurons in Rexed laminae V to VIII (T-cells). Their action here is purely facilitatory. Furthermore, neurons in lamina III of Rexed have a presynaptic inhibitory effect on both the small and large fiber systems projecting upon laminae V to VIII.

The gate control theory may be summarized as follows.

The ongoing activity which precedes a stimulus is carried solely by the small fiber system and tends to keep the gate open and ready to receive new impulses.

A superimposed peripheral stimulus will activate both the small and large fiber systems. The discharge from the latter initially fires the tract neurons (T-cells) in laminae V to VIII through the direct facilitatory route, then partially closes the gate through its action on lamina III neurons (facilitation of presynaptic inhibition).

If the stimulus is prolonged, the large fiber system adapts, resulting in a relative increase in small fiber system activity; the gate opens, further increasing activity in laminae V to VIII.

If, however, the large fiber system is activated by the proper stimulus (vibration), its activity increases and the gate tends to close, diminishing activity in Rexed laminae V to VIII.

The gating mechanism in the spinal cord is under the control of the brain. In this way, brain mechanisms concerned with attention, emotion, and memory can influence pain impulses in the spinal cord.

Present Concepts

The present status of our understanding of pain mechanisms can be summarized by the following observations.

The pain receptor is not specific for pain stimuli but is specialized. Below a certain threshold, a noxious or painful stimulus will elicit responses from free nerve endings. Intense stimulation, however, will elicit responses from all types of receptors.

Pain impulses are conducted via the small A-delta fibers and C-fibers (peripheral nerve). The larger A-beta fibers also play a role in pain mechanisms.

The spinal cord posterior horn is a center for integration of pain mechanisms. It integrates activity arriving from the periphery with that arriving from cortical and subcortical regions.

Pain impulses are conducted in the neuraxis via two major pathways. These are a direct (neospinothalamic and trigeminothalamic) pathway and an indirect, multisynaptic (spinoreticulothalamic) pathway.

The direct ascending pathway projects upon posterior nuclei of the thalamus (ventral posterolateral, ventral posteromedial, and posterior group), whereas the multisynaptic pathway projects upon the intralaminar nuclei of the thalamus.

The cortical projection areas include the primary somethestic cortex of the parietal lobe, the frontal cortex, and the limbic lobe. The parietal cortex is concerned with the appreciation of the sharp, well-localized type of pain; the frontal cortex is concerned with intellectual appreciation and affective reaction; and the limbic lobe is concerned with the memory of painful experience and the emotional reaction to pain. Pain can be appreciated at subcortical levels, primarily in the thalamus.

Abnormalities in Pain Sensation

Definitions

Several abnormalities of pain sensation are encountered in clinical practice. The most common are the following.

Analgesia   This is a specific absence of pain in a certain cutaneous area. All other modalities of sensation are otherwise intact.

Anesthesia   This is a total loss of all sensation (including pain) in a cutaneous area.

Hyperalgesia   This is a state of increased sensitivity to painful stimuli.

Hyperpathia   This is a state of increased sensitivity in which pain has an unpleasant, distressing quality.

Dysesthesia   This is a continuous burning or pricking sensation not necessarily associated with pain.

Paresthesia   This is a feeling of tingling or pins and needles.

Syndromes

Phantom Limb Pain   Following amputation of a limb or part of a limb, many patients remain conscious of the amputated part. Some patients even try to use the amputated part and often experience sensation in it. This consists of the sensation of tingling, of heat and cold, or of heaviness. Some amputees describe burning, shooting, or crushing pains. These sensations are frequent following amputations that were associated with long-term pain. Phantom limb pain may subside spontaneously or may persist for years.

The basic mechanisms underlying phantom limb pain remain controversial. Pain pathways have been interrupted at the peripheral nerve level (neurectomy), dorsal root (rhizotomy), sympathetic chain (sympathectomy), and lateral funiculus (cordotomy) of the spinal cord without constant and lasting effects. The collected evidence points to the involvement of multiple areas (both peripheral and central) in the genesis of phantom limb pain. It is believed that abnormal inputs secondary to trauma of the limb or amputation change the pattern of information processing in the central nervous system, so that a closed, self-exciting neuronal loop is established in the posterior horn of the spinal cord which triggers impulses to the brain and gives rise to pain. The slightest irritation to the amputated limb further triggers this reverberating chain of active neurons and propagates the abnormal process for years. Although this theory is attractive, it fails to explain all the manifestations of the phantom limb syndrome.

Causalgia   This is a distressing, painful condition that follows abrupt and violent deformation of peripheral nerves, such as occurs in high velocity missile injury. Thus, it is typically seen in those wounded in combat. Causalgic pain is burning in character and is elicited after even the most gentle touch to the injured area. The pain is so distressing that patients with causalgia try to protect the injured limb by covering it or even by immobilizing it. Like the phantom limb pain, attempts at relief of causalgic pain by sectioning the peripheral nerve, the dorsal root or the spinal cord, by placing lesions in the somatosensory cortex, or even by amputating the affected limb have met with as much failure as success. The evidence again points toward abnormal activity at multiple levels of the nervous system, both peripheral and central.

Neuralgia   Neuralgias are characterized by severe, unremitting, recurring pain in the distribution of a spinal or cranial nerve. The pain is lightning or burning in quality and is usually precipitated by stimulation of the cutaneous area supplied by the nerve. In trigeminal neuralgia, the pain is lightning and stabbing in character, paroxysmal, and triggered by eating, talking, or brushing the teeth. It is limited to the sensory distribution of the trigeminal nerve in the face.

In herpetic neuraliga, a disorder associated with infection of the dorsal root ganglion and the adjacent sensory root by herpes zoster virus, the pain is distressingly burning (hyperpathic) in the distribution of the affected sensory root.

All of the above pain syndromes share the following characteristics.

Pain can be triggered by both noxious (painful) and non-noxious peripheral stimuli.

Although the peripheral input from receptors is an essential element in the genesis of pain, the role of other factors seems to be of equal importance. These factors include sympathetic activity, auditory and visual inputs, anxiety, and emotional disturbances. All of these factors probably act upon a disturbed central neural process to modify the peripheral input.

Pain persists long after the pathologic process that triggered the pain subsides. This may suggest the existence of an abnormal, reverberating, self-perpetuating central neuronal pool that perpetuates this pain. It may also suggest a memory mechanism for pain.

Pain may be triggered from areas not in the vicinity of the original pathologic process.

Pain is usually resistant to all known methods of treatment. Although various modes of treatment may afford relief for a period of time, pain frequently recurs with its original intensity.

Relief of Pain

Methods for relief of pain can be grouped into three categories: pharmacologic agents, ablation procedures, and stimulation procedures. The last two have been used in the treatment of intractable pain after failure of pharmacologic agents to provide relief.

Pharmacologic Agents

Several analgesic and anesthetic agents have been used over the years to relieve pain. These agents may act on one site (*e.g.*, receptor, dorsal horn, etc.) or on multiple sites. Aspirin, for example, seems to exert its analgesic effect upon the receptor site as well as centrally. Nitrous oxide in analgesic doses seems to exert an effect upon the midbrain reticular formation. Anesthetic blocks of trigger points, sensitive skin areas, peripheral nerves, or sympathetic ganglia have also been used in an attempt to reduce the total sensory input to the spinal cord.

Ablation Procedures

Besides sectioning of peripheral nerves (neurectomy) and the dorsal root (rhizotomy) in the treatment of phantom limb pain and causalgia, surgeons have attempted to section the central pain pathways to relieve intractable pain. The interruption of these central pathways has been attempted at different levels of the neuraxis. Unfortunately, pain either is not abolished or recurs after a period of time.

Spinal Cord The pain-conducting pathways in the spinal cord have been interrupted by sectioning the anterolateral part of the spinal cord (anterolateral cordotomy). To be effective, the section should be performed bilaterally a few segments apart. The sectioning technique has been perfected so that it can be done by a needle electrode introduced percutaneously into the spinal cord under X-ray screen visualization (percutaneous cordotomy). Once the electrode is in place, a radiofrequency lesion is placed while the patient is sedated but awake.

The pain-conducting pathways have also been interrupted as they cross in the anterior white commissure of the spinal cord (spinal commissurotomy).

Medulla Oblongata Interruption of the descending tract of the trigeminal nerve in the medulla oblongata (trigeminal tractotomy) is done to relieve the pain encountered in cancer and neuralgias. The approach to the trigeminal tract can be an open one or a closed one using a needle electrode accurately localized. The tract should be sectioned below the obex to preserve touch sensibility over the face.

Pons Interruption of the pain-conducting pathways in the pons has recently been attempted using the stereotaxic technique, but the results are discouraging. In one series, the mortality rate was high. Further studies to perfect this approach are in progress.

Midbrain Earlier attempts at open interruption of the spinothalamic pathway in the midbrain have been virtually abandoned due to high mortality. Interruption of the pathway through a stereotaxic approach has been successful and continues to be used.

Thalamus Stereotaxic lesions have been placed in the posterior thalamus (thalamotomy) to relieve intractable pain. The lesion is usually aimed at the intralaminar nuclei, but often involves part of the medial and lateral nuclear groups. The mechanism by which thalamotomy relieves pain remains controversial. It may be due to interruption of the slow conducting, multisynaptic reticulothalamic pathways or to the alteration of thalamic neuronal mechanisms in such a way as to inhibit the spinal interneuronal pool. To be effective, thalamotomies must be bilateral. Lesions have also been placed in the internal medullary lamina (thalamolaminotomy) and the pulvinar nucleus with good results.

Cerebral Cortex Lesions of both the prefrontal cortex (prefrontal lobectomy or lobotomy) and the cingulum (cingulumotomy) have been attempted to relieve pain. The effect of such lesions has been to abolish the affective and emotional aspects of pain, thus reducing the suffering of the patient.

Stimulation Procedures

Stimulation procedures to relieve pain are relatively recent. They were prompted by the discovery of Melzack and Wall of gating mechanisms in the spinal cord and the role of large fiber activation in inhibiting pain mechanisms. Since then, several stimulation techniques have been used at different levels of the neuraxis to relieve pain.

Peripheral Nerve Peripheral nerves have been stimulated through the transcutaneous approach for relief of pain with excellent results, especially in patients with peripheral nerve injury. This method has also been used to test patient tolerance of stimulators prior to spinal cord implantation of an electrode.

Spinal Cord Stimulation of the posterior column through intradurally implanted electrodes has been used to relieve pain. The patient can usually select the frequency and voltage which gives him the most relief from pain. In some patients, a curious phenomenon has been noted of gradual reduction and ultimate disappearance of the pain following cessation of the stimulation. The initial high rate (50 to 80%) of success in posterior column stimulation usually drops to 25% or less.

Midbrain Earlier reports of stimulus-produced analgesia following stimulation of the periaqueductal gray matter in animals have been confirmed in man.

Thalamus Stimulation electrodes have been placed in the posteroventral medial nucleus (PVM) to relieve facial pain. The mechanism of action of such stimulation remains controversial. It is believed, however, to effect its action locally, at the thalamic level, by exerting an inhibitory effect upon the intralaminar nuclei. Stimulation electrodes have also been placed in the posteroventral lateral nucleus with good results.

Internal Capsule The internal capsule is believed to contain descending cortical fibers that are inhibitory to the thalamus. Stimulators placed in the internal capsule have been effective in the relief of pain. Their mechanism of action is most likely through enhancement of the descending inhibitory fiber system.

Septal Area Stimulation of the septal area in the region anterior and lateral to the columns of the fornix has been effective in the relief of pain. This method is no longer in general use because patients treated with this method develop a rage reaction.

Acupuncture

Acupuncture refers to the technique of placing needles into specific areas of the skin to cure various disorders. In China, acupuncture has been used to induce a state of profound analgesia for surgical procedures. Acupuncture has also been effective in relief of pain in many patients. The analgesia and relief of pain are effected by twirling the needles for a prolonged period of time. Although the exact mechanism of action of acupuncture analgesia is not fully understood, it is most probably due to hyperstimulation of peripheral neural pathways that will ultimately close the gating mechanism in the spinal cord and thus interefere with the conduction of pain.

The site of insertion of needles for operative acupuncture analgesia remains an enigma. Needles are inserted in the pinna of each ear for stomach operations and in the wrists for thyroid operations. These placements are obviously not consistent with known segmental neural organization. It is conceivable, however, that specific areas of the skin have a heightened input into the reticular formation, which may be instrumental in the production of the observed analgesia. Experimental evidence has shown that electrical stimulation of certain areas in the reticular formation can produce analgesia in large segments of the body.

Although acupuncture is currently being used as a method of pain relief, many questions related to it remain unanswered.

References

Bishop, B.: Pain: Its Physiology and Rationale for Management. Part II. Analgesic Systems of the CNS. Phys Ther 60 (1980) 21–23.

Duggan, A.W.: Enkephalins as Transmitters in the Central Nervous System. Circ Res 46 (1980) I-49–I-153.

Kerr, F.W.L.: An Overview of Neural Mechanisms of Pain. Neurosci Res Program Bull 16 (1978) 30–65.

Kubek, M.J.; Wilber, J.F.: Regional Distribution of Leucine-Enkephalins in Hypothalamic and Extrahypothalamic Loci of the Human Nervous System. Neurosci Lett 18 (1980) 155–161.

Meyerson, B.A.; Boëthius, J.; Carlsson, A.M.: Percutaneous Central Gray Stimulation for Cancer Pain. Appl Neurophysiol 41 (1978) 57–65.

Sherman, J.E.; Liebeskind, J.C.: An Endorphinergic Centrifugal Substrate of Pain Modulation: Recent Findings, Current Concepts and Complexities. In: Pain. Research Publication of Association for Research in Nervous and Mental Disease, No. 58, pp. 191–204, Ed. by J.J. Bonica. Raven Press, New York, 1980.

Snyder, S.H.: Peptide Neurotransmitter with Possible Involvement in Pain Perception. In: Pain. Research Publication of Association for Research in Nervous and Mental Disease, No. 58, pp. 233–243, Ed. by J.J. Bonica. Raven Press, New York, 1980.

21

Higher Brain Functions

Hemisphere Specialization

The concept of cerebral dominance has undergone significant modification in recent years, primarily because of studies on patients with unilateral brain damage. The older concept which assigned to the left hemisphere a dominant role in higher cerebral function, with the right hemisphere being subordinate to the dominant hemisphere, has been replaced by a new concept of hemisphere specialization, which implies that each hemisphere is in some way dominant for the execution of specific tasks. According to this new concept, the left hemisphere is dominant, or specialized, for comprehension and expression of language, whereas the right hemisphere is specialized for complex nonverbal perceptual tasks and for some aspects of visual and spatial perception. Thus, lesions of the left hemisphere are associated with disorders of language (aphasia or dysphasia), whereas lesions of the right hemisphere are associated with impairment of visuospatial and visuoconstructive skills. Patients with right hemisphere lesions are more likely to show such manifestations as constructional apraxia (inability to construct or draw figures and shapes), dressing apraxia, denial of the left side of the body (denial that their left side is part of their body), and hemineglect (visual and spatial neglect of the left side of their space including their own parts). Some of the deficits associated with left and right hemisphere lesions are discussed below.

Language

Language is defined as the ability of the individual to communicate through the use of symbols. A disorder in language function (aphasia or dysphasia) includes disturbances in the ability to comprehend (decoding) and/or program (coding) the symbols necessary for communication. Aphasia is most

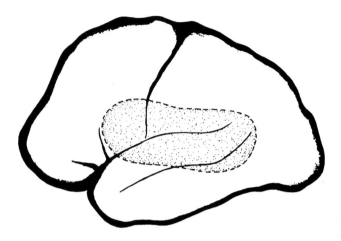

21–1 Schematic diagram showing the perisylvian core area concerned with language.

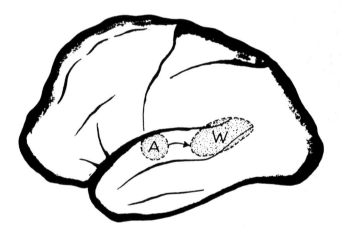

21–2 Schematic diagram showing transmission of auditory symbols from the primary auditory cortex (*A*) to Wernicke's area (*W*) for comprehension.

frequently encountered in cortical lesions in the left hemisphere, although it may occur in subcortical lesions. The cortical area of the left hemisphere invariably involved in aphasia is a central core surrounding the sylvian fissure (Fig. 21–1). The perisylvian core area is surrounded by a larger region in which aphasia occurs less frequently.

The sequence of complex cortical activities during the production of language may be simplified as follows. When a word is heard, the output from the primary auditory area (Heschl's gyrus) is conveyed to an adjacent

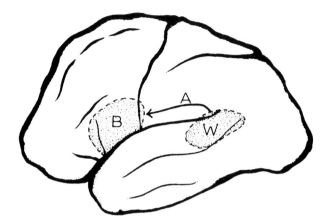

21-3 Schematic diagram showing transmission of comprehended words from Wernicke's area (*W*) via the arcuate fasciculus (*A*) to Broca's area (*B*) for speech.

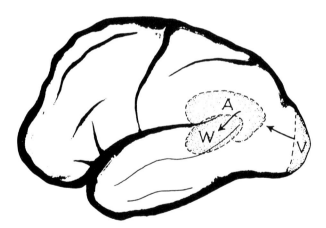

21-4 Schematic diagram showing transmission of output from the primary visual area (*V*) to the angular gyrus (*A*) where the auditory form of the word is elicited from Wernicke's area (*W*).

cortical area (Wernicke's area) where the word is comprehended (Fig. 21–2). If the word is to be spoken, the comprehended pattern is transmitted via the arcuate fasciculus from Wernicke's area to Broca's area of speech in the inferior frontal gyrus (Fig. 21–3). If the word is to be read, the output from the primary visual area in the occipital cortex is transmitted to the angular gyrus, which in turn arouses the corresponding auditory form of the word in Wernicke's area (Fig. 21–4).

For didactic purposes, aphasia is classified into Broca's, Wernicke's, conduction, transcortical, anomic, global, and pure word-deafness. The different varieties of aphasia can be classified into those with abnormal repetition (Broca's, Wernicke's, and conduction aphasias), those in which repetition is preserved (transcortical and anomic aphasias), and total aphasia (global).

Broca's aphasia is also known as nonfluent, anterior, motor, or expressive aphasia. This type of aphasia is characterized by a decreased and labored language output of 10 words or less per minute, during which the patient utilizes facial grimaces, body posturing, deep breaths, and hand gestures to aid output; characteristically, small grammatical words and the endings of nouns and verbs are omitted, resulting in telegraphic speech. The speech output is thus unmelodic and dysrhythmic (dysprosody). In spite of the above limitations in verbal output, the speech often conveys considerable information. These patients are unable to repeat what has been said to them. Although Broca's aphasia is usually attributed to a lesion in Broca's area of the frontal lobe, recent correlations of aphasic speech with lesions seen on computerized tomography (CT scan) have shown that the lesion is frequently larger than Broca's area and involves the insula and the insulolenticular area. Since the temporal lobe is intact in these patients, auditory comprehension is usually intact.

Wernicke's aphasia is also known as fluent, posterior, sensory, or receptive aphasia. In contrast to Broca's aphasia, the quantity of output in this type ranges from low normal to supernormal with an output in most patients of 100 to 150 words per minute. Speech is produced with little or no effort, articulation and phrase length are normal, and the output is melodic. Pauses to search for a meaningful word are frequent and substitution within language (paraphasia) is common; this may be substitution of a syllable (literal paraphasia), phonemic substitution of a word (kench for wrench), (verbal paraphasia), semantic substitution (knife for fork), or substitution of a meaningless nonsense word (neologism). If a word is not readily available, the patient may attempt to describe it and the description may necessitate yet another description, resulting in a meaningless output (circumlocution). Paraphasias may also occur in Broca's aphasia, but these are articulatory errors, in contrast to those in Wernicke's aphasia, which are true substitutions. In spite of the fluent nature of speech output in Wernicke's aphasia, little information is conveyed (empty speech). As in Broca's aphasia, patients with Wernicke's aphasia are unable to repeat what is said to them. Wernicke's aphasia is attributed to a lesion in Wernicke's area in the posterior temporal lobe.

Conduction aphasia is characterized by fluent paraphasic speech, intact comprehension, poor naming, and repetition. Classically, patients with conduction aphasia cannot read out loud because of paraphasic intervention. Writing usually involves the use of incorrect letters in words. Pathology in these patients is usually located in the posterior perisylvian region and interrupts the output from Wernicke's area to Broca's area via the arcuate fasciculus. Recent reports suggest that conduction aphasia may result from lesions deep to the insula affecting the extreme capsule.

Transcortical aphasia has been subdivided into motor, sensory, and mixed types. All are characterized by preserved repetition. In transcortical motor aphasia, verbal output is nonfluent and comprehension is intact, but writing is invariably abnormal. Pathology in this type of aphasia is located in the dominant frontal lobe in the neighborhood of Broca's area. In transcortical sensory aphasia, speech output is fluent and paraphasic, comprehension is poor and there are associated difficulties in reading and writing. Pathology in such cases is usually in the border zone between the temporal and parietal lobes in the neighborhood of Wernicke's area. Mixed transcortical aphasia, also known as isolation of the speech area, is characterized by nonfluent speech output, poor comprehension, and inability to name, read, or write. Pathology in these patients usually spares the perisylvian core region but involves the surrounding border zone or watershed area, which is supplied by the most distal tributaries of the middle cerebral artery.

Anomic aphasia, also known as amnestic or nominal aphasia, is characterized primarily by word-finding difficulty. Verbal output is fluent and empty with little or no paraphasia, comprehension is relatively normal, and repetition is intact. Anomic aphasia is often a sequela of any type of recovering aphasia. Although common, this type of aphasia is the most difficult to localize.

Global aphasia is a severe form of aphasia in which all the major functions of language (verbal output, comprehension, repetition, naming, reading, and writing) are severely impaired. Pathology is invariably extensive, involving much of the dominant hemisphere in the middle cerebral artery territory.

Pure word-deafness, also known as verbal auditory agnosia, is characterized by poor comprehension of spoken language and by poor repetition with intact comprehension of written language, naming, writing, and spontaneous speech. The lesion in this type of disorder either affects the primary auditory area or disconnects this area from Wernicke's area. This syndrome is pure in the sense that it is not associated with other aphasic symptoms.

Ideomotor Apraxia

Ideomotor apraxia is the inability to carry out, on verbal command, an activity that can be performed perfectly well spontaneously. It is implied that this "inability" is not due to comprehension, motor, or sensory defects. Thus, a patient with ideomotor apraxia will not be able to carry out a verbal command to walk, stop, salute, open a door, stick out the tongue, etc.

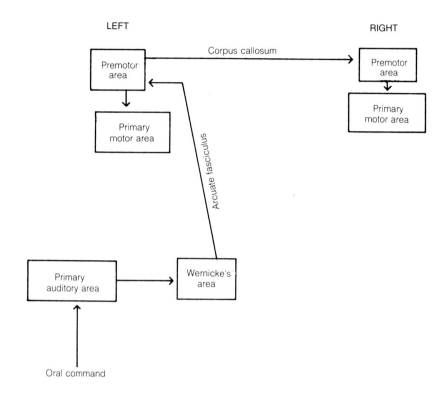

21-5 Schematic diagram showing the pathways involved in carrying out a motor skill in response to an oral command.

To appreciate the pathophysiology of ideomotor apraxia, it should be understood that for a skilled task to be performed, several events must take place. For example, the command to walk, if oral, reaches the primary auditory area and is relayed to the left auditory association cortex (Wernicke's area) for comprehension. Wernicke's area is connected to the ipsilateral premotor area (motor association cortex, area 6) via the arcuate fasciculus. The motor association area on the left side is connected to the primary motor cortex (area 4) on the left side. When the person is asked to carry out a command with the left hand, the information is relayed from the left premotor area to the right premotor area (via the anterior part of the corpus callosum) and from there to the right primary motor area, which controls movements of the left side of the body (Fig. 21-5). Based on the above anatomic connections, three clinical varieties of ideomotor apraxia have been recognized: parietal, in which the lesion is in the anterior-inferior parietal lobe of the dominant hemisphere; sympathetic, in which the lesion is in the left premotor area; and callosal, in which the lesion is in the anterior part of the corpus callosum.

Visuoconstructive Apraxia

Visuoconstructive apraxia, also known as constructional apraxia, is the inability of the individual to put together or articulate component parts to form a single shape or figure, such as assembling blocks to form a design or drawing four lines to form a shape. It implies a defect in perceiving spatial relationships among the component parts. Visuoconstructive apraxia was originally described in lesions of the left (dominant) posterior parietal area. Subsequently it was shown that this type of apraxia is more prevalent and severe in right hemisphere parietal lesions.

Alexia (Acquired Dyslexia)

Alexia is the acquired inability to comprehend written language. It occurs in an individual who loses the ability to read normally following brain damage. It is thus a distinct entity different from developmental dyslexia, which is an inability to learn to read normally from childhood. There are two major types of alexia: pure alexia (alexia without agraphia, pure word-blindness) and alexia with agraphia (parietal alexia).

In pure alexia, the defect in comprehension may manifest itself in an inability to read letters (literal alexia) or words (verbal alexia) or may be global with a total inability to read either letters or words (global alexia). The anatomic substrate of pure alexia is usually a lesion in the left primary visual area coupled with another lesion in the splenium of the corpus callosum (Fig. 21–6). The lesion in the left visual area prevents visual stimuli entering the left hemisphere from reaching the left (dominant) angular gyrus, which is necessary for comprehension of written language. The lesion in the splenium of the corpus callosum prevents visual stimuli entering the intact right visual area from reaching the left angular gyrus. Writing is normal in this type of alexia, but the patient cannot read what he writes. Cases have been described of pure alexia without a splenial lesion. In such cases, one deep lesion in the left occipitotemporal region isolates both occipital cortices from the left speech area in the angular gyrus.

In alexia with agraphia, there is a defect in both reading comprehension and writing. The reading disorder is usually verbal (inability to read words). The writing difficulty is usually severe. The anatomic substrate of this type

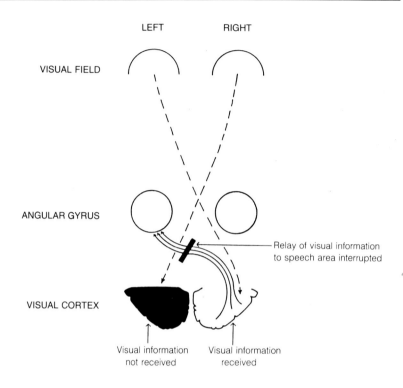

21–6 Schematic diagram showing the neural substrate of the syndrome of pure alexia without agraphia.

of alexia is a lesion in the dominant angular gyrus, hence the name parietal alexia.

Agnosia

Agnosia is the inability of the individual to recognize perceived sensory information. Implied in this definition is an intact sensory processing of the input, clear mental state, and intact naming ability. The concept of agnosia has been severely criticized by many authors and anatomic localization of the different varieties of agnosia has not yet been resolved.

Agnosia is often modality-specific: visual, auditory, and tactile.

Visual agnosias include visual object agnosia (inability to recognize objects presented visually), visual color agnosia (inability to recognize colors), prosopagnosia (inability to recognize faces, including one's own face, cars, types of trees, etc.), picture agnosia, and simultanagnosia (inability to recognize the whole, although parts of the whole are correctly appreciated).

Auditory agnosia is the inability to recognize sounds in the presence of otherwise adequate hearing. It includes auditory verbal agnosia (inability to recognize spoken language or pure word-deafness), auditory sound agnosia (inability to recognize nonverbal sounds such as animal sounds, sound of running water, sound of a bell, etc.), and sensory amusia (inability to recognize music).

Tactile agnosia is the inability to recognize objects in the tactile modality. The distinction between tactile agnosia and astereognosia is not clear. It includes amorphognosia (impaired recognition of size and shape of objects), ahylognosia (impaired discrimination of quality of objects, such as weight, texture, density), and asymbolia (impaired recognition of the identity of an object in the absence of amorphognosia and ahylognosia). Asymbolia is used by some authors to refer to tactile agnosia.

Callosal Syndrome

The disconnection of the right from the left hemisphere by lesions in the corpus callosum results in the isolation of each hemisphere in such a way that each has its own learning processes and memories which are inaccessible to the other hemisphere. The following are some of the effects seen in such patients.

Visual Effects

Each hemisphere retains its own visual images and memories, but only the left hemisphere is able to communicate, because of the callosal disconnection, what it sees through speech or writing.

Hemialexia

Patients are unable to read material presented in the left hemifield. This occurs when the splenium of the corpus callosum is involved in the lesion. Such visually presented material reaches the right occipital cortex but cannot be comprehended because the splenial lesion interferes with transmission of the visual image to the left (dominant) angular gyrus (Fig. 21–7).

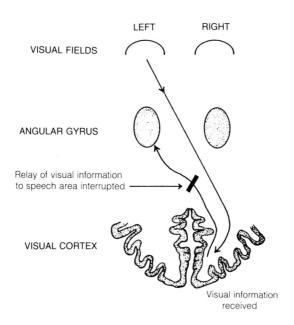

21–7 Schematic illustration of the mechanism of hemialexia.

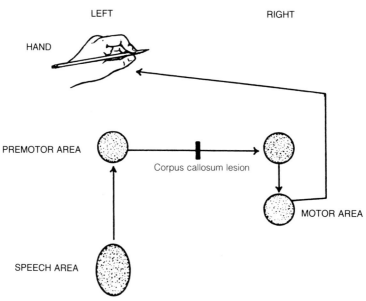

21–8 Schematic diagram illustrating the mechanism of unilateral (left) ideomotor apraxia.

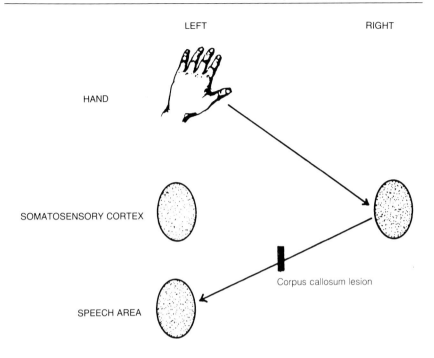

21–9 Simplified schematic diagram showing the anatomic substrate of unilateral (left) tactile anomia.

Unilateral (Left) Ideomotor Apraxia

In response to verbal commands, patients are unable to carry out with the left hand some behavior which is readily carried out with the right hand. The verbal command is adequately received by the left (dominant) hemisphere but, because of the callosal disconnection, it cannot reach the right hemisphere which controls left hand movement.

Unilateral (Left) Agraphia

Patients with callosal lesions are unable to write using their left hand (Fig. 21–8).

Unilateral (Left) Tactile Anomia

Patients with callosal disconnection are unable, with eyes closed, to name or describe an object placed in the left hand, although they readily name the same object in the right hand. The object placed in the left hand is correctly perceived in the right somatosensory cortex but cannot be identified because of the callosal lesion which disconnects the right parietal cortex from the left (dominant) hemisphere (Fig. 21–9).

Left Ear Extinction

Patients with callosal lesions show left ear extinction when sounds are simultaneously presented to both ears (dichotic listening). Sounds presented to the left ear reach the right temporal cortex but, because of the callosal disconnection, are not relayed to the left temporal cortex (dominant) for comprehension.

There is evidence to suggest functional specialization of different segments of the corpus callosum. Thus, lesions in the posterior part of the corpus callosum (splenium) are associated with hemialexia, lesions of the anterior part are associated with left ideomotor apraxia, and lesions of the middle part are associated with left hand agraphia; lesions in the middle and posterior parts result in left hand tactile anomia.

Musical Faculty

With the allocation of specific functions to each hemisphere, the question has arisen as to which hemisphere is specialized for music. In this context, one should separate musical perception from musical execution and should consider both the naive listener and the professional. Whereas a naive listener perceives music in its overall melodic contour, the professional perceives music as a relation between musical elements (language). With this type of analysis, it is conceivable that the naive listener perceives music in the right hemisphere whereas the professional perceives music in the left hemisphere. On the other hand, musical execution (singing) seems to be a function of the right hemisphere irrespective of musical knowledge and training.

Learning and Memory

The role of the nervous system in learning and memory has been studied using behavioral experiments (Pavlovian conditioning and problem maze), neurosurgical techniques (ablation of selective areas of the brain), electrophysiologic methods (neural pathways and mechanisms), biochemical studies (role of RNA and other proteins), neuropharmacologic approach (effect of drugs on synaptic transmission and on intracellular processes), and studies on humans with memory deficit (amnesia). The processes of learning and memory seem to depend upon two distinct changes: an electrical membrane event of a temporary nature and a more stable, permanent change in the chemistry of the nervous system. The discovery that DNA and RNA can act as codes for synaptic transmission has led to the theory that these substances are responsible for learning and for transforming short-term memories into permanent stores.

It is generally acknowledged that there are three types of memory; these are 1) immediate, 2) short-term, and 3) long-term. These are characterized by the duration of recall in each type. The duration of recall in immediate memory is a matter of seconds. An example of this is the recall of names of persons or telephone numbers within seconds. Short-term memory may be recalled for minutes to hours, as occurs in the recall of recent events. Long-term memory can be recalled months or years after it has been stored. Pathologic processes in the brain may affect one type of memory and spare others. Older people lose the ability to recall what they ate earlier in the day but can recall, with the minutest details, an experience they had many years earlier. People who suffer head trauma in car accidents are unable to recall what transpired, for minutes to hours, before the accident, but the recall of older memories remains intact. There are indications for anatomic specialization of each type of memory. The anatomic substrate for immediate memory seems to involve the appropriate primary sensory area as well as the corresponding association cortex. Ablation of the primary auditory and the adjacent association auditory cortices will abolish the immediate recall of auditory memory. Damage to the temporal lobe (involving the hippocampus) is usually associated with recent (short-term) memory loss. Such a deficit rarely if ever occurs following unilateral hippocampal lesions; it is more often encountered following bilateral lesions. Short-term memory is also lost in patients with thiamine deficiency (Wernicke-Korsakoff syndrome), in which the mamillary bodies are affected. The mamillary bodies are connected with the hippocampus and the defect in short-term memory can be explained by the interruption of the mamillohippocampal pathway. Although the role of the hippocampus in recent memory has been emphasized in the literature, it should be stated that the damage to the hippocampus, in all human cases reported, also involved adjacent parts of the hippocampal gyrus. In addition, cases have been reported with congenital maldevelopment of the hippocampus without concomitant loss of recent memory. There is mounting evidence to suggest that the dorsomedial nucleus of the thalamus plays an important role in recent memory.

In contrast to immediate and short-term memory, long-term memory does not seem to be discretely localized to specific cortical areas, but rather is related to the integrity of the total cerebral cortex and possibly subcortical structures as well. Diseases which may involve the cerebral cortex in a diffuse manner, like the presenile dementias (Alzheimer's disease), have as a part of their manifestations the loss of long-term memory.

Repeated stimulation of a cortical area has been shown to establish a reverberating circuit that will continue to have rhythmic action potentials for minutes after cessation of the stimulus. Furthermore, repeated use of a synapse has been shown to give rise to the phenomenon of post-tetanic potentiation in which the synaptic potentials are increased. The above two mechanisms (reverberating circuits and post-tetanic potentiation) have been invoked in the genesis of immediate memory. It is of interest to note in this connection that the hippocampus is known to show particularly long post-tetanic potentiation.

Immediate memory may be explained as a transient electrical alteration at the synapse; longer lasting short-term and long-term memory may be explained as an actual physical or chemical alteration of the synapse. Several such alterations have been described in different experimental situations and include changes in the number and size of synaptic terminals as well as their chemical composition. Changes in the postsynaptic neurons have also been invoked. Such changes in the pre- or postsynaptic components of the synapse have been thought to facilitate the transmission of impulses at the synapse and thus establish a memory code or ingram.

Several biochemical studies have suggested a role for protein and RNA in memory mechanisms. Evidence for this has been obtained from 1) experiments in which protein and RNA syntheses were either increased or blocked by drugs, 2) measurement of protein and RNA content of stimulated neuronal systems, and 3) experiments in which learned tasks were presumably transferred from the trained animal to the untrained animal after injection of RNA or protein from the brains of the trained subjects.

References

Albert, M.L.: Alexia. In: Clinical Neuropsychology, pp. 59–91, Ed. by K.M. Heilman and E. Valenstein. Oxford University Press, Inc., New York, 1979.

Benson, D.F.: Aphasia. In: Clinical Neuropsychology, pp 22–58, Ed. by K.M. Heilman and E. Valenstein. Oxford University Press, Inc., New York, 1979.

Benson, D.F.: Aphasia, Alexia, and Agraphia. Clinical Neurology and Neurosurgery Monographs, Vol. 1, Ed. by G.H. Glaser. Churchill Livingstone Inc., New York, 1979.

Benton, A.: Visuoperceptive, Visuospatial, and Visuoconstructive Disorders. In: Clinical Neuropsychology, pp. 186–232, Ed. by K.M. Heilman and E. Valenstein. Oxford University Press, Inc., New York, 1979.

Bogen, J.E.: The Callosal Syndrome. In: Clinical Neuropsychology, pp. 308–359, Ed. by K.M. Heilman and E. Valenstein. Oxford University Press, Inc., New York, 1979.

Butters, N.: Amnesic Disorders. In: Clinical Neuropsychology, pp. 439–474, Ed. by K.M. Heilman and E. Valenstein. Oxford University Press, Inc., New York, 1979.

Damasio, A.R.: Notes on the Anatomical Basis of Pure Alexia and of Color Anomia. In: Aphasia, Assessment and Treatment, pp. 126–131, Ed. by M. Taylor and S. Höök. Almqvist & Wiksell International, Stockholm, 1978.

Damasio, H.; Damasio, A.R.: The Anatomical Basis of Conduction Aphasia. Brain 103 (1980) 337–350.

Funkenstein, H.H.: Approaches to Hemispheric Asymmetries. In: Current Neurology, Vol. 1, pp. 336–359, Ed. by H.R. Tyler and D.M. Dawson. Houghton Mifflin, Medical Division, Boston, 1978.

Heilman, K.M.: Apraxia. In: Clinical Neuropsychology, pp. 159–185, Ed. by K.M. Heilman and E. Valenstein. Oxford University Press, Inc., New York, 1979.

Kertesz, A.; Harlock, W.; Coates, R.: Computer Tomographic Localization, Lesion Size and Prognosis in Aphasia and Nonverbal Impairment. Brain Language 8 (1979) 34–50.

Mazzochi, F.; Vignolo, L.A.: Localisation of Lesions in Aphasia: Clinical-CT Scan Correlations in Stroke Patients. Cortex 15 (1979) 627–654.

Rubens, A.B.: Agnosia. In: Clinical Neuropsychology, pp. 233–267, Ed. by K.M. Heilman and E. Valenstein. Oxford University Press, Inc., New York, 1979.

Warrington, E.K.; Shallice, T.: Word-Form Dyslexia. Brain 103 (1980) 99–112.

Yamadori, A.; Osumi, Y.; Ikeda, H.; Kanazawa, Y.: Left Unilateral Agraphia and Tactile Anomia. Disturbances Seen after Occlusion of the Anterior Cerebral Artery. Arch. Neurol 37 (1980) 88–91.

22

Major Sensory and Motor Pathways

Major Sensory Pathways

Pathway for Conscious Proprioception (Fig. 22–1)

The pathway for kinesthesia (position and vibration sense) and discriminative touch (well-localized touch and two-point discrimination) is the posterior column-medial lemniscus system.

The receptors for this system are in joint capsules and in other locations and include Pacinian corpuscles. Impulses arising in the receptors travel via the thickly myelinated large nerve fibers that enter the spinal cord as the medial division of the posterior (dorsal) root and occupy the posterior funiculus of the spinal cord. Those arising below the sixth thoracic spinal segment form the medial part of the posterior funiculus (gracile tract). Those arising above the sixth thoracic segment form the lateral part of the posterior funiculus (cuneate tract). Fibers in the gracile and cuneate tracts project upon neurons in the posterior column nuclei of the medulla oblongata (nuclei gracilis and cuneatus). Axons of neurons in the posterior column nuclei (second order neurons) decussate in the tegmentum of the medulla oblongata (internal arcuate fibers) to form the medial lemniscus, which ascends throughout the medulla oblongata, pons, and midbrain to terminate upon neurons of the ventral posterolateral nucleus (VPL) of the thalamus. Axons of neurons in this thalamic nucleus (third order neurons) project upon the terminal station of this pathway in the somesthetic (primary sensory) cortex of the parietal lobe.

493

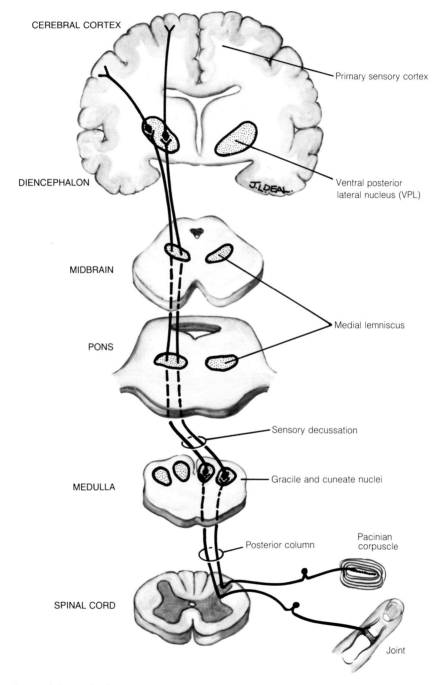

22–1   Schematic diagram of the pathway for kinesthesia and discriminative touch.

Lesions of the posterior column-medial lemniscus system are manifested clinically by the following signs.

1. Inability to identify position of the limb in space with eyes closed. Such patients are unable to tell whether a joint is in a position of flexion or extension.
2. Inability to identify objects placed in the hands, such as keys or coins, from their shape, size, and texture with eyes closed.
3. Loss of two-point discrimination. Such patients are unable to recognize two simultaneously applied stimuli to the skin when the two stimuli are separated by the minimal necessary distance for their proper identification as two stimuli.
4. Inability to perceive vibration when a vibrating tuning fork is applied to a bony prominence.
5. Inability to maintain steady standing posture when eyes are closed and feet are placed close together (Romberg test). Such patients begin to sway and may fall when they close their eyes, which eliminates visual compensation.

The role of the posterior column system in the control of pain is discussed in the chapter on the spinal cord.

Pathways for Nonconscious Proprioception

Nonconscious proprioception is mediated via the two spinocerebellar tracts (Figs. 22–2 and 22–3); these are posterior (dorsal) and anterior (ventral).

The posterior spinocerebellar tract conveys impulses from the muscle spindle and Golgi tendon organ. Such impulses travel via groups Ia, Ib, and II nerve fibers, enter the spinal cord in the medial, thickly myelinated, large diameter fiber portion of the posterior root, and project upon the ipsilateral nucleus dorsalis of Clarke and the accessory cuneate nucleus. Axons of neurons in the nucleus dorsalis of Clarke (second order neurons) form the posterior spinocerebellar tract, which ascends in the lateral funiculus of the spinal cord and the medulla oblongata to reach the cerebellum via the inferior cerebellar peduncle (restiform body). Axons of neurons in the accessory cuneate nucleus form the cuneocerebellar tract, which reaches the cerebellum via the restiform body.

The anterior spinocerebellar tract conveys impulses from the Golgi tendon organ via Ib afferents. Incoming fibers project upon neurons in the posterior horn of the spinal cord (laminae V to VII). Axons of neurons in these laminae decussate to the contralateral lateral funiculus to form the anterior spinocerebellar tract, which ascends throughout the spinal cord, medulla oblongata, pons, and midbrain, loops backward to join the superior cerebellar peduncle (brachium conjunctivum), and enters the cerebellum. The spinocerebellar pathways convey to the cerebellum infor-

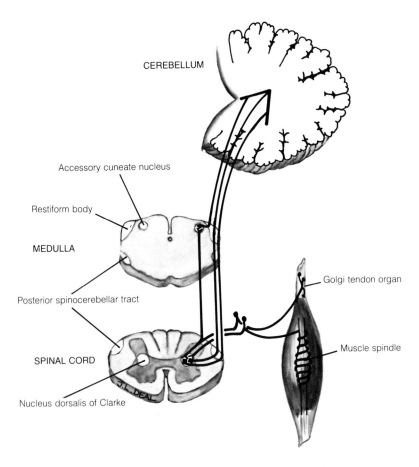

CEREBELLUM

Accessory cuneate nucleus

Restiform body

MEDULLA

Golgi tendon organ

Posterior spinocerebellar tract

Muscle spindle

SPINAL CORD

Nucleus dorsalis of Clarke

22–2 Schematic diagram of the posterior spinocerebellar pathway.

mation about activity of muscles and progress of motion for coordination of movement.

Lesions of the spinocerebellar pathways (as occur in hereditary spinocerebellar degeneration) result in incoordinate movement. Such patients tend to walk with a wide base, stagger, and frequently fall.

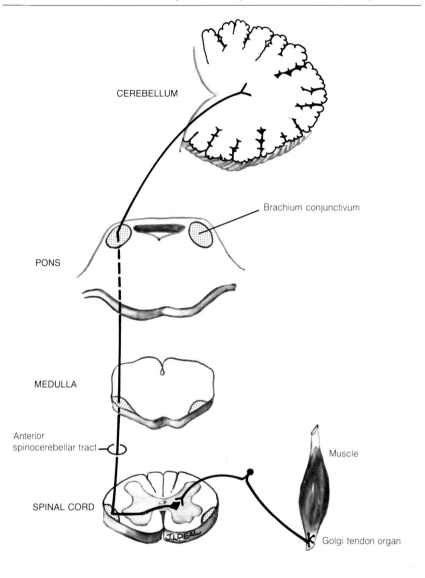

22–3   Schematic diagram of the anterior spinocerebellar pathway.

Pathway for Pain and Temperature

Small diameter, unmyelinated, or thinly myelinated fibers conveying pain and thermal sensations (Fig. 22–4) enter the spinal cord via the lateral division of the dorsal (posterior) root. Within the spinal cord they ascend for one or two segments and project upon neurons in several laminae in the posterior horn. From tract neurons in laminae II and V to VIII, axons cross in the anterior white commissure and form the lateral spinothalamic tract in the lateral funiculus. Sacral fibers are laterally placed and cervical fibers are more medially placed in the tract. The spinothalamic tract ascends throughout the spinal cord and brain stem to project upon neurons in the ventral posterolateral nucleus (VPL) of the thalamus. Axons of VPL neurons project to the somesthetic cortex.

Lesions of the spinothalamic tract result in diminution or loss of pain and thermal sense contralateral to the lesion. When the tract is affected in the spinal cord, the sensory deficit begins one or two segments below the level of the lesion.

The spinothalamic tract may be sectioned surgically (cordotomy) for the relief of intractable pain.

Major Motor Pathways

Cortical Origin

Corticospinal (Pyramidal) Tract (Fig. 22–5)   This is the single most important descending tract. From its origin in the cerebral cortex, it descends through all levels of the neuraxis except the cerebellum. It arises primarily from pyramidal neurons in the sensory motor cortex and passes through the internal capsule, cerebral peduncle, basis pontis, and the pyramids of the medulla oblongata. In the caudal medulla, about 75 to 90% of the fibers decussate through the motor or pyramidal decussation to form the lateral corticospinal tract in the lateral funiculus of the spinal cord. About 8% of pyramidal fibers remain uncrossed and form the anterior corticospinal tract in the anterior funiculus of the spinal cord. Fibers in the anterior corticospinal tract decussate at segmental spinal levels. In the final analysis, therefore, roughly about 98% of fibers in the pyramidal tract are crossed. The remaining 2% of the fibers remain ipsilateral and form the tract of Barnes. Pyramidal tract fibers influence alpha motor neurons directly or via interneurons. They facilitate flexor motor neurons and inhibit extensor motor neurons. The pyramidal tract is important in the initiation of voluntary motor activity. Lesions of this tract result in paralysis. If the lesion is above the level of the motor decussation, the paralysis is contra-

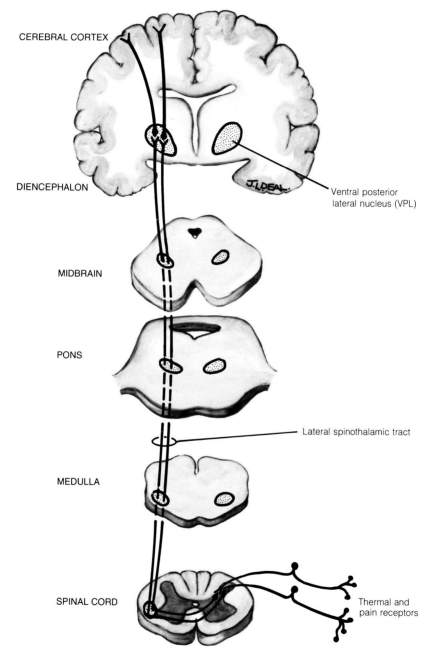

22–4 Schematic diagram of the pathway for specific pain and temperature sensations.

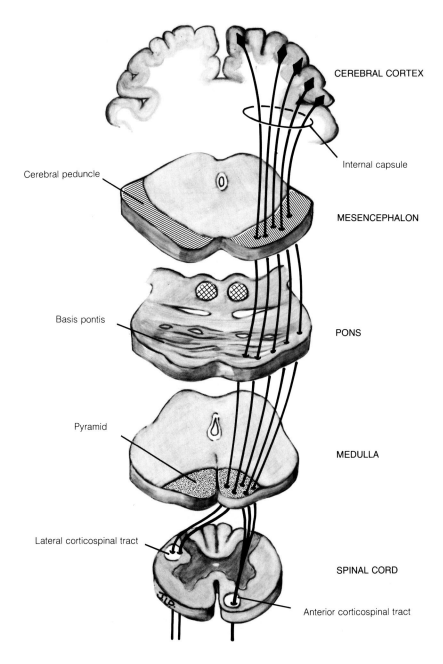

22-5 Schematic diagram of the corticospinal pathway.

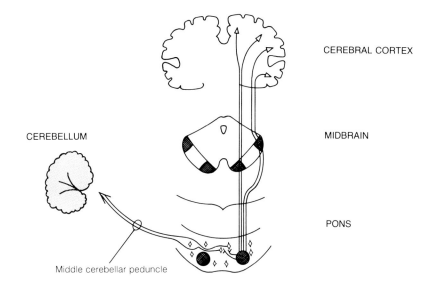

22–6 Schematic diagram of the corticopontocerebellar pathway.

lateral to the site of the lesion. In lesions of the pyramidal tract below the decussation, the paralysis is ipsilateral to the site of the lesion.

Corticopontocerebellar Tract (Fig. 22–6). This tract constitutes by far the largest component of the cortically originating descending fiber system. It is estimated to contain approximately 19 million fibers, in contrast to the pyramidal tract, which contains approximately one million fibers. The tract originates from wide areas of the cerebral cortex, but primarily from the primary sensory and motor cortices, and descends in the internal capsule, cerebral peduncle, and basis pontis, from which its fibers project upon pontine nuclei. Second order neurons from pontine nuclei cross to the contralateral side of the basis pontis, enter the middle cerebellar peduncle (brachium pontis), and project upon the cerebellum. The corticopontocerebellar tract is one of several pathways by which the cerebral cortex influences the cerebellum. It plays a role in the rapid correction of movement. Lesions of the corticopontocerebellar pathway will result in ataxia.

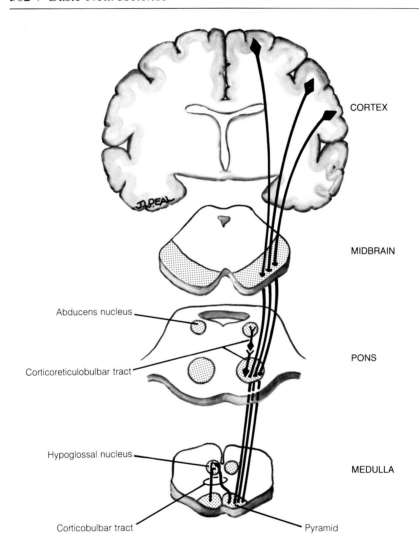

22–7 Schematic diagram of the corticobulbar pathway.

Corticobulbar Tract (Fig. 22-7)   Corticobulbar fibers originate from the same areas in the cerebral cortex that give rise to the corticospinal tract. They descend in the genu of the internal capsule, cerebral peduncle, basis pontis, and pyramid, but do not reach the spinal cord. They project, at different levels of the neuraxis, upon cranial nerve nuclei. Some corticobulbar fibers project directly upon cranial nerve nuclei (trigeminal, facial, and hypoglossal); the majority, however, project upon reticular nuclei before reaching the cranial nerve nuclei. Thus, the latter system is known as the corticoreticulobulbar tract. The majority of cranial nerve nuclei receive bilateral cortical input. Interruption of the corticobulbar or the corticoreticulobulbar fiber system results in paresis (weakness) of the muscles supplied by the corresponding cranial nerve nucleus. This condition is known as pseudobulbar palsy.

Other Corticofugal Tracts   These include the corticothalamic, corticostriate, and corticohypothalamic tracts, which serve as feedback mechanisms from the cortex to these sites.

Subcortical Origin

These tracts arise from the midbrain, pons, and medulla oblongata.

Midbrain   The major motor pathway from the midbrain is the rubrospinal tract (Fig. 22-8). The rubrospinal tract originates from neurons in the caudal part of the red nucleus, crosses in the ventral tegmental decussation of the midbrain, and descends in the midbrain, pons, medulla, and the spinal cord, where it occupies a position in the lateral funiculus in close proximity to the lateral corticospinal tract. The rubrospinal tract is considered an indirect corticospinal tract. Like the corticospinal, the rubrospinal tract facilitates flexor motor neurons and inhibits extensor motor neurons.

Pons   The major motor pathways emanating from the pons are the lateral vestibulospinal and pontine reticulospinal tracts.

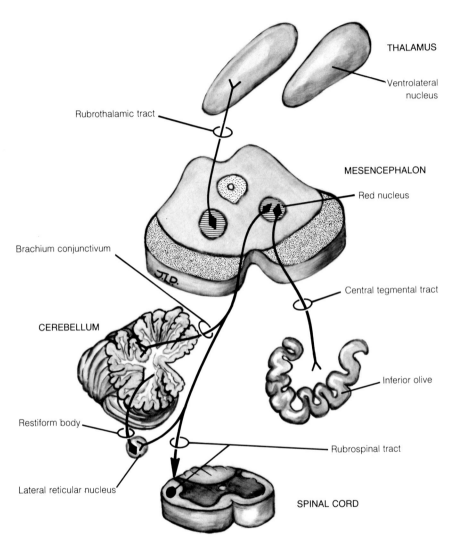

THALAMUS

Ventrolateral
nucleus

Rubrothalamic tract

MESENCEPHALON

Red nucleus

Brachium conjunctivum

Central tegmental tract

CEREBELLUM

Inferior olive

Restiform body

Rubrospinal tract

Lateral reticular nucleus

SPINAL CORD

22–8   Schematic diagram of the major efferent connections of the red nucleus.

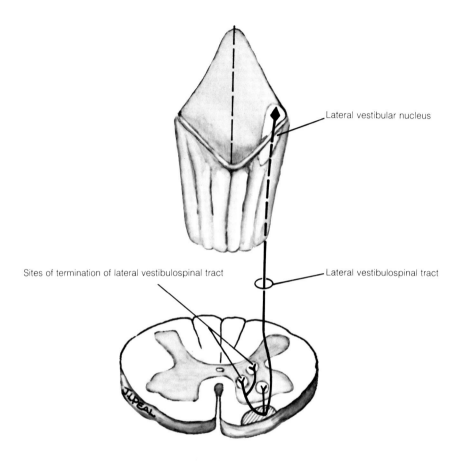

22–9　Schematic diagram of the lateral vestibulospinal pathway.

Lateral Vestibulospinal Tract (Fig. 22–9).　The lateral vestibulospinal tract originates from the lateral vestibular nucleus and descends ipsilaterally in the pons, medulla, and spinal cord, where it occupies a position in the lateral funiculus. The lateral vestibulospinal tract facilitates extensor motor neurons and inhibits flexor motor neurons.

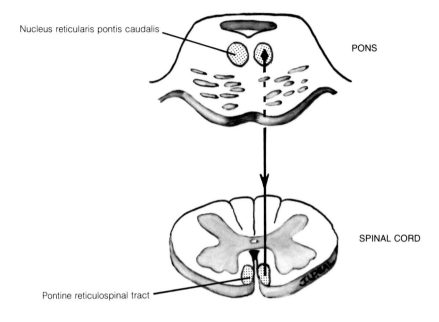

22–10 Schematic diagram of the pontine reticulospinal pathway.

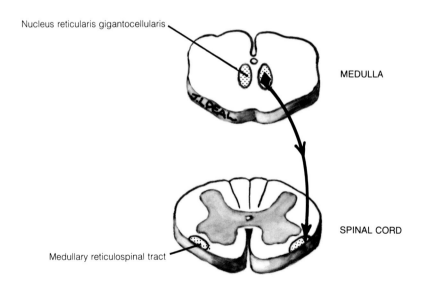

22–11 Schematic diagram of the medullary reticulospinal pathway.

Pontine Reticulospinal Tract (Fig. 22–10)   The pontine reticulospinal tract arises mainly from the medial group of pontine reticular nuclei (nuclei reticularis pontis caudalis and oralis), descends primarily ipsilaterally through the pons and medulla oblongata, and occupies a position in the anterior funiculus of the spinal cord. It facilitates extensor motor neurons and inhibits flexor motor neurons.

Medulla Oblongata (Fig. 22–11)   The major descending pathway from the medulla oblongata is the medullary reticulospinal tract. It arises mainly from the medial (central) group of medullary reticular nuclei (nucleus reticularis gigantocellularis), descends primarily ipsilateral to its site of origin, and occupies a position in the lateral funiculus of the spinal cord. It facilitates flexor motor neurons and inhibits extensor motor neurons.

Atlas of Brain and Spinal Cord

The following is a series of photomicrographs of coronal, parasagittal, and horizontal sections of brain and of coronal sections of spinal cord stained by either the Weigert or Weil method. The magnification of each photomicrograph is indicated. Selective levels are presented to aid the student in the neuroanatomy laboratory.

Coronal Sections

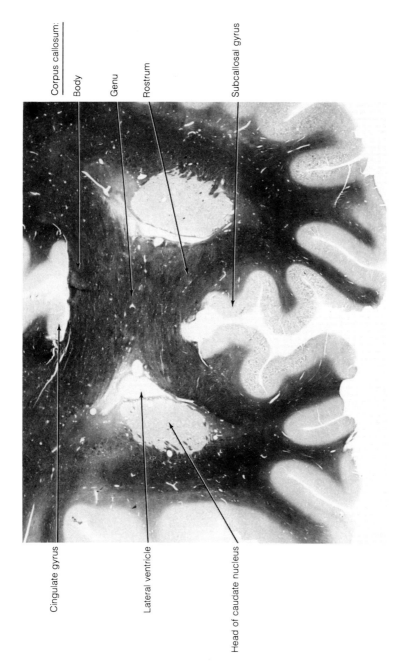

Corpus callosum:

Body

Genu

Rostrum

Subcallosal gyrus

Cingulate gyrus

Lateral ventricle

Head of caudate nucleus

A–1   Corpus callosum (×2).

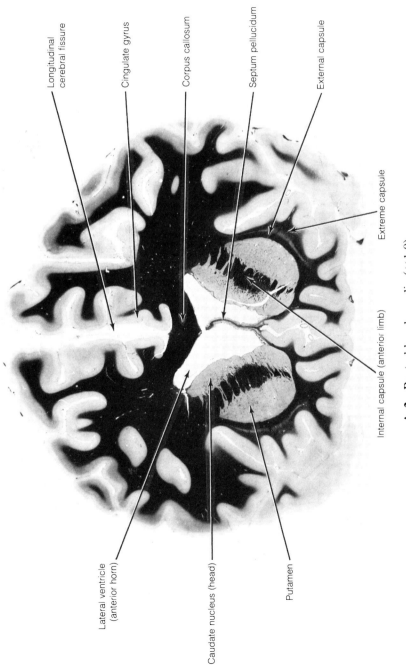

Longitudinal cerebral fissure

Cingulate gyrus

Corpus callosum

Septum pellucidum

External capsule

Extreme capsule

Internal capsule (anterior limb)

Lateral ventricle (anterior horn)

Caudate nucleus (head)

Putamen

A–2 Rostral basal ganglia ($\times 1.0$).

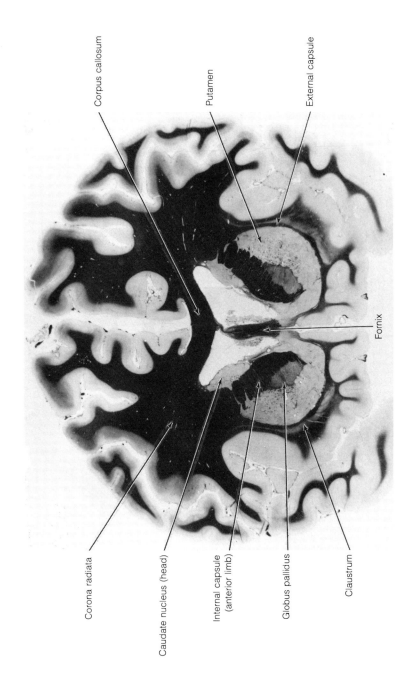

A–3 Rostral basal ganglia (×1.3).

Corpus callosum

Putamen

External capsule

Fornix

Corona radiata

Caudate nucleus (head)

Internal capsule (anterior limb)

Globus pallidus

Claustrum

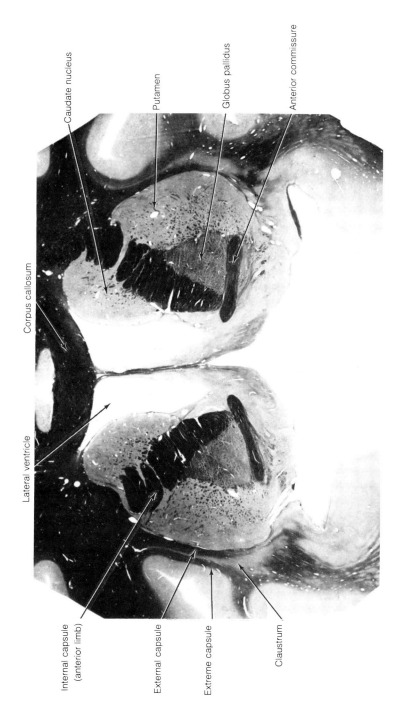

Caudate nucleus

Putamen

Globus pallidus

Anterior commissure

Corpus callosum

Lateral ventricle

Internal capsule
(anterior limb)

External capsule

Extreme capsule

Claustrum

A–4   Anterior commissure (×1.75).

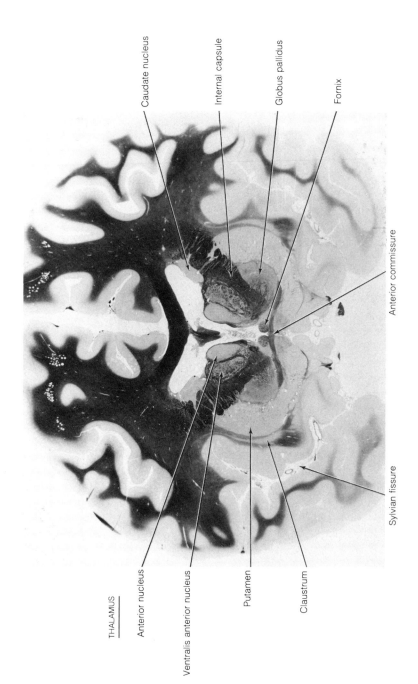

Caudate nucleus

Internal capsule

Globus pallidus

Fornix

Anterior commissure

A–5 Rostral diencephalon (×1.3).

Sylvian fissure

THALAMUS

Anterior nucleus

Ventralis anterior nucleus

Putamen

Claustrum

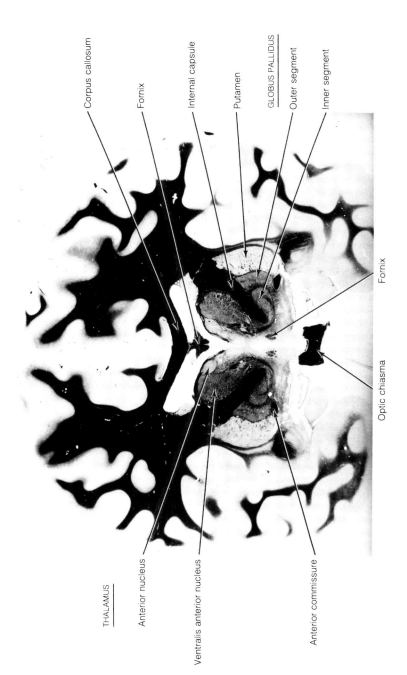

Corpus callosum

Fornix

Internal capsule

Putamen

GLOBUS PALLIDUS
Outer segment

Inner segment

Fornix

Optic chiasma

THALAMUS

Anterior nucleus

Ventralis anterior nucleus

Anterior commissure

A–6 Level of optic chiasma (×0.9).

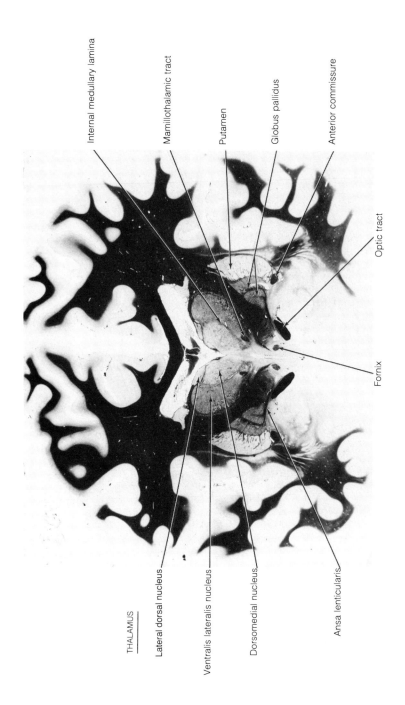

Internal medullary lamina

Mamillothalamic tract

Putamen

Globus pallidus

Anterior commissure

Optic tract

Fornix

Ansa lenticularis

Dorsomedial nucleus

Ventralis lateralis nucleus

Lateral dorsal nucleus

THALAMUS

A–7 Level of optic tract (×1.2).

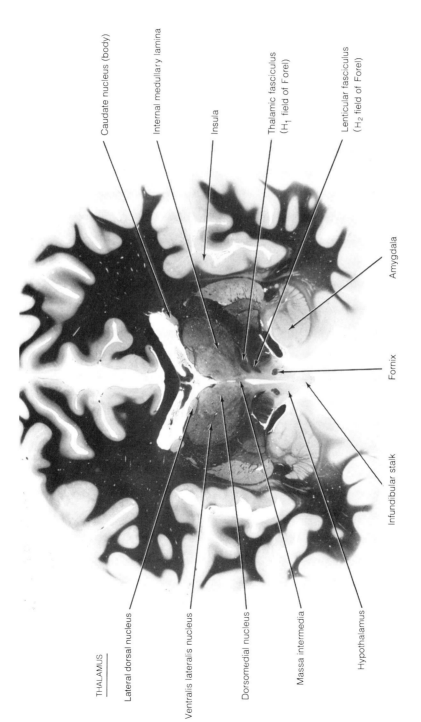

Caudate nucleus (body)

Internal medullary lamina

Insula

Thalamic fasciculus
(H₁ field of Forel)

Lenticular fasciculus
(H₂ field of Forel)

Amygdala

Fornix

Infundibular stalk

Hypothalamus

Massa intermedia

Dorsomedial nucleus

Ventralis lateralis nucleus

Lateral dorsal nucleus

THALAMUS

A–8 Level of posterior thalamus (×1.2).

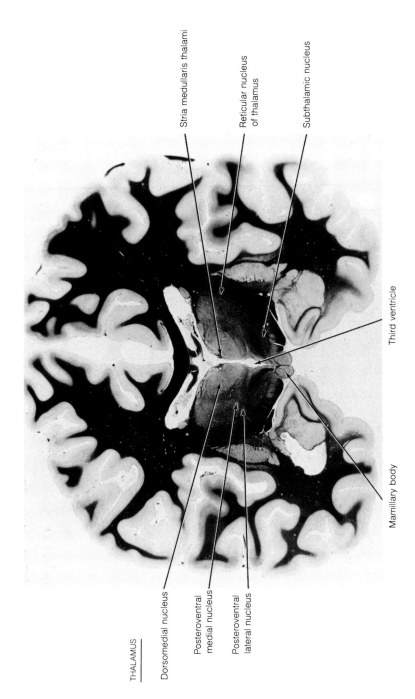

Stria medullaris thalami

Reticular nucleus of thalamus

Subthalamic nucleus

Third ventricle

Mamillary body

THALAMUS

Dorsomedial nucleus

Posteroventral medial nucleus

Posteroventral lateral nucleus

A–9 Level of mamillary body (× 1.1).

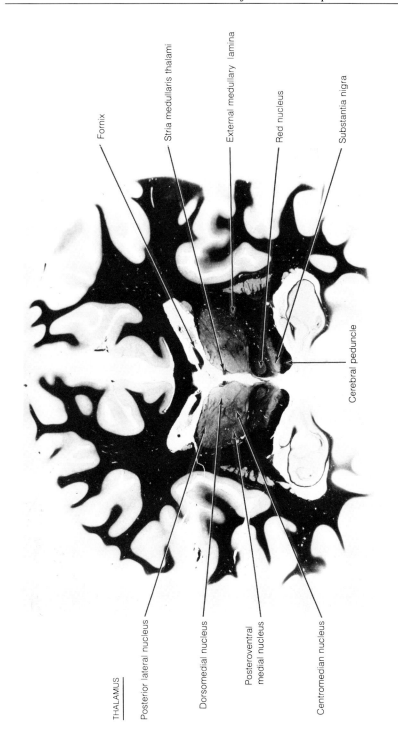

A–10 Level of diencephalic-rostral mesencephalic junction (× 1.2).

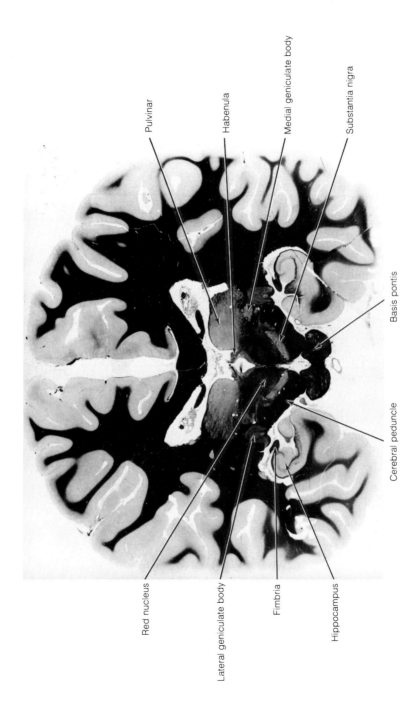

A–11 Level of diencephalic-caudal mesencephalic junction (×1.1).

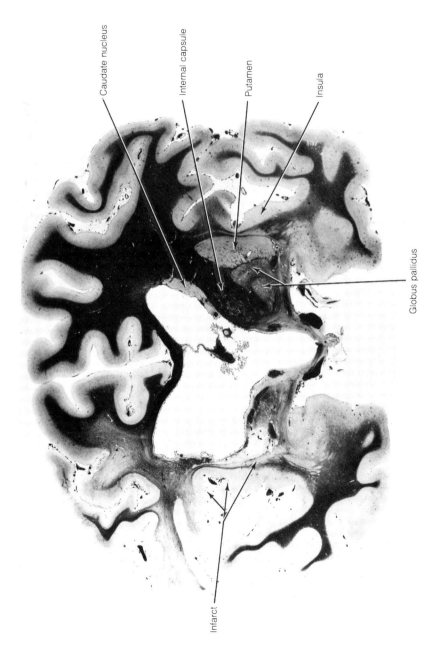

Caudate nucleus

Internal capsule

Putamen

Insula

Globus pallidus

Infarct

A–12 Infarct in area of distribution of middle cerebral artery (×1.1).

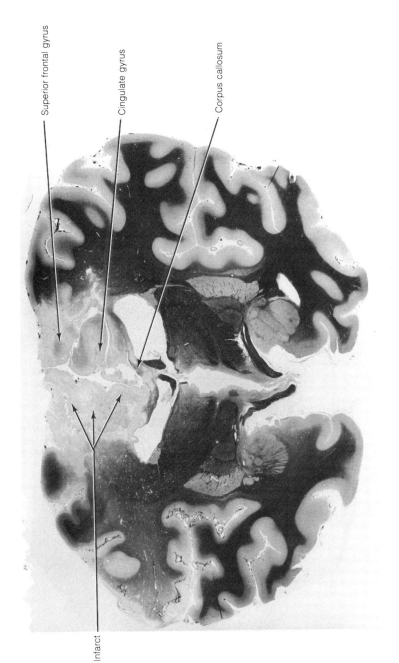

Superior frontal gyrus

Cingulate gyrus

Corpus callosum

Infarct

A–13 Infarct in area of distribution of anterior cerebral artery (×1.0).

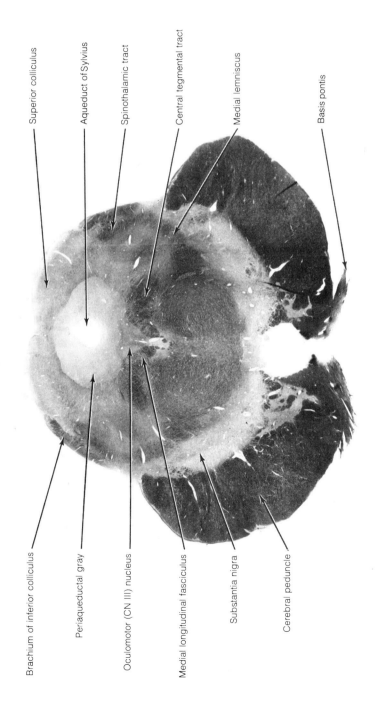

Superior colliculus

Aqueduct of Sylvius

Spinothalamic tract

Central tegmental tract

Medial lemniscus

Basis pontis

Brachium of inferior colliculus

Periaqueductal gray

Oculomotor (CN III) nucleus

Medial longitudinal fasciculus

Substantia nigra

Cerebral peduncle

A–14 Mesencephalon, caudal superior colliculus (×3.3).

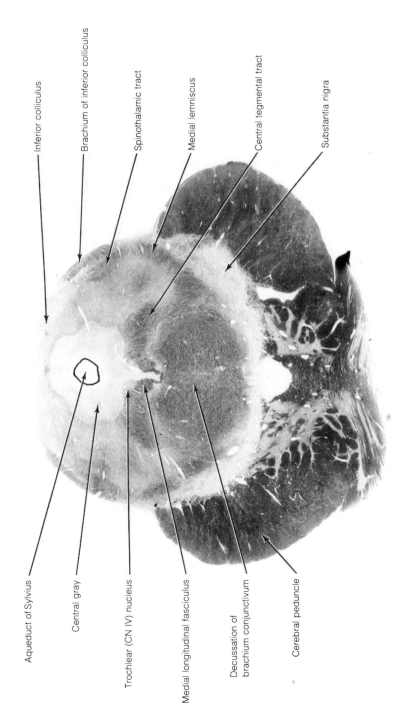

Inferior colliculus

Brachium of inferior colliculus

Spinothalamic tract

Medial lemniscus

Central tegmental tract

Substantia nigra

Aqueduct of Sylvius

Central gray

Trochlear (CN IV) nucleus

Medial longitudinal fasciculus

Decussation of brachium conjunctivum

Cerebral peduncle

A–15 Mesencephalon, inferior colliculus (×3.2).

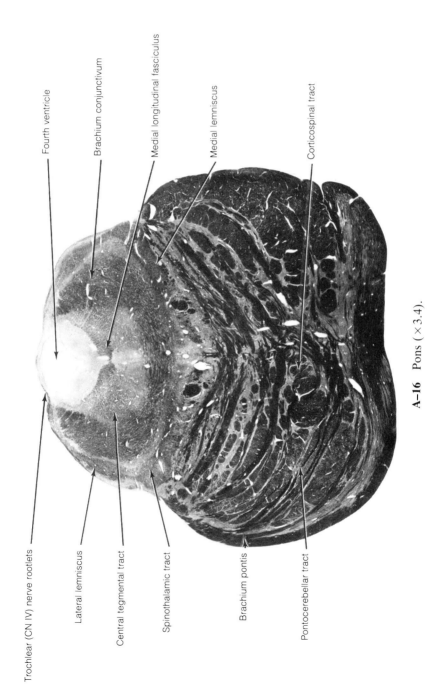

Fourth ventricle

Brachium conjunctivum

Medial longitudinal fasciculus

Medial lemniscus

Corticospinal tract

Trochlear (CN IV) nerve rootlets

Lateral lemniscus

Central tegmental tract

Spinothalamic tract

Brachium pontis

Pontocerebellar tract

A–16   Pons (×3.4).

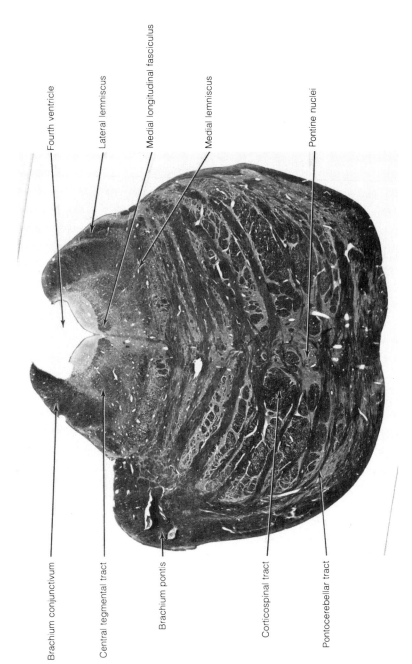

Fourth ventricle

Lateral lemniscus

Medial longitudinal fasciculus

Medial lemniscus

Pontine nuclei

Brachium conjunctivum

Central tegmental tract

Brachium pontis

Corticospinal tract

Pontocerebellar tract

A–17 Pons (×3.0).

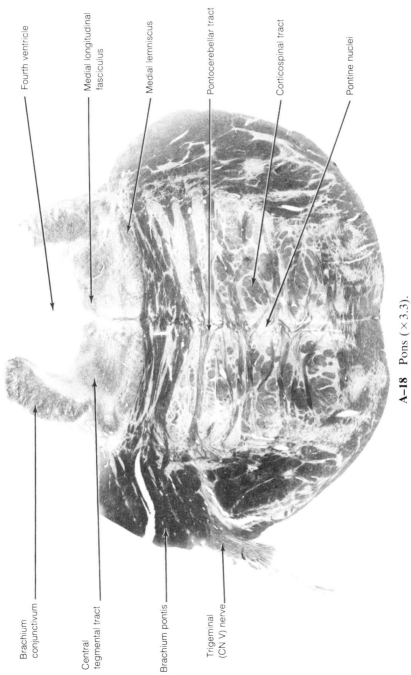

Fourth ventricle

Medial longitudinal fasciculus

Medial lemniscus

Pontocerebellar tract

Corticospinal tract

Pontine nuclei

Brachium conjunctivum

Central tegmental tract

Brachium pontis

Trigeminal (CN V) nerve

A–18 Pons (×3.3).

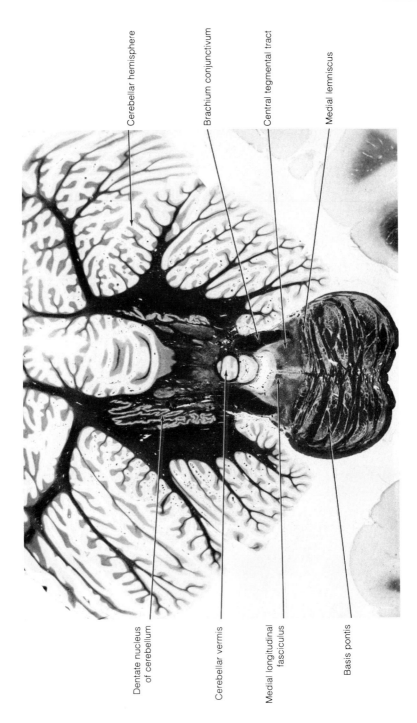

Cerebellar hemisphere

Brachium conjunctivum

Central tegmental tract

Medial lemniscus

Dentate nucleus of cerebellum

Cerebellar vermis

Medial longitudinal fasciculus

Basis pontis

A–19 Level of pons and cerebellum ($\times 2.0$).

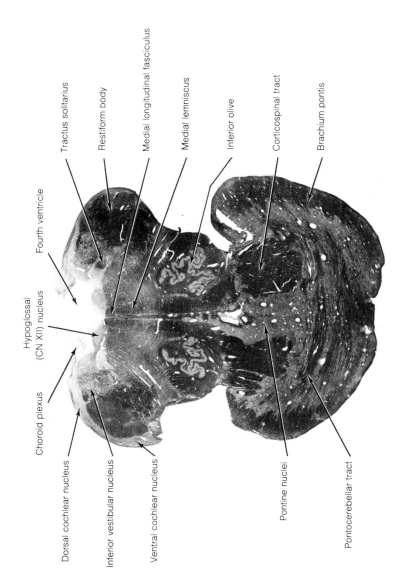

Tractus solitarius

Restiform body

Medial longitudinal fasciculus

Medial lemniscus

Inferior olive

Corticospinal tract

Brachium pontis

Fourth ventricle

Hypoglossal (CN XII) nucleus

Choroid plexus

Dorsal cochlear nucleus

Inferior vestibular nucleus

Ventral cochlear nucleus

Pontine nuclei

Pontocerebellar tract

A–20 Pontomedullary junction (×3.0).

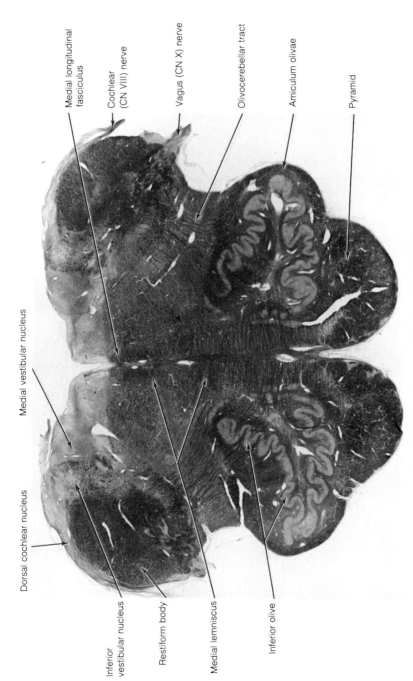

Medial longitudinal fasciculus

Cochlear (CN VIII) nerve

Vagus (CN X) nerve

Olivocerebellar tract

Amiculum olivae

Pyramid

Medial vestibular nucleus

Dorsal cochlear nucleus

Inferior vestibular nucleus

Restiform body

Medial lemniscus

Inferior olive

A–21 Medulla oblongata, inferior olive ($\times 6.5$).

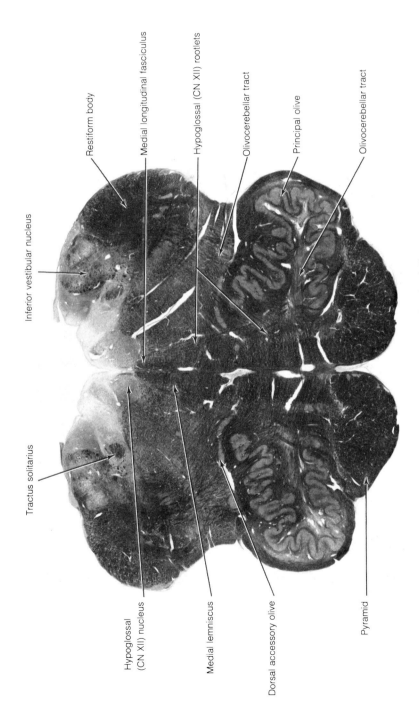

Inferior vestibular nucleus

Restiform body

Medial longitudinal fasciculus

Hypoglossal (CN XII) rootlets

Olivocerebellar tract

Principal olive

Olivocerebellar tract

Tractus solitarius

Hypoglossal (CN XII) nucleus

Medial lemniscus

Dorsal accessory olive

Pyramid

A–22 Medulla oblongata, inferior olive (×6.3).

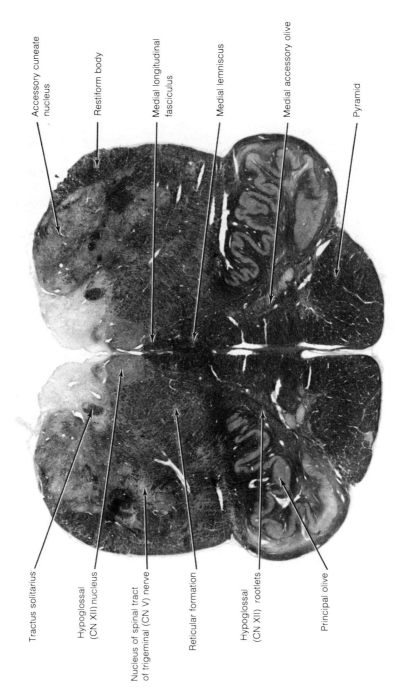

Accessory cuneate nucleus

Restiform body

Medial longitudinal fasciculus

Medial lemniscus

Medial accessory olive

Pyramid

Tractus solitarius

Hypoglossal (CN XII) nucleus

Nucleus of spinal tract of trigeminal (CN V) nerve

Reticular formation

Hypoglossal (CN XII) rootlets

Principal olive

A–23 Medulla oblongata, inferior olive ($\times 7.0$).

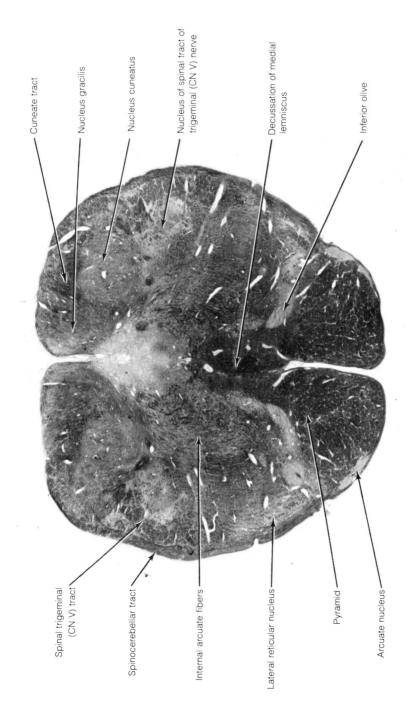

Cuneate tract

Nucleus gracilis

Nucleus cuneatus

Nucleus of spinal tract of trigeminal (CN V) nerve

Decussation of medial lemniscus

Inferior olive

Spinal trigeminal (CN V) tract

Spinocerebellar tract

Internal arcuate fibers

Lateral reticular nucleus

Pyramid

Arcuate nucleus

A–24 Medulla oblongata, sensory decussation (×6.8).

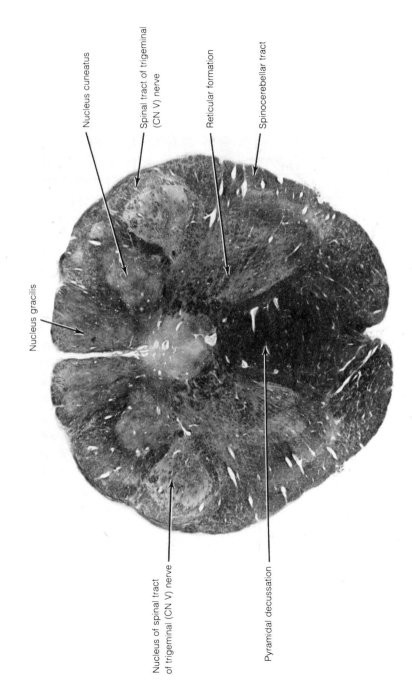

A–25 Medulla oblongata, pyramidal decussation (×7.7).

Nucleus cuneatus

Spinal tract of trigeminal (CN V) nerve

Reticular formation

Spinocerebellar tract

Nucleus gracilis

Nucleus of spinal tract of trigeminal (CN V) nerve

Pyramidal decussation

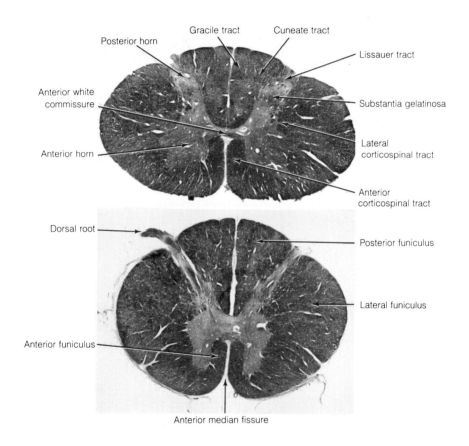

A–26   Cervical spinal cord ($\times 6.0$).

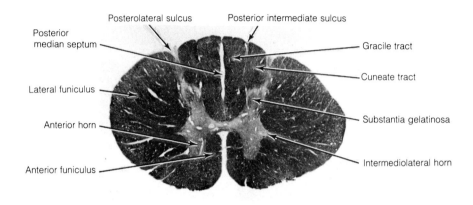

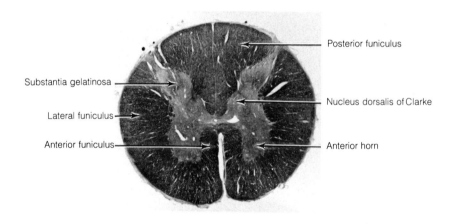

A-27 Thoracic spinal cord and lumbar spinal cord (×6.3).

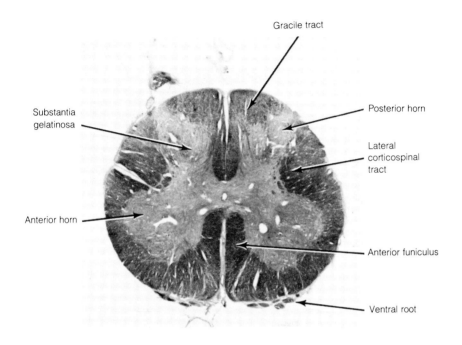

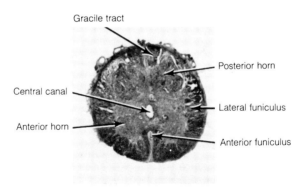

A–28   Sacral spinal cord ($\times 7.1$); coccygeal spinal cord ($\times 8.0$).

Parasagittal Sections

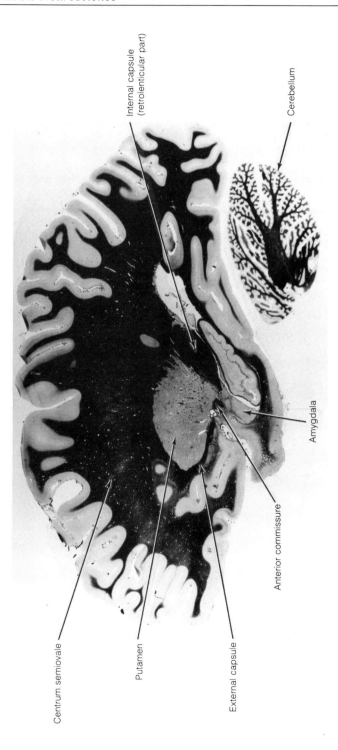

A–29 Section through putamen (×1.0).

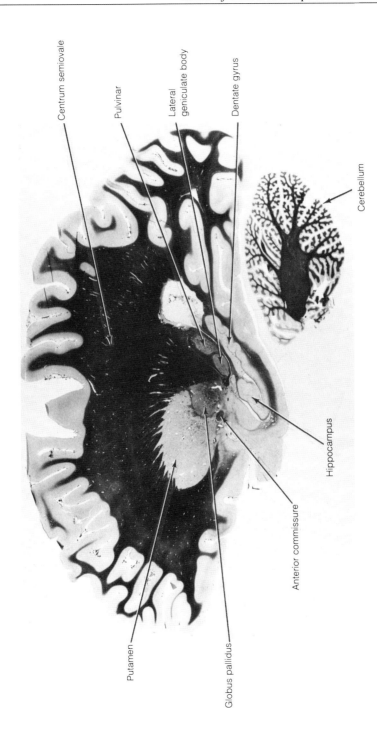

Centrum semiovale

Pulvinar

Lateral geniculate body

Dentate gyrus

Cerebellum

Hippocampus

Anterior commissure

Putamen

Globus pallidus

A–30 Section through lenticular nucleus (×1.0).

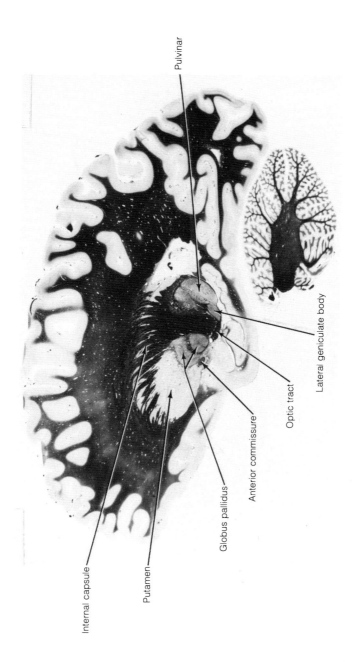

A–31 Section through lenticular nucleus and lateral geniculate body (×1.0).

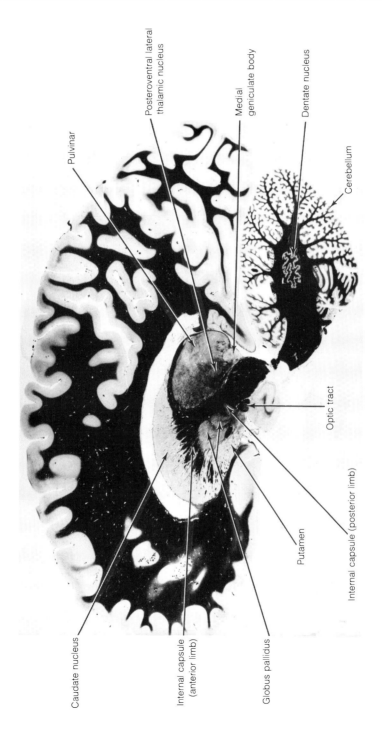

Pulvinar

Posteroventral lateral thalamic nucleus

Medial geniculate body

Dentate nucleus

Cerebellum

Caudate nucleus

Internal capsule (anterior limb)

Globus pallidus

Putamen

Internal capsule (posterior limb)

Optic tract

A–32   Section through corpus striatum (×1.0).

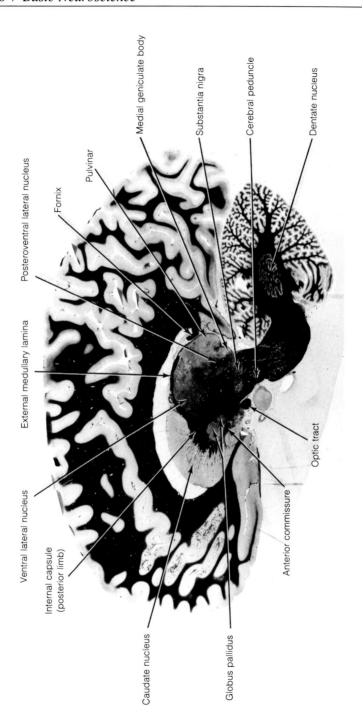

A–33 Section through cerebral peduncle (×1.0).

Medial geniculate body

Substantia nigra

Cerebral peduncle

Dentate nucleus

Pulvinar

Fornix

Posteroventral lateral nucleus

External medullary lamina

Ventral lateral nucleus

Internal capsule
(posterior limb)

Caudate nucleus

Globus pallidus

Anterior commissure

Optic tract

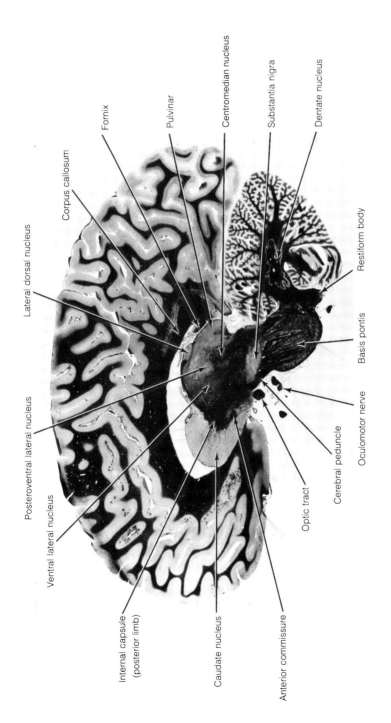

A–34   Section through oculomotor nerve (×1.0).

Centromedian nucleus

Substantia nigra

Dentate nucleus

Fornix

Pulvinar

Corpus callosum

Restiform body

Lateral dorsal nucleus

Basis pontis

Posteroventral lateral nucleus

Oculomotor nerve

Ventral lateral nucleus

Cerebral peduncle

Internal capsule
(posterior limb)

Optic tract

Caudate nucleus

Anterior commissure

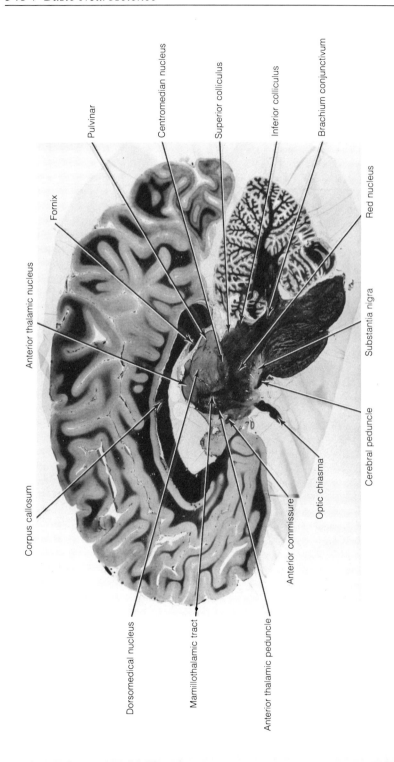

Corpus callosum

Anterior thalamic nucleus

Fornix

Pulvinar

Centromedian nucleus

Superior colliculus

Inferior colliculus

Brachium conjunctivum

Red nucleus

Substantia nigra

Cerebral peduncle

Optic chiasma

Anterior commissure

Anterior thalamic peduncle

Mamillothalamic tract

Dorsomedical nucleus

A–35 Section through medial thalamus (×1.0).

Horizontal Sections

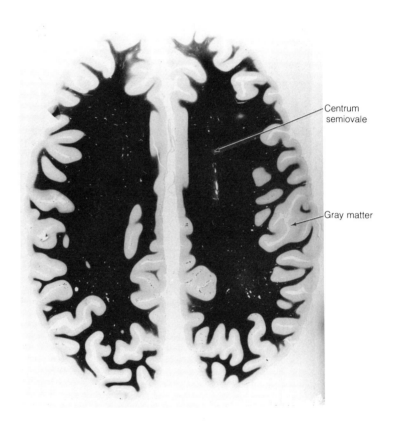

Centrum
semiovale

Gray matter

A–36 Section through centrum semiovale (× 1.0).

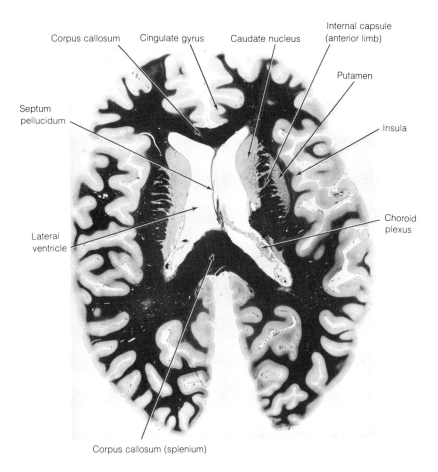

Corpus callosum   Cingulate gyrus   Caudate nucleus   Internal capsule (anterior limb)

Putamen

Septum pellucidum

Insula

Lateral ventricle

Choroid plexus

Corpus callosum (splenium)

A–37   Section through striatum ($\times 1.0$).

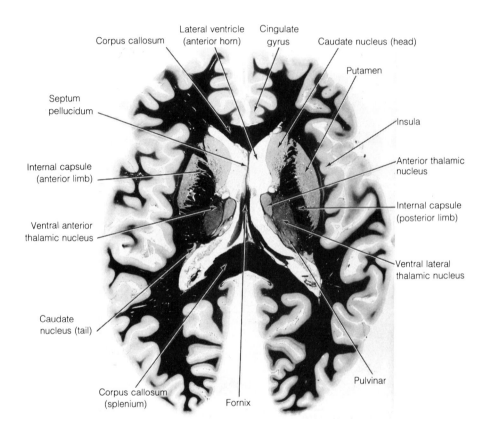

A–38 Section through striatum and thalamus (× 1.1).

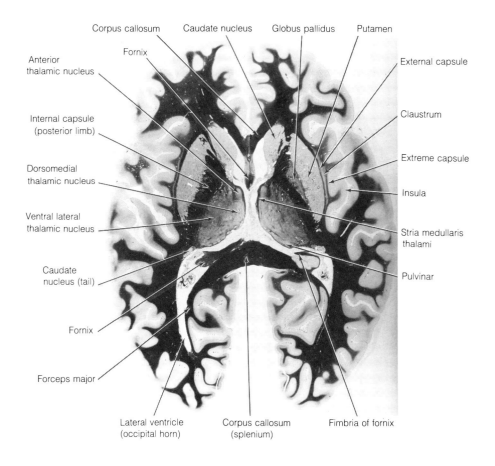

Corpus callosum Caudate nucleus Globus pallidus Putamen

Anterior
thalamic nucleus

Fornix

External capsule

Internal capsule
(posterior limb)

Claustrum

Dorsomedial
thalamic nucleus

Extreme capsule

Insula

Ventral lateral
thalamic nucleus

Stria medullaris
thalami

Caudate
nucleus (tail)

Pulvinar

Fornix

Forceps major

Lateral ventricle
(occipital horn)

Corpus callosum
(splenium)

Fimbria of fornix

A–39   Section through thalamus (× 1.0).

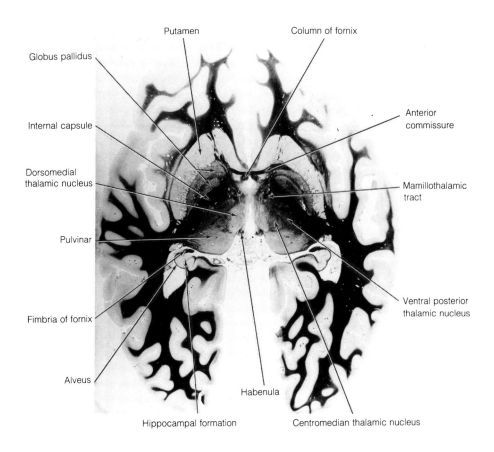

A–40   Section through posterior thalamus ($\times 1.1$).

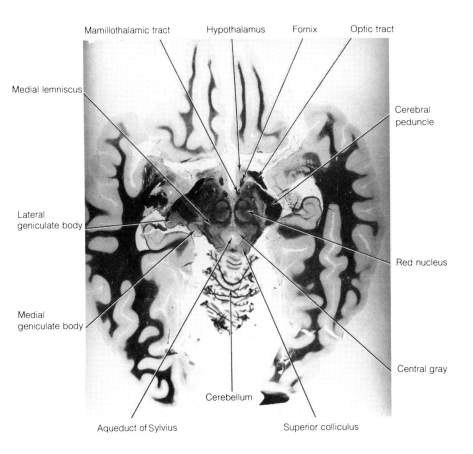

Mamillothalamic tract   Hypothalamus   Fornix   Optic tract

Medial lemniscus

Cerebral peduncle

Lateral geniculate body

Red nucleus

Medial geniculate body

Central gray

Cerebellum

Aqueduct of Sylvius   Superior colliculus

A–41   Section through midbrain and hypothalamus (× 1.1).

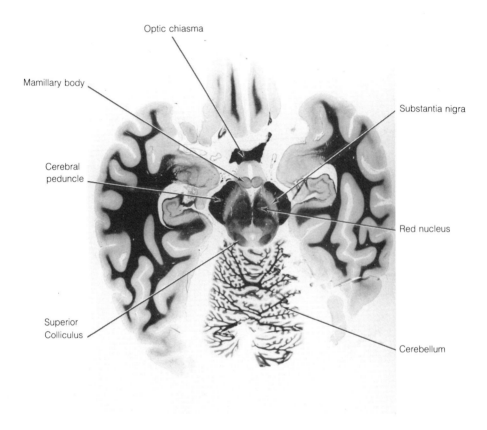

Optic chiasma

Mamillary body

Substantia nigra

Cerebral peduncle

Red nucleus

Superior Colliculus

Cerebellum

A–42 Section through optic chiasma (× 1.0).

Bibliography

Afifi, A.K.; Bahuth, N.B.; Kaelber, W.W.; Mikhael, E.; Nassar, S.: The Cortico-Nigral Fiber Tract. An Experimental Fink-Heimer Study in Cats. J Anat 118 (1974) 469–476.

Aidley, D.J.: The Physiology of Excitable Cells. Cambridge University Press, Cambridge, 1971.

Alami, S.Y.; Afifi, A.K.: Cerebrospinal Fluid Examination. In: Laboratory Medicine, Vol. 4, pp. 1–26, Ed. by G.J. Race. Harper & Row, Hagerstown, 1973.

Alksne, J.F.; Lovings, E.T.: The Role of the Arachnoid Villus in the Removal of Red Blood Cells from the Subarachnoid Space. J Neurosurg 36 (1972) 192–200.

Angaut-Petit, D.: The Dorsal Column System: II. Functional Properties and Bulbar Relay of the Postsynaptic Fibers of the Cat's Fasciculus Gracilis. Exp Brain Res 22 (1975) 471–493.

Angevine, J.B.; Cotman, C.W.: Principles of Neuroanatomy. Oxford University Press, New York, 1981.

Astruc, J.: Corticofugal Connections of Area 8 (Frontal Eye Fields) in Macaca Mulata. Brain Res 33 (1971) 241–256.

Bak, I.J.; Baker, R.; Choi, W.B.; Precht, W.: Electron Microscopic Investigation of the Vestibular Projection to the Cat Trochlear Nuclei. Neuroscience 1 (1976) 477–482.

Barr, M.L.; Kiernan, J.A.: The Human Nervous System, Ed. 4. Harper & Row, Hagerstown, 1983.

Benson, D.F.; Geschwind, N.: The Alexias. In: Handbook of Clinical Neurology, Vol. 4, pp. 112–140, Ed. by P.J. Vinken and G.W. Bruyn. North-Holland Publishing Co., Amsterdam, 1969.

Benson, D.F.; Sheremata, W.A.; Bouchard, R.; Segarra, J.M.; Price, D.; Geschwind, N.: Conduction Aphasia. A Clinicopathological Study. Arch Neurol 28 (1973) 339–346.

Benton, A.L.; Joynt, R.J.: Early Descriptions of Aphasia. Arch Neurol 3 (1960) 205–222.

Bergman, R.A.; Afifi, A.K.: Atlas of Microscopic Anatomy. W.B. Saunders Co., Philadelphia, 1974.

Bergman, R.A.; Johns, R.J.; Afifi, A.K.: Ultrastructural Alterations in Muscle from Patients with Myasthenia Gravis and the Eaton-Lambert Syndrome. Ann NY Acad Sci 183 (1971) 88–122.

Bertrand, G.; Blundell, J.; Musella, R.: Electrical Exploration of the Internal Capsule and Neighbouring Structures during Stereotaxic Procedures. J Neurosurg 22 (1965) 333–343.

Bishop, B.: Pain: Its Physiology and Rationale for Management. Part III. Consequences of Current Concepts of Pain Mechanisms Related to Pain Management. Phys Ther 60 (1980) 24–27.

Bodian, D.: Neuron Junctions. A Revolutionary Decade. Anat Rec 174 (1972) 73–84.

Bradley, P.B. (Ed.): Methods in Brain Research. John Wiley & Sons, London, 1975.

Brodal, A.: The Cranial Nerves. Blackwell Scientific Publications, Oxford, 1962.

Brodal, A.: Cerebrocerebellar Pathways. Acta Neurol Scand Suppl 51 (1972) 153–196.

Brodal, A.: Neurological Anatomy in Relation to Clinical Medicine, Ed. 3. Oxford University Press, London, 1981.

Brown, A.G.: Subcortical Mechanisms Concerned in Somatic Sensations. Br Med Bull 33 (1977) 121–128.

Carpenter, M.B.: Core Text of Neuroanatomy, Ed. 2. The Williams & Wilkins Co., Baltimore, 1978.

Carpenter, M.B.; McMasters, R.E.: Lesions of the Substantia Nigra in the Rhesus Monkey. Efferent Fiber Degeneration and Behavioral Observations. Am J Anat 114 (1964) 293–319.

Carpenter, M.B.; Pierson, R.J.: Pretectal Region and the Pupillary Light Reflex. An Anatomical Analysis in Monkey. J Comp Neurol 149 (1973) 271–300.

Cervero, F.; Iggo, A.; Ogawa, H.: Nociceptor-Driven Dorsal Horn Neurones in the Lumbar Spinal Cord of the Cat. Pain 2 (1976) 5–24.

Chusid, J.G.: Correlative Neuroanatomy and Functional Neurology, Ed. 15. Lange Medical Publications, Los Altos, 1973.

Conlee, J.W.; Kane, E.S.: Descending Projections from the Inferior Colliculus to the Dorsal Cochlear Nucleus in the Cat. An Autoradiographic Study. Neuroscience 7 (1981) 161–178.

Cooper, I.S.: Neuroanatomic Structures Subserving Posture. In: Involuntary Movement Disorders, pp. 16–49, Ed. by I.S. Cooper. Hoeber, New York, 1969.

Cooper, K.E.: Temperature Regulation and the Hypothalamus. Br Med Bull 22 (1966) 238–242.

Corvaja, N.; Grofová, I. Pompeiano, O.; Walberg, F.: The Lateral Reticular Nucleus in the Cat. I. An Experimental Anatomical Study of Its Spinal and Supraspinal Afferent Connections. Neuroscience 2 (1977) 537–553.

Cotman, C.W.: Neuronal Plasticity. Raven Press, New York, 1978.

Courville, J.; Faraco-Cantin, F.: On the Origin of the Climbing Fibers of the Cerebellum. An Experimental Study in the Cat with an Autoradiographic Tracing Method. Neuroscience 3 (1978) 797–809.

Cowan, W.M.; Hall, Z.W.; Kandel, E.R. (Eds.): Annual Review of Neuroscience, Vol. 1. Annual Reviews Inc., Palo Alto, 1978.

Crelin, E.S.: Development of the Nervous System. Ciba Clin Symp 26, No. 2 (1974).

Crosby, E.C.; Humphrey, T.; Lauer, E.W.: Correlative Anatomy of the Nervous System. The Macmillan Co., New York, 1962.

Curtis, B.A.; Jacobson, S.; Marcus, E.M.: An Introduction to the Neurosciences. W.B. Saunders Co., Philadelphia, 1972.

Daube, J.R.; Sandok, B.A.; Reagan, T.J.; Westmoreland, B.F.: Medical Neurosciences. An Approach to Anatomy, Pathology and Physiology by Systems and Levels. Little, Brown and Co., Boston, 1978.

DeArmond, S.J.; Fusco, M.M.; Dewey, M.M.: A Photographic Atlas. Structure of the Human Brain, Ed. 2. Oxford University Press, New York, 1976.

Destombes, J.; Gogan, P.; Rouviere, A.: The Fine Structure of Neurones and Cellular Relationships in the Abducens Nucleus in the Cat. Exp Brain Res 35 (1979) 249–267.

Dunkerley, G.B.: A Basic Atlas of the Human Nervous System. F.A. Davis Co., Philadelphia, 1975.

Eccles, J.C.: The Understanding of the Brain. McGraw-Hill Book Co., New York, 1972.

Eliasson, S.G.; Prensky, A.L.; Hardin, W.B.: Neurological Pathophysiology. Oxford University Press, London, 1974.

Englander, R.N.; Netsky, M.C.; Adelman, L.S.: Location of Human Pyramidal Tract in the Internal Capsule: Anatomic Evidence. Neurology 25 (1975) 823–826.

Evarts, E.V.: Contrast between Activity of Precentral and Postcentral Neurons of Cerebral Cortex during Movement in the Monkey. Brain Res 40 (1972) 25–31.

Feltz, P.: Persistence of Caudate Unitary Responses to Nigral Stimulation after Destruction and Functional Impairment of Striatal Dopaminergic Terminals. Brain Res 43 (1972) 595–600.

Fitzsimons, J.T.: The Hypothalamus and Drinking. Br Med Bull 22 (1966) 232–237.

Fix, J.D.; Punte, C.S.: Atlas of Human Brain Stem and Spinal Cord. University Park Press, Baltimore, 1981.

Frederiks, J.A.M.: The Agnosias. Disorders of Perceptual Recognition. In: Handbook of Clinical Neurology, Vol. 4, pp. 13–47, Ed. by P.J. Vinken and G.W. Bruyn. North-Holland Publishing Co., Amsterdam, 1969.

Fuxe, K.; Hökfelt, T.; Jonsson, G.; Ungerstedt, U.: Fluoresence Microscopy in Neuroanatomy. In: Contemporary Research Methods in Neuroanatomy, pp. 275–314, Ed. by W.J.H. Nauta and S.O.E. Ebbesson. Springer-Verlag New York Inc., New York, 1970.

Ganong, W.F.: The Nervous System. Lange Medical Publications, Los Altos, 1977.

Geschwind, N.: Language and the Brain. Sci Am 226, No. 4 (1972) 76–83.

Gillilan, L.A.: The Correlation of the Blood Supply to the Human Brain Stem with Clinical Brain Stem Lesions. J Neuropath Exp Neurol 23 (1964) 78–108.

Gilroy, J.; Meyer, J.S.: Medical Neurology. The Macmillan Co., London, 1969.

Gloning, K.; Hoff, H.: Cerebral Localization of Disorders of Higher Nervous Activity. Clinical, Anatomical and Physiological Aspects. In: Handbook of Clinical Neurology, Vol. 3, pp. 22–47, Ed. by P.J. Vinken and G.W. Bruyn. North-Holland Publishing Co., Amsterdam, 1969.

Gomez, D.G.; Potts, G.; Deonarine, V.: Arachnoid Granulations of the Sheep. Arch Neurol 30 (1974) 169–175.

Grabow, J.D.; Ebersold, M.J.; Albers, J.W.; Schima, E.M.: Cerebellar Stimulation for the Control of Seizures. Mayo Clin Proc 49 (1974) 759–774.

Graybiel, A.M.: The Thalamocortical Projection of the So-Called Posterior Nuclear Group. A Study with Anterograde Degeneration Methods in the Cat. Brain Res 49 (1973) 229–244.

Greenblatt, S.H.: Alexia without Agraphia or Hemianopsia. Brain 96 (1973) 307–316.

Growdon, J.H.; Winkler, G.F.; Wray, S.H.: Midbrain Ptosis. A Case with Clinicopathologic Correlation. Arch Neurol 30 (1974) 179–181.

Guillery, R.W.: Light- and Electron-Microscopical Studies of Normal and Degenerating Axons. In: Contemporary Research Methods in Neuroanatomy, pp. 77–105, Ed. by W.J.H. Nauta and S.O.E. Ebbesson. Springer-Verlag New York Inc., New York, 1970.

Guyton, A.C.: Textbook of Medical Physiology, Ed. 4. W.B. Saunders Co., Philadelphia, 1971.

Guyton, A.C.: Structure and Function of the Nervous System. W.B. Saunders Co., Philadelphia, 1972.

Ha, H.; Liu, C.N.: Cell Origin of the Ventral Spinocerebellar Tract. J Comp Neurol 133 (1968) 185–206.

Haines, D.E.: Neuroanatomy. An Atlas of Structures, Sections and Systems. Urban & Schwarzenberg, Inc., Baltimore, 1983.

Hansen, R.N.; Horn, J.: Functional Aspects of Cerebellar Signs in Clinical Neurology. Acta Neurol Scand Suppl 51 (1972) 219–246.

Harris, G.W.; Reed, M.: Hypothalamic Releasing Factors and the Control of Anterior Pituitary Function. Br Med Bull 22 (1966) 266–272.

Heimer, L.: Selective Silver-Impregnation of Degenerating Axoplasm. In: Contemporary Research Methods in Neuroanatomy, pp. 106–131, Ed. by W.J.H. Nauta and S.O.E. Ebbesson. Springer-Verlag New York Inc., New York, 1970.

Henriksson, N.G.; Pfaltz, C.R.; Torok, N.; Rubin, W.: A Synopsis of the Vestibular System. Sandoz Ltd., Basel, 1972.

Hökfelt, T.; Kellerth, J.-O.; Nilsson, G.; Pernow, B.: Experimental Immunohistochemical Studies on the Localization and Distribution of Substance P in Cat Primary Sensory Neurons. Brain Res 100 (1975) 235–252.

Horel, A.: The Neuroanatomy of Amnesia: A Critique of the Hippocampal Memory Hypothesis. Brain 101 (1978) 403–445.

Hornykiewicz, O.: Dopamine in the Basal Ganglia. Br Med Bull 29 (1973) 172–178.

Hosobuchi, Y.; Adams, J.E.; Linchitz, R.: Pain Relief by Electrical Stimulation of the Central Gray Matter and Its Reversal by Naloxone. Science 197 (1977) 183–186.

Hultborn, H.; Mori, K.; Tsukahara, N.: Cerebellar Influence on Parasympathetic Neurones Innervating Intra-Ocular Muscles. Brain Res 159 (1978) 269–278.

Igarashi, S.; Sasa, M., Takaori, S.: Feedback Loop between Locus Coeruleus and Spinal Trigeminal Nucleus Neurons Responding to Tooth Pulp Stimulation in the Rat. Brain Res Bull 4 (1979) 74–83.

Ingram, W.R.: A Review of Anatomical Neurology. University Park Press, Baltimore, 1976.

Isaacson, R.L.: The Limbic System. Plenum Press, New York, 1974.

Jordan, L.M.; Kenshalo, D.R., Jr.; Martin, R.F.; Haber, L.H.; Willis, W.D.: Two Populations of Spinothalamic Tract Neurons with Opposite Responses to 5-Hydroxytryptamine. Brain Res 164 (1979) 342–346.

Kaelber, W.W.; Afifi, A.K.: Nigro-Amygdaloid Fiber Connections in the Cat. Am J Anat 148 (1977) 129–135.

Kaelber, W.W.; Mitchell, C.L.; Yarmat, A.J.; Afifi, A.K.; Lorens, S.A.: Centrum Medianum-Parafascicularis Lesions and Reactivity to Noxious and Non-Noxious Stimuli. Exp Neurol 46 (1975) 282–290.

Karp, J.S.; Hurtig, H.I.: "Locked-In" State with Bilateral Midbrain Infarcts. Arch Neurol 30 (1974) 176–178.

Kemp, J.M.; Powell, T.P.S.: The Cortico-Striate Projection in the Monkey. Brain 93 (1970) 525–546.

Kennedy, G.C.: Food Intake, Energy Balance and Growth. Br Med Bull 22 (1966) 216–220.

Kerr, F.W.L.: The Ventral Spinothalamic Tract and Other Ascending Systems of the Ventral Funiculus of the Spinal Cord. J Comp Neurol 159 (1975) 335–356.

Kiernan, J.A.; Berry, M.: Neuroanatomical Methods. In: Methods in Brain Research, pp. 1–77, Ed. by P.B. Bradley. John Wiley & Sons Ltd., London, 1975.

Künzle, H.: Autoradiographic Tracing of the Cerebellar Projections from the Lateral Reticular Nucleus in the Cat. Exp Brain Res 22 (1975) 255–266.

Lance, J.W.; McLeod, J.G.: A Physiological Approach to Clinical Neurology, Ed. 2. Butterworth & Co., Ltd., London, 1977.

Lhermitte, F.; Gautier, J.C.: Aphasia. In: Handbook of Clinical Neurology, Vol. 4, pp. 84–104, Ed. by P.J. Vinken and G.W. Bruyn. North-Holland Publishing Co., Amsterdam, 1969.

Livett, B.G.: Histochemical Visualization of Adrenergic Neurons. Br Med Bull 29 (1973) 93–99.

Livingston, K.E.: Anatomical Bias of the Limbic System Concept. Arch Neurol 24 (1971) 17–21.

Llinas, R.R.: The Cortex of the Cerebellum. Sci Am 232 (1975) 56–71.

Manter, J.T.; Gatz, A.J.: Essentials of Clinical Neuroanatomy and Neurophysiology, Ed. 4. F.A. Davis Co., Philadelphia, 1973.

Mark, R.: Memory and Nerve Cell Connections. Clarendon Press, Oxford, 1974.

Melzack, R.: The Puzzle of Pain. Basic Books, Inc., New York, 1973.

Miller, R.A.; Burack, E.: Atlas of the Central Nervous System in Man, Ed. 2. The Williams & Wilkins Co., Baltimore, 1977.

Miller, R.A.; Strominger, N.L.: Efferent Connections of the Red Nucleus in the Brain Stem and Spinal Cord of Rhesus Monkey. J Comp Neurol 152 (1973) 327–346.

Minckler, J.: Introduction to Neuroscience. C.V. Mosby Co., St. Louis, 1972.

Mitchell, G.A.G.: The Essentials of Neuroanatomy. Churchill Livingstone, London, 1971.

Morest, D.K.: Experimental Study of the Projections of the Nucleus of the Tractus Solitarius and the Area Postrema in the Cat. J Comp Neurol 130 (1967) 277–300.

Mountcastle, V.B. (Ed.): Medical Physiology, Ed. 13, Vol. 1. C.V. Mosby Co., St. Louis, 1974.

Nakamura, Y.; Mizuno, N.; Konish, A.; Sato, M.: Synaptic Reorganization of the Red Nucleus after Chronic Deafferentation from Cerebellorubral Fibers. An Electron Microscope Study in the Cat. Brain Res 82 (1974) 298–301.

Norgren, R.; Leonard, C.M.: Taste Pathways in Rat Brain Stem. Science 173 (1971) 1139–1140.

Norman, S.: Diagnostic Categories for the Patient with a Right Hemisphere Lesion. Am J Nurs 79 (1979) 2126–2130.

Norman, S.; Baratz, R.: Understanding Aphasia. Am J Nurs 79 (1979) 2135–2138.

O'Leary, J.L.; Dunsker, S.B.; Smith, J.M.; Inukai, J.; O'Leary, M.: Termination of the Olivocerebellar System in the Cat. Arch Neurol 22 (1970) 193–206.

Oxbury, J.M.: The Right Hemisphere and Hemispheric Disconnection. In: Recent Advances in Clinical Neurology, No. 1, pp. 1–22, Ed. by W.B. Matthews. Churchill Livingstone, Edinburgh, 1975.

Pandya, D.N.; Hallett, M.; Mukherjee, S.K.: Intra- and Interhemispheric Connections of the Neocortical Auditory System in the Rhesus Monkey. Brain Res 14 (1969) 49–65.

Pandya, D.N.; Karol, E.A.; Heilbronn, D.: The Topographical Distribution of Interhemispheric Projections in the Corpus Callosum of the Rhesus Monkey. Brain Res 32 (1971) 31–43.

Pandya, D.N.; Kuypers, H.G.J.M.: Cortico-Cortical Connections in the Rhesus Monkey. Brain Res 13 (1969) 13–36.

Patton, H.D.; Sundsten, J.W.; Crill, W.E.; Swanson, P.D.: Introduction to Basic Neurology. W.B. Saunders Co., Philadelphia, 1976.

Peele, T.L.: The Neuroanatomic Basis for Clinical Neurology, Ed. 2. McGraw-Hill Book Co., New York, 1961.

Perl, E.R.: Organization of Aδ and C Fiber Input in the Dorsal Horn. Neurosci Res Program Bull 16 (1978) 65–82.

Powell, E.W.; Hatton, J.B.: Projections of the Inferior Colliculus in Cat. J Comp Neurol 136 (1969) 183–192.

Powell, T.P.S.: The Somatic Sensory Cortex. Br Med Bull 33 (1977) 129–135.

Raisman, G.: Neural Connexions of the Hypothalamus. Br Med Bull 22 (1966) 197–201.

Richardson, D.E.; Akil, H.: Pain Reduction by Electrical Brain Stimulation in Man. Part 1: Acute Administration in Periaqueductal and Periventricular Sites. J Neurosurg 47 (1977) 178–183.

Roberts, M.; Hanaway, J.: Atlas of the Human Brain in Sections. Lea & Febiger, Philadelphia, 1970.

Rockstein, M. (Ed.): Development and Aging in the Nervous System. Academic Press, New York, 1973.

Rose, S.: The Conscious Brain. Alfred A. Knopf, New York, 1973.

Ross. E. D.; Stewart, R. M.: Akinetic Mutism from Hypothalamic Damage: Successful Treatment with Dopamine Agonists. Neurology 31 (1981) 1435–1439.

Ruch, T. C.; Patton, H. D. (Eds.): Physiology and Biophysics. W. B. Saunders Co., Philadelphia, 1965.

Ruch, T. C.; Patton, H. D.; Woodbury, J. W.; Towe, A. L.: Neurophysiology. W. B. Saunders Co., Philadelphia, 1961.

Schadé, J. P.; Ford, D. H.: Basic Neurology. An Introduction to the Structure and Function of the Nervous System.

Elsevier Publishing Co., Amsterdam, 1965.

Schadé, J. P.; Ford, D. H.: Atlas of the Human Brain. Elsevier Publishing Co., Amsterdam, 1966.

Scheibel, M. E.; Davies, T. L.; Scheibel, A. B.: On Thalamic Substrates of Cortical Synchrony. Neurology (Minneap) 23 (1973) 300–304.

Shipps, F. C.; Jones, J. M.; D'Agostino, A.: Atlas of Brain Anatomy for C. T. Scans, Ed. 2. Charles C Thomas, Springfield, Illinois, 1977.

Sindou, M.; Quoex, C.; Baleydier, C.: Fiber Organization at the Posterior Spinal Cord Rootlet Junction in Man. J Comp Neurol 153 (1974) 15–26.

Sisson, W. B.: Physiology of Choroid Plexus and Studies of Cerebrospinal Fluid. Bull Los Angeles Neurol Soc 34 (1969) 256–265.

Skinner, H. A.: The Origin of Medical Terms, Ed. 2. The Williams & Wilkins Co., Baltimore, 1961.

Smith, A. D.: Release of Noradrenaline from Sympathetic Nerves. Br Med Bull 29 (1973) 123–129.

Strub, R. L.; Black, F. W.: The Mental Status Examination in Neurology, pp. 39–61. F. A. Davis Co., Philadelphia, 1977.

Sundt, T. M.: The Cerebral Autonomic Nervous System. Mayo Clin Proc 48 (1973) 127–137.

Sweet, W. H.: Pain Modulation. The Human Experience. Neurosci Res Program Bull 16 (1978) 148–155.

Szabo, J.: Distribution of Striatal Afferents from the Mesencephalon in the Cat. Brain Res 188 (1980) 3–21.

Tripathi, R. C.: Ultrastructure of the Arachnoid Mater in Relation to Outflow of Cerebrospinal Fluid. A New Concept. Lancet II (1973) 8–11.

Truex, R. C.; Carpenter, M. B.: Human Neuroanatomy, Ed. 6. Williams & Wilkins Co., Baltimore, 1969.

Valverde, F.: The Golgi Method. A Tool for Comparative Structural Analyses. In: Contemporary Research Methods in Neuroanatomy, pp. 12–31, Ed. by W. J. H. Nauta and S. O. E. Ebbesson. Springer-Verlag New York Inc., New York, 1970.

Victor, M.; Adams, R. D.; Collins, G. H.: The Wernicke-Korsakoff Syndrome. F. A. Davis; Philadelphia, 1971.

Vogt, M.: Functional Aspects of Catecholamines in Central Nervous System. Br Med Bull 29 (1973) 168–172.

Walberg, F.: Axoaxonic Contacts in the Cuneate Nucleus; Probable Basis for Presynaptic Depolarization. Exp Neurol 13 (1965) 218–231.

Wall, P. D.: The Gate Control Theory of Pain Mechanisms. A Re-Examination and Re-Statement. Brain 101 (1978) 1–18.

Warrington, E. K.: Constructional Apraxia. In: Handbook of Clinical Neurology, Vol. 4, pp. 67–83, Ed. by P. J. Vinken and G. W. Bruyn. North-Holland Publishing Co., Amsterdam, 1969.

Warwick, R.: Williams, P. L.: Gray's Anatomy, Ed. 35. W. B. Saunders Co., Philadelphia, 1973.

Watson, C.: Basic Human Neuroanatomy. An Introductory Atlas. Little, Brown and Co., Boston, 1974.

Watson, R. T.; Heilman, K. M.; Miller, B. D.; King, F. A.: Neglect after Mesencephalic Reticular Formation Lesions. Neurology 24 (1974) 294–298.

Webster, K. E.: Somaesthetic Pathways. Br Med Bull 33 (1977) 113–120.

Weinstein, E. A.; Friedland, R. P. (Eds.): Hemi-Inattention and Hemisphere Specialization. Advances in Neurology, Vol. 18. Raven Press, New York, 1977.

Weiss, L. (Ed.): Histology. Cell and Tissue Biology, Ed. 5. Elsevier Biomedical, New York, 1983.

Willis, W. D., Jr.; Grossman, R. G.: Medical Neurobiology, Ed. 2. C. V. Mosby Co., St. Louis, 1977.

Young, D. W.; Gottschaldt, K.-M.: Neurons in the Rostral Mesencephalic Reticular Formation of the Cat Responding Specifically to Noxious Mechanical Stimulation. Exp Neurol 51 (1976) 628–636.

Zuleger, S.; Staubesand, J.: Atlas of the Central Nervous System in Sectional Planes. Urban & Schwarzenberg. Baltimore, 1977.

Index

Z